Diagnostic Imaging of Emerging Infectious Diseases

Pu-Xuan Lu • Bo-Ping Zhou
Editors

Diagnostic Imaging of Emerging Infectious Diseases

PEOPLE'S MEDICAL PUBLISHING HOUSE

Springer

Editors
Pu-Xuan Lu
Department of Radiology
Shenzhen Third People's Hospital Guangdong
Shenzhen
China

Bo-Ping Zhou
Department of Infection
Shenzhen Third People's Hospital Guangdong
Shenzhen
China

ISBN 978-94-017-7362-1 ISBN 978-94-017-7363-8 (eBook)
DOI 10.1007/978-94-017-7363-8

Library of Congress Control Number: 2015954244

Springer Dordrecht Heidelberg New York London

Printed on acid-free paper

Springer Science+Business Media B.V. Dordrecht is part of Springer Science+Business Media (www.springer.com)

Foreword I

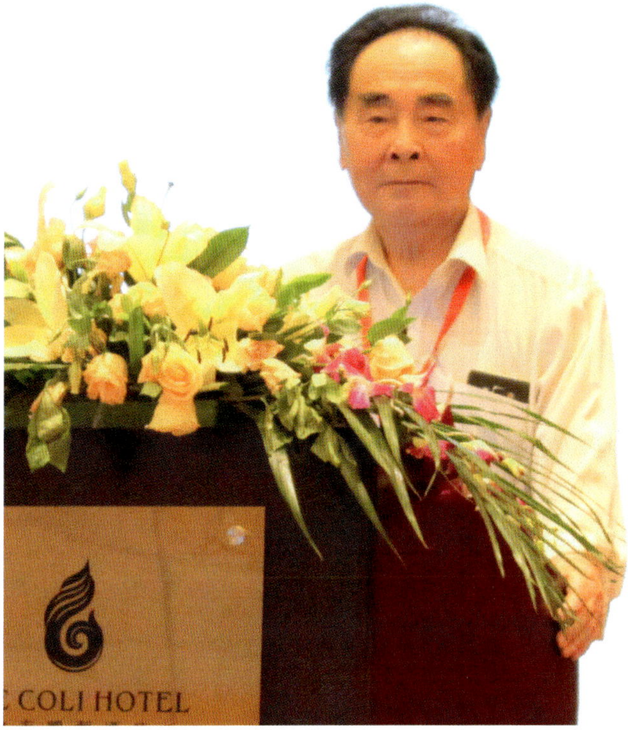

Epidemics of severe acute respiratory syndrome (SARS) in 2003 and sporadic prevalence of human avian influenza around 2006 make people fully realize the great threats of emerging infectious diseases (EIDs) on human health, society, and economy. In the coming twenty-first century, the prevention and treatment of EIDs are expected to remain a crucial task in public health for countries around the world.

Professor Lu Puxuan and Professor Zhou Boping are among the pioneers in China dedicated to clinical diagnosis and treatment of EIDs. Their remarkable exploration and contribution in imaging detection and diagnosis of EIDs have laid a solid foundation for this book entitled *Clinical Diagnostic Imaging of Emerging Infectious Diseases*. This book is the first monograph domestically and internationally on the clinics of EIDs. It compiled the valuable experience and research outcomes of over 80 clinical workers and researchers from frontline combat of EIDs that start in China and have heavy impacts around the world such as SARS and human avian influenza. This book details the pathological changes and clinical imaging diagnosis of EIDs and the imaging diagnosis and differential diagnosis of EID-related complications. Complete with detailed and authentic data, this book is focused and highly practicable, which yields high academic value for clinical reference. It will serve well for basic, clinical, and preventive medical workers and relevant administrators, even the public. I am hereby very glad to recommend this book.

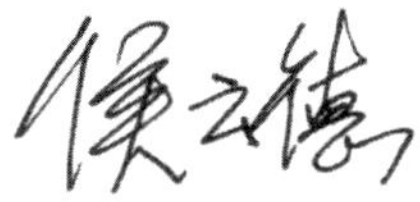

Beijing
March 2014

Hou Yunde
Academician of Chinese Academy of Engineering

Foreword II

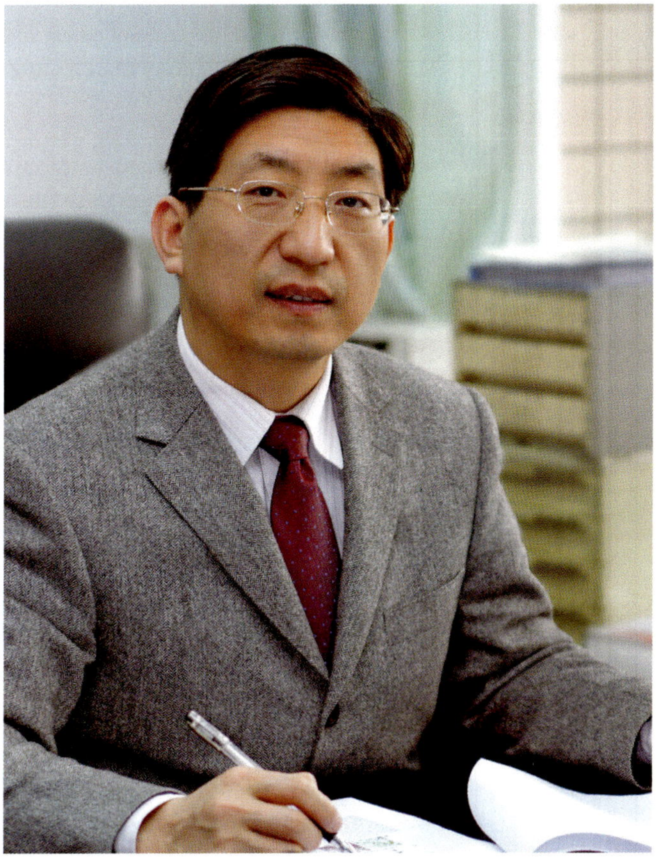

Over the past 30 years, approximately 40 emerging infectious diseases (EIDs) have appeared, with at least one EID each year. Severe acute respiratory syndrome (SARS), type A (H1N1) influenza, and human avian influenza (H5N1, H7N9) are the most globally challenging EIDs in the past 10 years. Their uncertain and unpredictable etiology leaves us unable to launch specific preventive measures, derive early and accurate diagnosis, and realize effective control, thus resulting in wide prevalence and high mortality with serious impacts on social stability and economic development.

The *Clinical Diagnostic Imaging of Emerging Infectious Diseases* compiled by Professor Lu Puxuan and Professor Zhou Boping of Shenzhen Third People's Hospital is the first monograph domestically and internationally on EIDs. This book summarizes the valuable experience and research outcomes of clinical workers and researchers from frontline combat of EIDs that start in China and have great impacts around the world such as SARS and human avian influenza and elaborates the pathophysiological and pathological changes and clinical imaging diagnosis of EIDs and the imaging diagnosis and differential diagnosis of EID-related complications. Meanwhile, it also presents an introduction of the etiology, epidemiology, and clinical diagnosis of EIDs.

This book is rich, novel, focused, and highly practicable, which demonstrates great reference value for basic, clinical, and preventive medical staff, administrators, and medical students. It is of great significance for popularizing the clinical knowledge of examination, diagnosis, prevention, and treatment of EIDs among the public so as to improve the diagnosis and treatment of EIDs.

I had the privilege of reading this book in advance. Deeply impressed by its academic significance and value, I hereby strongly recommend it.

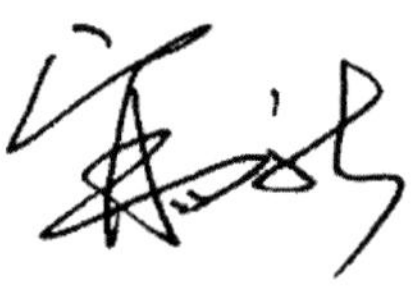

Beijing
March 2014

Zeng Yixin
President of Peking Union Medical College
Academician of Chinese Academy of Sciences

Preface

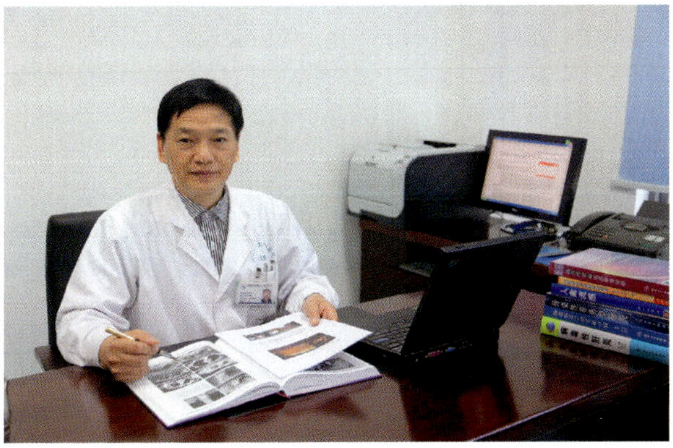

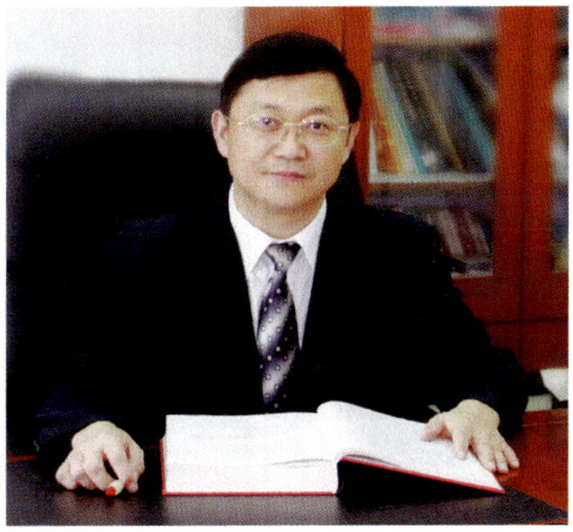

Emerging infectious diseases (EIDs) comprise new, emerging, or drug-resistant infectious diseases; its incidence in human populations is found on continual rise or indicated likely to further increase. Over the past 30 years, approximately 40 EIDs have appeared, with at least one EID occurring each year. Fifty percent of these infections are viral, and 75 % are of animal origin. In the past 10 years, SARS and highly pathogenic avian influenza EIDs have cast the greatest threats around the world. Due to the uncertainty and unpredictability of EIDs, people cannot immediately reach decisions and take measures for specific prevention, early diagnosis, and effective control, thus resulting in high mortality and severe impacts on social stability and economic development. EIDs have become a major global public health concern.

At present, the predominant emerging infectious diseases have not been fully elucidated. Therefore, for healthcare professionals, particularly those dedicated to clinics, pathology, and medical imaging of infectious diseases, it is of great importance to understand and study the clinics, pathology, imaging diagnosis, and differential diagnosis of emerging infectious diseases. Besides, radiographic examinations have great values in EID diagnosis, differential diagnosis, treatment efficacy assessment, and prognostic evaluation. Hence, based on the clinical experience and research outcomes from first-line combat of EIDs, we compile this *Clinical Diagnostic Imaging of Emerging Contagious Diseases*.

This book is divided into 8 chapters with 51 sections. It covers seven emerging infectious diseases with high incidence and mortality that pose enormous effects on human, including severe acute respiratory syndrome (SARS), human avian influenza (H5N1, H7N9), hand-foot-mouth disease, type A (H1N1) influenza, acquired immune deficiency syndrome (AIDS), viral hepatitis and tuberculosis (TB). This book elaborates the pathogenesis and pathology of emerging infectious diseases (EIDS), imaging techniques and rational selection of these techniques for EIDS, EID'S presentations and characteristics on imaging, and diagnosis and differential diagnosis of EID-related complications with imaging techniques. Meanwhile, considering that EIDs are special and partly unknown, some sections are devoted to the introduction of etiology, epidemiology, pathophysiology, clinical symptoms and signs, laboratory tests, clinical diagnosis, and differential diagnosis, as well as prevention, treatment, and prognosis of EIDs. In this way, we hope readers may understand relevant clinical knowledge of EIDs besides the pathological changes, imaging examinations, and diagnosis of EIDs, thus popularizing knowledge about EID examinations and diagnosis among the extensive healthcare professionals.

The content of this book is rich, novel, focused, and well illustrated. Besides, the over 600 precious pathological and imaging pictures make it more informative and unique. With high practical value, this clinical monograph on EIDs boasts reference value for both staff in basic medicine, clinical medicine, preventive medicine, administrators, and medical students.

We would like to express our sincere gratitude to Professor Zeng Yixin, President of Peking Union Medical College and academician of Chinese Academy of Sciences (CAS), and Professor Hou Yunde, academician of Chinese Academy of Engineering (CAE), for their great support and concern on this book. It is our honor to invite both of them to preface this book.

In light of the extensive coverage of this book, many problems of EIDs in basic, clinical, and preventive medicine still remain unresolved. Though this book has been carefully compiled by more than 80 professors and experts engaged in EID frontline clinics and researches, there may still be some omission. Along with lapse of time, researches about EIDs will go deeper, and some scientific problems will be gradually unveiled and solved. Meanwhile, new infectious diseases may occur or break out. Therefore, we gratefully welcome any critique, correction, addition, and improvement.

Shenzhen, China Pu-Xuan Lu
Shenzhen, China Bo-Ping Zhou

Editors

Chief Editors:
Pu-Xuan Lu, Bo-Ping Zhou

Editors (in alphabetic order)
Qi An
Jianbo Chen, Xinchun Chen, Guanxun Cheng, Yutian Chong
Qunyi Deng, Yingying Deng, Changfeng Dong
Mutong Fang, Tiejian Feng
Yungen Gan, Yang Ge, Honghan Gong, Jizhou Gou, Yujuan Guan
Qing He, Jian He, Yulin He, Yanan Hu, Ting Huang, Hua Huang, Wenxian Huang, Shaobiao Huang, Xiangrong Huang
Zhenwei Lang, Xiaohua Le, Bing Li, Guobao Li, Hanying Li, Hongjun Li, Jianming Li, Jingjing Li, Jiafu Lin, Dechun Liu, Guohui Liu, Jinxin Liu, Yan Liu, Yingxia Liu, Zhi Liu, Mingwu Lou, Jian Lu, Xingxian Lu
Wei Ma, Xiaoming Mao
Shanxing Ou
Cheng Peng, Xiaohui Peng
Chen Qiu
Xiangui Ran
Yuxin Shi, Wangshui Shan, Ziling Sha
Xiaoping Tang
Chenglin Wang, Haopeng Wang, Hui Wang, Shaoqin Wang, Jinqing Wang, Yixiang Wang, Shipin Wu, Xiaobing Wu
Yong Xiao, Cheng Xu, Jin Xu, Rengen Xu
Demin Yan, Gendong Yang, Guang Yang, Guilin Yang, Guoan Yang, Ruxin Ye, Weiye Yu, Hong Yuan, Jing Yuan
Hongmei Zhang, Fan Zhang, Peize Zhang, Qianqian Zhang, Weiren Zhang, Xiangmei Zhang, Zhiyong Zhang, Guanglu Zhao, Guangyu Zhao, Guangping Zheng, Feiqun Zheng, Lei Zhou, Yushen Zhou, Wenke Zhu, Ying Zhu, Hongwu Zeng, Jianfeng Zeng, Yue Zeng, Qingsi Zeng, Zheng Zeng, Xunhua Zhong

Acknowledgement

The Shenzhen No. 3 People's Hospital, Guangdong Medical College, Shenzhen, China
Shenzhen City People's Hospital
You'an hospital, Capital Medical University, Beijing, China
Public Health Clinical Center, Shanghai, China
The Eighth People's Hospital in Guangzhou
Shenzhen CDC
The First Affiliated Hospital of Nanchang University
The Chinese University of Hong Kong, Prince of Wales Hospital
Chronic Diseases Hospital in Shenzhen City China's
Military Academy of Medical Sciences, Microbial Institute of Epidemic
The Third Affiliated Hospital of Zhongshan University
Shenzhen Children's Hospital
Shenzhen Yantian District People's Hospital
Tuberculosis Prevention and Control of Hospital in Heilongjiang Province
The Fourth People's Hospital of Guangxi Nanning
Peking University Shenzhen Hospital
The Second People's Hospital of Fuyang city in Anhui Province
The Second People's Hospital of Jiangxi Province, China
Women's Hospital of Zhejiang University School of Medicine
Changzhou No. 2 People's Hospital
The First Hospital of Nanchang
Affiliated Hospital of North Sichuan Medical College
The First Affiliated Hospital of Guangzhou Medical University
General Hospital of Guangzhou Military Command of PLA
Longgang Central Hospital of ShenZhen
Medical Emergency Center of BaoShan Distrct, ShangHai, China

Contents

1 Introduction of Emerging Infectious Diseases

Pu-Xuan Lu, Bo-Ping Zhou, Yang Gui-Lin, and An Qi

1.1 Definition of Emerging Infectious Diseases (EIDs)

Emerging infectious diseases (EIDs) refer to contagious diseases newly appeared, or with drug resistance, whose incidences have been rapidly increasing and are likely to further rise in the future. EIDs are usually discovered in three ways. Firstly, some existing diseases are ascertained as EIDs due to the recent discovery of pathogens. Secondly, previously considered noninfectious diseases are identified contagious as a result of new etiological findings. Thirdly, new infectious diseases are incurred by various complicated reasons such as evolution of pathogens. Due to their uncertainty and unpredictability, EIDs could result in high mortality and great impacts on social stability and economic development as people are unable to react immediately and take specific preventive or control measures. Therefore, EIDs have become a major public health problem worldwide. Cases in point are the epidemics of SARS in 2003 and H7N9 avian influenza around 2006, which have eloquently demonstrated their great threats to human health, society, and economy. In the coming twenty-first century, contagious diseases are expected to remain as a crucial public health concern for countries around the world.

1.2 Classification of EIDs

At present, more than 40 kinds of EIDs have been found worldwide, and over 30 kinds have been reported successively in China. EIDs can be classified into the following five categories.

1.2.1 EIDs Caused by New Pathogens

Such contagious diseases did not exist in the past and newly emerge due to new pathogens such as AIDS, severe acute respiratory syndrome (SARS), human infection with highly pathogenic avian influenza H5N1, influenza A (HlN1), and human infection with avian influenza H7N9.

1.2.2 EIDs Caused by New Variant Strains

Such diseases are caused by new variants mutated from existing pathogenic microorganisms. For example, current study suggests that *Vibrio cholera* O_{139} may be the result of genetic mutation of O_1 serogroup.

1.2.3 Newly Acknowledged EIDs

Some existing diseases are not recognized as EIDs until recently, such as hepatitis D and E, legionnaire's disease, and Lyme disease.

1.2.4 Existing Noncontagious Diseases Redefined as EIDs

Some existing diseases considered noninfectious are found contagious in recent years, such as peptic ulcer caused by *H. pylori* and T-cell leukemia.

Pu-Xuan Lu (✉)
Department of Radiology, Shenzhen Third People's Hospital
Guangdong, Shenzhen, China
e-mail: lupuxuan@126.com

Bo-Ping Zhou
Department of Infection, Shenzhen Third People's Hospital
Guangdong, Shenzhen, China
e-mail: zhoubp@hotmail.com

Yang Gui-Lin • An Qi
The Shenzhen No.3 People's Hospital, Guangdong College,
Shenzhen, China

P.-X. Lu, B.-P. Zhou (eds.), *Diagnostic Imaging of Emerging Infectious Diseases*, DOI 10.1007/978-94-017-7363-8_1

1.2.5 EIDs Endemic in Some Places

Contagious diseases endemic in some places become prevalent in new places and then are generally considered as EIDs, such as West Nile virus (WNV) that was once popular in Middle East and Europe and broke out in the USA in 2012.

1.3 Epidemiology of EIDs

1.3.1 Prevalence Characteristics

Pandemic and subject to multiple influential factors. For example, diseases like Lyme disease, Legionnaires' disease, and peptic ulcer disease are globally distributed, SARS appears in 32 countries and regions, and BSE rages over 22 European countries.

Highly contagious and complex in dissemination routes. EIDs like Ebola hemorrhagic fever, SARS, West Nile encephalitis, and mad cow disease are all highly contagious through various channels.

Fast transmission with severe damages. AIDS, described as super cancer and the top killer in twentieth century, has been spreading across the world in an astonishing speed since diagnosed in 1981. In 2003, both the outbreak of SARS in spring and the highly pathogenic avian influenza H5N1 after mid-December caused casualties and huge economic losses. SARS, human avian influenza, and influenza HlN1 have all become rampant worldwide in a short time. Besides, convenient transportation and close international contacts also facilitate their spread.

Zoonotic. More than three quarters of EIDs are zoonotic and closely related to animals. Researches by *Jones et al.* revealed that 60.3 % EIDs were zoonotic, with 71.8 % caused by wild animals, such as human avian influenza and Ebola virus.

Difficult to prevent, diagnose, and treat due to the varied pathogens. Pathogens of EIDs mainly encompass viruses, bacteria, rickettsia, and chlamydia, predominantly viruses which are highly elusive and infectious.

Free of natural immunity in human populations. With strong variability, the viruses of EIDs are able to escape the immune barrier and develop resistance to drugs in new hosts as the environment changes. Therefore, people have no immunity to EIDs.

1.3.2 Influential Factors

Biological factors. Pathogenic microorganisms may mutate to adapt new environment. Therefore, nonpathogenic strains may become pathogenic, and attenuated strains become virulent, or evolve into new pathogens, thus giving rise to EIDs. Pathogens may generate numerous mutant strains by acquisition, recombination, or transfer of genes in a short time, part of which may develop into new pathogens of contagious diseases.

Natural factors. Global warming has changed the geographical distribution of vector insects and increased their reproduction speed and invasiveness. As a result, breeding time of pathogens outside human bodies is curtailed, making insect-borne contagious diseases more frequent.

Social factors. Deforestation, construction of dams, and other human activities can change the ecological environment. Additionally, population movement, sexual promiscuity, drug abuse, and other bad behaviors may cause and spread contagious diseases.

1.4 Clinical and Imaging Characteristics of EIDs

1.4.1 Clinical Signs of Infectious Diseases

Similar to other contagious diseases, EIDs progress through four periods: incubation period, prodromal period, period of apparent manifestation, and convalescent period.

1.4.1.1 Incubation Period

This period commences from the invasion of pathogens into human body and ends upon the appearance of clinical symptoms.

1.4.1.2 Prodromal Period

This period spans from onsets to manifestation of evident symptoms. Clinical manifestations are usually nonspecific and shared by all EIDs, such as headache, fever, fatigue, and muscle soreness. It commonly lasts 1–3 days.

1.4.1.3 Period of Apparent Manifestation

After prodromal period, some patients with acute contagious diseases enter the period of apparent manifestation. During this period, all the signs and symptoms of the infectious diseases usually fully manifest.

1.4.1.4 Convalescent Period

When human immunity grows to a certain extent, the pathophysiological changes would come to an end, and patients' symptoms and signs basically disappear, which is clinically called convalescent period. Some diseases can reoccur, and some may cause sequelae.

1.4.2 Clinical Imaging Characteristics of EIDs

Clinical imaging diagnosis is of great significance for the diagnosis, differential diagnosis, and efficacy evaluation of EIDs.

1.4.2.1 Necessary Imaging Examinations and Protection Should Be Carried Out for EIDs

In light of the strong infectiveness and variability of EIDs, imaging data are needed for their clinical diagnosis, differential diagnosis, treatment evaluation, and prognosis.

1.4.2.2 Basic Imaging Presentations of EIDs Are Ground-Glass Opacity and Pulmonary Consolidation Shadows

Mostly caused by viruses, EIDs have mainly such pulmonary imaging changes as rapid occurrence of ground-glass opacity and (or) pulmonary consolidation. Cavity and cystic changes can also be seen in some cases.

1.4.2.3 Dynamic Imaging Visualizes Rapid Changes of Lesions

For some patients, imaging presentations and clinical symptoms and signs are not consistent. For example, the imaging findings may be serious, while clinical symptoms are mild.

1.4.2.4 Lesion Absorption Is Slow

For example, the pulmonary interstitial fibrosis lesions of patients with human avian influenza H5N1 may procrastinate for several years.

1.4.2.5 Complications May Occur

During convalescent period, absorption of lesions is slow and imaging changes such as interlobular septal thickening and interstitial hyperplasia may be observed. For example, pulmonary fibrosis may be left in some SARS patients with severe pulmonary injuries after recovery as the absorption of pulmonary lesions take a long time. Moreover, patients with SARS or avian influenza H7N9 may be complicated with avascular necrosis of femoral head.

1.5 Measures and Strategies Against EIDs

1.5.1 A Disease Surveillance Network Should Be Erected and Ameliorated

Efforts shall be made to strengthen the surveillance of EIDs from organization system, personnel, equipment, and technological competence. By monitoring and investigation, we could timely detect new sources of infection or new pathogens and influential factors and take prompt and effective measures to rein in their spread and contagion. A global coordinated information platform for EIDs prevention and control shall be established and improved where countries shall timely communicate epidemic situation of EIDs and share experience for EIDs prevention and control so as to block large-scale spreading.

1.5.2 Improvement of Public Health Infrastructure and Training of Relevant Personnel

Public health infrastructure is fundamental to support public health preventive measures and to assess public health status. The high quality training of public health practitioners plays an vital role for the control of infectious diseases. Faced with the threats of emerging infectious, public health professionals should strengthen their training, and establish team culture to evaluate epidemiology of infectious diseases, thereby in the face of emerging infectious diseases outbreaks reasonable measures can be taken in an orderly manner to control the situation.

1.5.3 Scientific Research About EIDs Should Be Reinforced and Research and Development of Vaccines and New Drugs Accelerated

1. Conduct epidemiological studies to clarify the epidemic stages, characteristics, and influential factors of EIDs, so as to provide scientific evidences for formulation of prevention countermeasures
2. Accelerate the research and development of vaccines
3. Speed up the research of diagnostic reagents to form experimental methods for rapid diagnosis of EIDs
4. Carry out studies on pathogenic mechanism and early warning techniques for EIDs
5. Accelerate the research and development of new drugs, especially antiviral drugs
6. Build a strain resource bank of pathogenic microorganisms

1.5.4 Relevant Laws and Regulations Targeted at EIDs Should Be Promulgated

Prevention and treatment in line with laws should be geared up and relevant laws and regulations be enacted.

1.5.5 Attention Should Be Paid to Public Education and Information Communication

Multidisciplinary studies in public health and journalism and communication should be launched to address social panics caused by the outbreak of contagious diseases.

1.5.6 The Ecological Balance Between Nature and Human Beings Should Be Maintained

Preservation of ecological balance and natural environment is the fundamental way to control and reduce zoonotic contagious diseases, therefore precluding EIDs from the source.

Further Reading

1. Shao JS, Lu HZ. Overview of EIDS researches [in Chinese]. J Diagn Concepts Pract. 2011;10(3):293–6.
2. Guan Y, Zheng BJ, He YQ, et al. Isolation and characterization of viruses related to the SARS coronavirus from animals in southern China. Science. 2003;302:276–8.
3. Liu DW, Zhang LM. Research contents and methods of EIDS [in Chinese]. Chi J Prev Med. 2007;8(4):478–80.
4. Lu PX, Zhou BP, Yuan MY, et al. Chest X-ray manifestations of SARS [in Chinese]. Chin J Radiol. 2003;37(8): 682–5.
5. Lu PX, Zhou BP, Yang GD, et al. Clinical characteristics and chest X-ray manifestations of severe SARS [in Chinese]. Chin J Emerg Med. 2003;12(7):437–9.
6. Cao Y, Zheng GP, Lu PX, et al. Study about indicators for beside radiogram and protection principles of influenza A (H1N1) [in Chinese]. Chin J Med. 2012;47(10):81–3.
7. Ma DQ. Role of imaging in diagnosis of human avian influenza [in Chinese]. Chin J Radiol. 2006;40(3):230.
8. Zhou BP, Tang XP, Lu PX, et al. SARS [in Chinese]. People's Medical Publishing House, Beijing; 2004.
9. Zhou BP, Li YM, Lu PX, et al. Human avian influenza [in Chinese]. Beijing: Science Press; 2007. p. 180–9.
10. Lu PX, Deng YY. Epidemiological characteristics and pulmonary imaging findings of human avian influenza [in Chinese]. Chin J Med Imag. 2010;16(5):431–4.
11. Lu PX, Zhou BP, et al. Chest clinical imaging diagnosis of AIDS [in Chinese]. Beijing: Science Press; 2012.
12. Zhou BP, Chun YT, et al. Viral hepatitis. People's Medical Publishing House, Beijing; 2011.
13. Zhou BP, Li CR, et al. EV-71Hand-foot-mouth disease. People's Medical Publishing House, Beijing; 2009.
14. Sun XD, Wang HY. The epidemic situation and t prevention and treatment strategies for EIDS [in Chinese]. Shanghai J Preventive Med. 2009;21(9):461–5.
15. Lin JD, Yang BB. The epidemic characteristics and countermeasures of EIDS [in Chinese]. China Trop Med. 2007;7(4):597–8.
16. Lu PX, Deng YY, Liu ST, Liu Y, Liu YX, Wang YX, Zhu WK, Le XH, Yu WY, Zhou BP. Correlation between imaging features of Pneumocystis Jiroveci Pneumonitis (PCP), CD(4) (+) T lymphocyte count, and plasma HIV viral load: a study in 50 consecutive AIDS patients. Quant Imaging Med Surg. 2012;2(2):124–9.
17. Lu PX, Deng YY, Yang GL, Liu WL, Liu YX, Huang H, Wang YX. Relationship between respiratory viral load and lung lesion severity: a study in 24 cases of pandemic H1N1 2009 influenza A pneumonia. J Thorac Dis. 2012;4(4):377–83.
18. Lu PX, Wang YX, Zhou BP, Ge Y, Zhu WK, Chen XC, Ran XG. Radiological features of lung changes caused by avian influenza subtype A H5N1 virus: report of two severe adult cases with regular follow-up. Chin Med J (Engl). 2010;123(1):100–4.

SARS

2

Bo-Ping Zhou, Pu-Xuan Lu, Qiu Chen, Tang Xiao-Ping, Guan Yu-Juan, Liu Jin-Xin, Lu Xing, Lang Zhen-Wei, and Chen Xin-Chun

2.1 Overview of SARS

2.1.1 Definition of SARS

Severe acute respiratory syndrome (SARS) is an acute respiratory tract infectious disease induced by SARS-CoV and mainly transmitted through the short-distance air droplets and close contact. Its main clinical characteristics is abrupt onset of the disease and the initial symptom is fever accompanied with systematic symptoms of headache, soreness and fatigue, and respiratory tract symptoms such as cough, chest dullness, and dyspnea. A few cases may progress to acute respiratory distress syndrome (ARDS). Due to its self-limiting feature, the prognosis is predominantly good but may be poor in severe cases, with mortality about 9.3 %. Some patients may develop such complications such as lung fibrosis and necrosis of the head of femur. On April 8, 2003, SARS was defined as a legal infectious disease by the Ministry of Heath of China.

Bo-Ping Zhou (✉)
Department of Infection, Shenzhen Third People's Hospital
Guangdong, Shenzhen, China
e-mail: zhoubp@hotmail.com

Pu-Xuan Lu
Department of Radiology, Shenzhen Third People's Hospital
Guangdong, Shenzhen, China
e-mail: lupuxuan@126.com

Qiu Chen
Shenzhen City People's Hospital, Shenzhen, China

Tang Xiao-Ping • Guan Yu-Juan • Liu Jin-Xin
The Eighth People's Hospital in Guangzhou, Guangzhou, China

Lu Xing • Chen Xin-Chun
The Shenzhen No.3 People's Hospital, Guangdong College, Shenzhen, China

Lang Zhen-Wei
Di'tan Hospital, Capital Medical University, Beijing, China

2.1.2 Discovery and Epidemic of SARS

2.1.2.1 The Discovery of the Disease

1. The first SARS case was reported around the world on January 2, 2003; a hospital in Heyuan city of Guangdong province hospitalized two patients' with severe pulmonary infection of unknown cause, which was the first traceable report of "SARS" around the global.
2. On February 28, 2003, SARS was first diagnosed by the WHO expert Carlor Urbani in Hanoi of Vietnam, who also named this new unexplained disease "*S*evere *A*cute *R*espiratory *S*yndrome" (SARS).

2.1.2.2 Control of SARS Epidemics

Following the emergence of SARS, WHO and governments around the world attached great importance and took consecutively effective control and prevention measures, which reined in the infection rapidly controlled in a short time.

On April 28, 2003, WHO eliminated Vietnam from the name list of the SARS-infected area, which made Vietnam the first to get rid of SARS outbreaks. Since then, numerous countries were also ticked off the list. On July 5, 2003, WHO announced to remove Taiwan of China from SARS-affected area list, which is also the last. At present, there is no SARS-affected area around the world, signaling the victory of global battle against SARS. By the end of September 26, 2003, there were in total 8,098 people infected and 774 deceased, with the mortality at 9.5 %.

2.2 Etiology

On April 16, 2003, a new coronavirus never seen was announced as the cause of SARS by WHO. It is the joint efforts of global scientists and biological scientific and technological advances that enabled establishment of international SARS research network, separation and identification of SARS coronavirus, and confirmation of SARS pathogenesis.

P.-X. Lu, B.-P. Zhou (eds.), *Diagnostic Imaging of Emerging Infectious Diseases*, DOI 10.1007/978-94-017-7363-8_2

2.2.1 Discovery of SARS Pathogen and Determination of Pathogenesis

2.2.1.1 Screening and Exclusion of Known Pathogens

Some Canadian laboratories excluded influenza virus A and B; para-influenza virus type 1, 2, and 3; adenovirus; and respiratory syncytial virus by scanning electron microscopy and direct fluorescent antibody test. They also conducted immunohistochemistry on the corpse tissues of dead patients about viruses including influenza virus A and B, respiratory syncytial virus, adenovirus, circovirus, Hantaan virus, measles virus, intestinal tract virus, and pneumonia mycoplasma and chlamydia, which showed negative. Scholars from German, France, America, Hong Kong, and Taiwan applied specific PCR tests targeted at corresponding pathogens to examine pneumonia mycoplasma, pneumonia chlamydia, human cytomegalovirus, circovirus, herpes virus, human coronavirus OC43 and 229E and Arenaviruses, Bunyavirus, Hantaan virus, Crimean-Congo hemorrhagic fever virus, which also indicated negative.

2.2.1.2 Separation and Identification of SARS Coronavirus

On March 21, 2003, Hong Kong University firstly separated and cultured coronavirus from the nasopharyngeal specimen of SARS patients by Vero cells, and then several laboratories of Canada and America disease center and SARS international coordination group also cultured coronavirus. On April 16, 2003, based on the aforementioned research findings, WHO declared a new coronavirus as the pathogen of SARS and named it as SARS coronavirus (SARS-CoV).

2.2.2 Physicochemical Characteristics of SARS Coronavirus

2.2.2.1 Morphologic Structure

SARS-CoV is a single-stranded and positive RNA virus belonging to the genus Coronavirus of Coronaviridae family of Nidovirales order. It bears great morphological resemblance with known human coronaviruses. Under the electric microscopes, SARS coronavirus presents with pleomorphic spherical particles with envelopes in Vero E6 cell in vitro and with a diameter of about 80–140 mm. It has distinct coronavirus morphological characteristics that rodlike surface projections about 20–40 nm long protrude outside viral envelope to form a corona. For separation and culture of viruses in Vero E6 cells, viral particles are mostly found in vacuoles inside cells under electric microscope, mainly hollow particle, and viruses outside cells observed with spikes.

2.2.2.2 Physicochemical Characteristics

The Coronavirus is mainly composed of nucleic acid, protein, carbonate, and lipid. SARS-CoV are relatively stable in human specimens and environment but relatively sensitive to chemical and physical factors. The viruses could be killed by exposure to ultraviolet rays for 60 min. As the envelope of SARS-CoV contains lipoids, they are sensitive to lipid solvents and could be inactivated by ether, chloroform, tween, 70 % ethyl alcohol, methanol, pancreatic enzymes, and ultraviolet rays. Ether could sterilize the virus completely under 4°Cafter 24 h, 75 % ethyl alcohol could deactivate virus after 5 min, and disinfectants containing chlorine may kill the virus aft.

2.3 Epidemiology

2.3.1 Overview of Epidemics

SARS is the first newly emerging infectious disease in the twenty-first century. Since the first case was detected in Guangdong on January 2, 2003, SARS spread to 29 countries at five states at an unprecedented speed with several months. According to the report of WHO, SARS epidemics was found in total 29 countries at five states (including Hong Kong and Taiwan of China) from January 2, 2003, to September 26, 2003. Since January 2, 2003, which infected 8,098 patients and caused 774 casualties. Besides, there were 5,327 patients in China mainland (including 1,002 medical workers) with 349 deaths; 1,755 patients in Hong Kong with 299 deaths; 346 patients in Taiwan with 37 deaths; 251 patients in Canada with 43 deaths; 238 patients in Singapore with 33 deaths; 63 patients in Vietnam with 5 deaths and 29 patients in America but without casualty. Meanwhile, SARS cases were reported in 24 provinces, municipalities under direct governance of central government and autonomous regions in China mainland, with 2,521 infection cases and 183 deaths in Beijing and 512 infection cases and 57 deaths in Guangdong.

2.3.2 Source of Infection

The main source of infection is SARS patients, and other infectious sources such as animals need to be further consolidated.

2.3.2.1 Symptomatic Patients

It is regarded that only symptomatic patients can effectively spread SARS-CoV.

2.3.2.2 Asymptomatic Patients

At present there still lacks clinical proof that asymptomatic SARS patients could spread SARS coronavirus.

2.3.2.3 Super-Spreader

Few cases are highly contagious and able to directly infect over 10 patients, who are called super-spreader. The five super-spreaders in Singapore have been found infecting 103 people. Such powerful infectiousness is attributable to the high viral load inside patients who could discharge abundant viruses via respiratory tract in a short time.

2.3.2.4 Animal Source of Infection

Specialists from the department of microbiology of Hong Kong University and Guangdong Provincial Disease Control and Prevention Center tested abundant SARS coronaviruses from the samples collected from civet cats sold in Guangzhou and Shenzhen, suggesting that the human SARS coronavirus might originate from civet cats.

2.3.3 Route of Spread

SARS virus is spread mainly through the respiratory tract and also spread by aerosol and droplet.

2.3.3.1 Droplet Spread

High level of SARS coronavirus could be detected in the throat swabs and sputum specimens of the patients in acute phase. Viruses discharged by patients via cough would exist in the air within certain radius, thus forming short-distance respiratory tract droplet spread. It is a main route of SARS dissemination.

2.3.3.2 Contact Spread

Indirect or direct contact spread could also spread SARS coronavirus. It could be spread through contact with the respiratory tract secretion or through the mouth and nose via contaminated hands and toys.

2.3.3.3 Aerosol Spread

As viruses proliferate abundantly in the respiratory tract, exfoliated cells containing infectious viruses could be expelled outside the body through patients' respiration, cough, and sneeze and suspend in the air, thus forming the aerosol of SARS virus. Cough and sneeze could greatly contribute to production of SARS virus aerosol.

2.3.4 Population Susceptibility

SARS is a new type of infectious diseases, and people effectively exposed to SARS pathogens are vulnerable.

2.3.4.1 Immunity After Illness

Present data reveal that SARS is an acute self-limiting infectious disease, and neutralizing antibodies to SARS could be detected 3 weeks after onset. However, the change patterns of neutralizing antibody titer have not been fully elucidated.

2.3.5 Epidemiological Characteristics

2.3.5.1 Characteristics of Time Distribution

The epidemics of SARS mainly take place in the winter and spring.

2.3.5.2 Characteristics of Area Distribution

SARS outbreaks are mainly concentrated at coastal tourism cities with prosperous economy, dense population, and convenient transport, particularly air transport. From the perspective of international geography, SARS primarily occurs in Southeastern countries or regions, including China mainland, Hong Kong, Taiwan, Singapore, and Vietnam.

2.3.5.3 Characteristics of Population Distribution

Analysis of the statistics of various countries shows that SARS onset is mainly recorded in young populations aged 20–50 years old, occupying around 80 % of the total.

2.4 Pathogenesis and Pathological Changes

2.4.1 Pathogenesis

SARS coronavirus (SARS-CoV), a mutant of Coronaviridae, is pathogenic to hosts in the following two aspects: firstly, viral infections could directly damage the structure and functions of infected cells and trigger cell apoptosis; secondly, immune reactions and release of various cytokines induced by viral infections could not only eliminate infectious pathogens but also may deal severe damages on histiocytes due to excessive immune reactions.

The member of Coronaviridae is a single-chain positive RNA virus, which taxonomically belongs to Nidovirales with Arteriviridae. The homological analysis of SARS-CoV structural protein amino-acid sequences shows that the main structural protein S (spike protein), M (membrane protein), N (nucleocapsid protein), and E (envelope protein) bear very low homology with other known coronaviruses, between 20 and 30 %. Besides, bioinformation analysis infers that SARS-CoV may also encode 5–9 nonstructural proteins of unknown functions. All these SARS-CoV specific proteins may play key roles in determining the viral virulence.

S-protein, existent on the viral surface in form of trimer, is the main component in constructing the coronal structure and major structural protein for the integration of virus and host cell receptors and fusion of viral envelope and cell membrane to enable invasion of viruses. After infection with sensitive cells, SARS-Cov could replicate enormously and release virions, which may disturb cell metabolism and directly result in injury of body tissues and cells.

In the early phase of the disease and in the continual progression phase, the active immune cells such as CD4+ and CD8+ T lymphocytes, NK cells, and DC cells are decreased prominently, to an extent positively correlated with severity of conditions and speed of progression. Besides, all dead patients are detected with irreversible significant decline. However, along with remission of conditions and entry into recovery phase, the number of aforementioned immune cells could be recovered to some extent, whose change presents distinct parallel correlation with disease evolution. Dynamic observations suggest that serum pre-inflammatory cytokine IL-6, IL-8, IL-16, and INF-α level of SARS patients could reach the peak at about second week of disease course, which relatively corresponds to the acute aggravation phase. All these consolidate the immune damage of SARS-CoV infections.

2.4.2 Pathological Changes

Autopsies of the over 20 patients who died after infected with SARS revealed that SARS is a disease detrimental to organs of the whole body, particularly lung tissue and immunity system. Primary pathologic changes can be classified into severe lung lesions, immune organ impairment, toxic changes of other organs, and secondary infections. The causes of death were as follows: (1) diffusive lung alveolar damages lead to progressive respiratory failure; (2) impairment of liver, kidney, heart, and several other organs may induce multiple organ failures and exacerbate conditions; (3) due to injury of immune organs particularly lymph nodes and spleen, the lymphocytes are decreased and immunity compromised, therefore resulting in secondary mycotic infections.

2.4.2.1 Lungs

Naked-Eye Observation

Lung tissues become swollen and heavier. According to domestic report, the left lung may reach 500–1480 g (average 811.4 g) and right lung 700–1125 g (average 869.3 g), with the total lung up to 1170–2605 g (average 1460.7 g). The lung tissues appear in dark red. Texture is hard, indicative of consolidation. The surface is relatively smooth and free of pleural adhesions. Lung tissues are observed with blood vessel dilation and congestion, spotted and patchy necrosis, and hemorrhagic infarct foci and focal compensatory emphysema. Sections of various lung lobes are visualized with outflows of light red or/and a few foamy blood-stained fluids. The trachea and bronchi are found with exudations of slight mucoid or blood-stained secretions. Pulmonary hilar lymph nodes are revealed with slight enlargement and pleural cavity without or with a few effusions.

Observation Under the Light Microscope

Microscopy reveals bilateral diffusive severe injuries of alveoli, characterized by acute exudative, hemorrhagic, and fibrinous inflammation. However, the injury may be inhomogeneous and diverse at different lung lobes and different parts of the same lobe. The characteristic change in early phase is pulmonary edema, with homogeneous pink serous or fibrinous effusions filling alveolar cavities as well as erythrocytes leakages in some cavities. The effusions from some alveolar cavities may condense to form thin-layer membranelike substance which adheres to alveolar walls, namely, formation of hyaline membrane (Fig. 2.1). Alveolar epithelia present with such diffusive injuries as degeneration and necrosis, with exfoliated or/and apoptotic type II alveolar epithelial cells observable in alveolar cavities, which are similar to changes of desquamative pneumonia (Fig. 2.2). Among them, some appear like apoptotic bodies. Partial regional type II alveolar epithelial cells and macrophages proliferate actively, with obvious increase of cell volume and distinct nucleolus. In some case, cells are detected fusing with each other to form syncytial monocytes and multinucleated giant cells (Fig. 2.3). The alveolar epithelia of some cases are examined with structures similar to viral inclusion bodies, mostly spherical and with eosinophilic staining, around which a transparent halo is visible (Fig. 2.4). Pulmonary interstitium and alveolar spaces are detected with

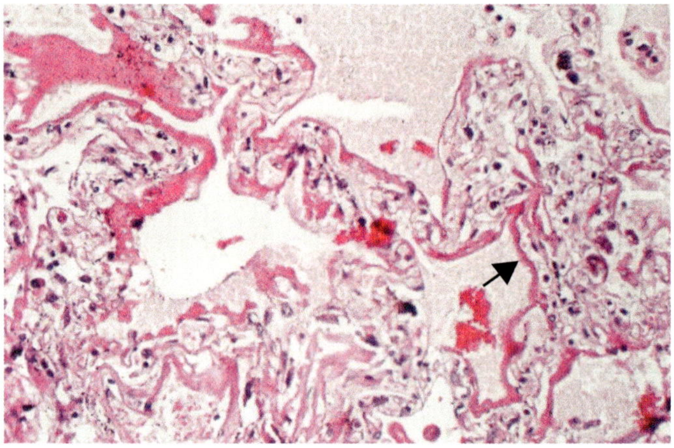

Fig. 2.1 Alveolar cavities were full of homogenous acidophilic effusions which condensed to form hyaline membranes (indicated by *arrow*) and attach to alveolar walls HE ×200

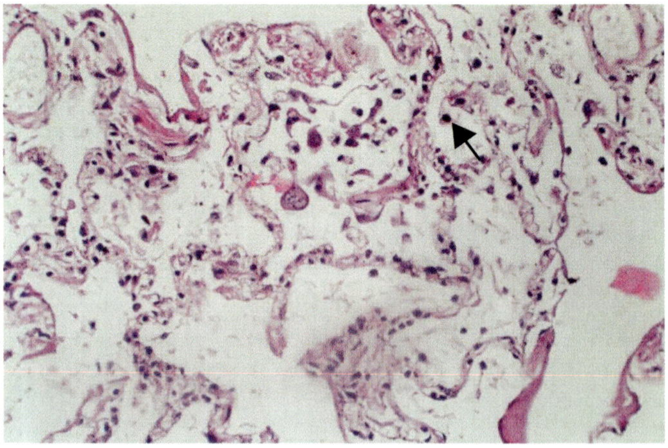

Fig. 2.2 Alveolar wall epithelial cells were disclosed with degeneration and necrosis, alveolar cavity with exfoliated type II alveolar epithelial cells (indicated by the *arrow*), and alveolar space with infiltration of a few lymphocytes and monocytes. HE ×200

high dilation and congestion of capillaries, swelling and exfoliation of epithelial cells, as well as widening of the latter, which present slight lymphocyte and monocyte infiltration, small vessel proliferation, and enlargement characteristic of vasculitis changes. Some regions are observed with pulmonary vascular embolism or fibrinous microthrombi in alveolar capillaries, while some alveolar capillary cavities manifest dilation but free of blood components. In addition, some patients are detected with lung tissue focal hemorrhage, compensatory emphysema, and small airway necrotizing inflammation and alveolar collapse or shrinkage. Patients with a disease course of over three weeks manifest fibroblast proliferation in alveolar septa, and individual cases demonstrate organization of fibrinous exudates from alveoli and fibroblast proliferation, which gives rise to glomeruloid structures, named "glomeruloid organizing pneumonia" (Fig. 2.5). The bronchial epithelial cells are revealed with exfoliation, scarce and exfoliated cilia, as well as structures similar to viral inclusions and squamous cell metaplasia at the inside. The bronchioli are detected with submucosal edema, inflammatory cell infiltration, and serous grandular hyperplasia with hyperactive secretion.

2.4.2.2 Immune Organs

Chest and Abdominal Lymph Nodes

Pulmonary hilar lymph nodes demonstrate light swelling and present different degrees of congestion, hemorrhagic necrosis, and decrease of innate lymphocytes under the microscope. Blood sinus in the lymph nodes presents with grave congestion and dilatation, lymphoid nodule atrophy or disappearance, prominently the cortex, and lymphatic tissue focal necrosis, accompanied by apoptosis of some lymphocytes (Fig. 2.6).

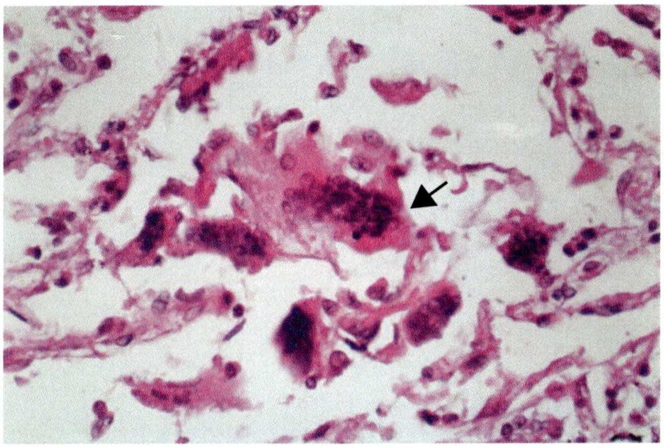

Fig. 2.3 Alveolar cavities were seen with multinucleated giant cells (indicated by the *arrow*). HE ×400

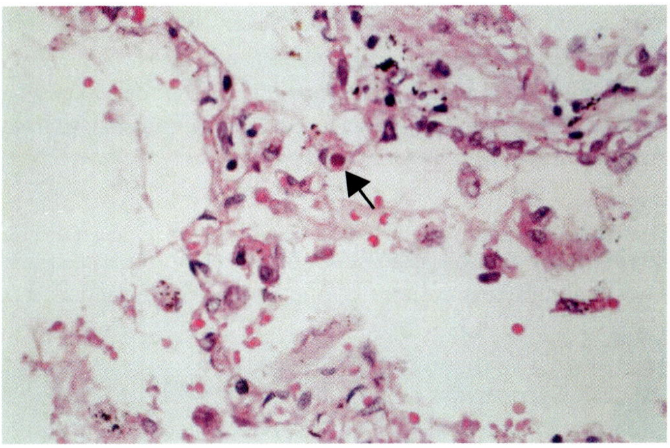

Fig. 2.4 Alveolar epithelial cells were detected with structures similar to viral inclusion bodies (indicated by the *arrow*), with spherical shape and acidophilic staining as well as transparent halo at the periphery. HE ×400

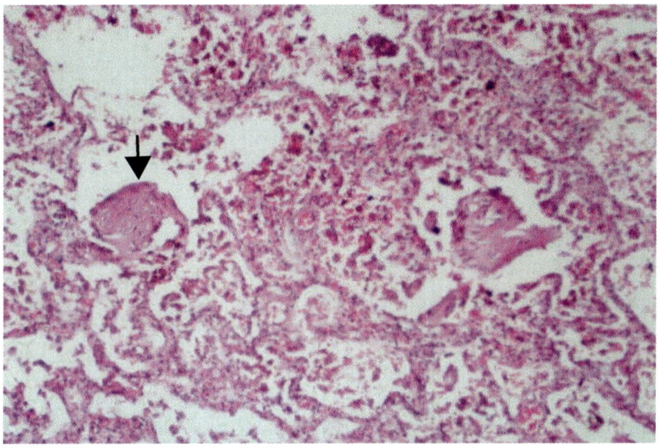

Fig. 2.5 Imaging visualized organization of fibrinous exudates from alveoli and proliferation of fibroblast to form similar glomerular structures (indicated by the *arrow*) HE ×200

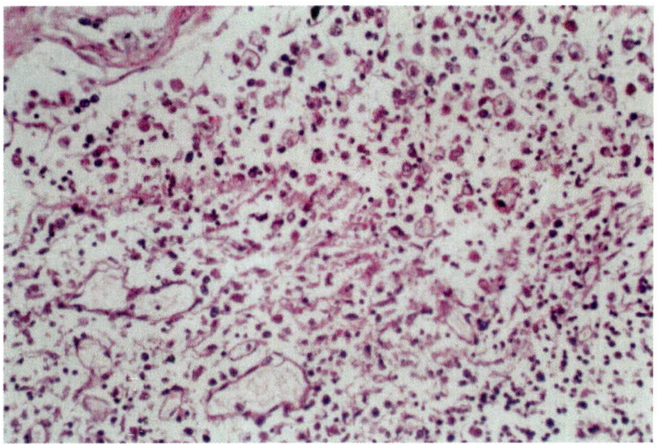

Fig. 2.6 Pulmonary hilar lymph nodes were seen with congestive necrosis and decrease of the innate lymphocytes and lymphoid nodules with atrophy and disappearance. HE ×400

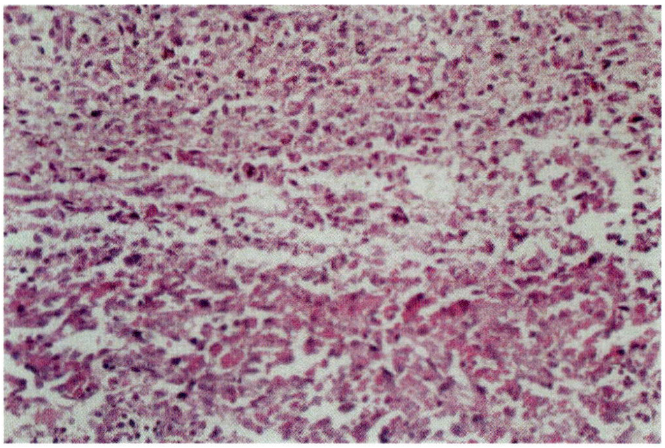

Fig. 2.7 The spleen was visualized with focal hemorrhagic necrosis and red pulp with sparse lymphocytes. HE ×200

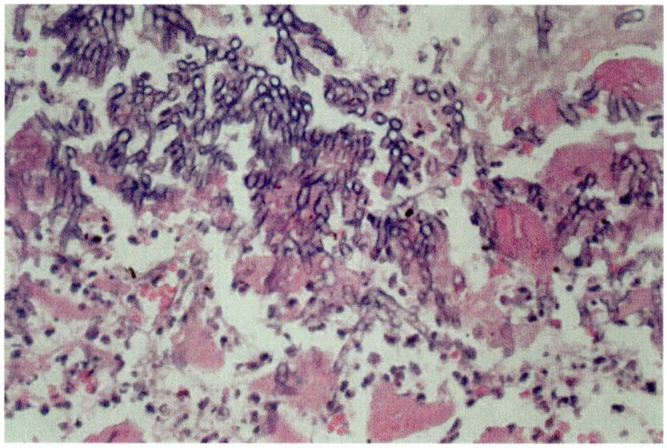

Fig. 2.8 SARS patient developed secondary pulmonary mycotic infection with dendritic hyphae. HE ×400 (Le Xiaohua Lu Jian Lang Zhenhua)

Spleen

The spleen mostly shrinks with soft texture, and has patchy and focal hemorrhage at the surface and sections. Splenic white pulp is detected obviously atrophic or absent, with central arterial wall thickened, endothelial cells swollen and partially shed, peripheral lymphatic sheath lymphocyte depleted greatly, and germinal center disappeared. Splenic corpuscle is observed with plasma protein sedimentation in central arterial walls, white pulp and marginal sinus lymph tissues with large patchy necrosis, and partial remaining lymphocytes with apoptosis. The splenic sinus inside red pulp is revealed with obvious congestion and focal hemorrhagic necrosis as well as proliferation of histiocytes (Fig. 2.7).

Bone Marrow

The number of hematopoietic cells in bone marrow declines, and granulocyte system and megakaryocytic system are relatively inhibited. Polychromatic erythroblasts present with small focal proliferation.

2.4.2.3 Other Main Organs

Tissues of the brain, liver, kidney, and heart demonstrate varying degrees of congestion, edema, degeneration, and necrosis as well as infiltration of a few lymphocytes.

2.4.2.4 Secondary Infection

Secondary bacterial pneumonia and fungal infection may occur (Fig. 2.8).

2.5 Clinical Manifestations

The initial symptom of SARS is frequently fever, accompanied by headache and general muscular and joint souring soreness, and often without nasal discharge, sore throat, and other upper respiratory tract catarrhal symptoms. Pulmonary signs are not obvious and signs and distinct systematic symptoms are inconsistent, which is typical to SARS. The clinical manifestations of SARS may vary, which can be divided into light type, common type, severe type, and atypical type, with the common type most commonly seen. Based on the clinical development, it could be divided into early phase, progression phase, and recovery phase.

2.5.1 Incubation Phase

Generally, the incubation phase lasts 2–14 days, with an average of 4–7 days and a median of 6 days, predominantly 2–10 days.

2.5.2 Symptoms

2.5.2.1 Fever

The initial symptom primarily is fever, mostly high fever, accounting for 94.4–100 %. Patient body temperature may reach 38–40 °C and 42 °C at the highest. The fever type varies, including remittent fever, irregular fever and continuous fever. The duration of fever is mostly 5–9 days.

2.5.2.2 Pain

It presents as headache, joint or/and systematic soreness, and chest pain. It is reported that the incidence of headache in SARS patients is 17–90 %.

2.5.2.3 Symptoms of T Respiratory System

Most SARS patients have cough, which is dry with scanty sputum. Generally SARS does not incur upper respiratory tract catarrhal symptoms. Severe cases may suffer from accelerated respiration, shortness of breath, or even acute respiratory distress syndrome, characterized by progressive dyspnea or even distress with respiratory frequency up to >20 times.

2.5.2.4 Palpitation and Chest Distress

Patients complain of heart beat or palpitation accompanied often by precordial discomfort. The incidence is 35–90 %.

2.5.2.5 Digestive System Symptoms

The incidence of diarrhea is reported mostly at 7–44 %, with single case up to 70 %.

2.5.3 Signs

One characteristic of SARS is severe symptoms and light signs. The signs are mostly not obvious or even absent.

2.5.3.1 Dyspnea

Dyspnea presents irregular respiratory frequency, depth, and rhythm. The incidence of dyspnea of SARS patients is 21–57 %. Severe patients may manifest nose fanning, orthopnea, and cyanosis, involvement of accessory respiratory muscles in respiration, as well as "three depression signs" upon inhalation.

2.5.3.2 Tachycardia

According to report, 11 % of typical patients and 14 % of severe patients have sinus tachycardia, and 2.3 % of SARS patients suffer from paroxysmal supraventricular tachycardia.

2.5.3.3 Pulmonary Signs

The pulmonary signs of SARS patients are frequently unobvious or absent in the early phase. Light moist rales may be audible (17–62 %). Patients may also demonstrate pulmonary consolidation sign and attenuated breath sounds. There may also be a few pleural effusions.

2.5.4 Classification

In light of conditions, it could be classified in clinics into light type, common (typical) type, severe type, and special (atypical) type.

2.5.5 Complications

2.5.5.1 Pulmonary Fibrosis

The follow-up visit of 267 SARS patients via X-ray and HRCT by Choi et al. found that about 3–4 % patients developed fibrotic changes of lung interstitium and shrinkage of lung volume.

2.5.5.2 Ischemic Necrosis of the Femoral Head

Application of glucocorticoids could to some extent alleviate lung injury of patients with severe infectious atypical pneumonia. However, long-term and abundant use of glucocorticoids may generate numerous side effects, and it is an undisputable fact that hormones may induce femoral head ischemic necrosis. Literature reports suggest that the incidence of femoral head ischemic necrosis is 5–25 %.

2.6 Laboratory Examinations

2.6.1 Blood Routine Examination

The white blood cell count remains within normal range in majority patients and may decrease in some patients (24.2 %). 95 % of severe patients without secondary infections are revealed with decreased total white blood cell, and normal neutrocyte and monocyte differential white blood cell count. However, 80 % initially diagnosed patients manifest a decrease of absolute lymphocyte count, suggestive of a tendency of gradual decline, and morphocytology change, with abnormal lymphocytes observable. 13.2–41 % patients are examined with thrombocytopenia. Many evidences prove that SARS-CoV could directly invade the immune system and act mainly on lymphocytic system, especially the T lymphocytes, which could lower peripheral blood lymphocytes. The peripheral blood white cell count is normal or decreased in most SARS patients, but CD3+, CD4+, and CD8+ T lymphocyte counts are distinctly lower compared with those of healthy population. The more severe the condition, the more drastically declined the T lymphocyte count.

2.6.2 Blood Gas Analysis

Blood gas analysis reveals hypoxemia of different degrees and commonly no carbon dioxide retention. Generally under 3–5 L/min oxygen uptake, patients with severe hypoxemia are measured of arterial partial pressure from oxygen (PaO_2) <70 mmHg or blood oxygen saturation (SpO_2) <93 %, or develop acute lung injury (ALI) or acute respiratory distress syndrome (ARDS).

2.6.3 Measurement of Peripheral Blood T Lymphocyte Subgroup

One of the main immunopathogenesis changes in SARS patients is insufficiency of T-lymphocyte-mediated specific cellular immunity, characterized by distinct damages of T lymphocytes and its subgroups, particularly $CD3^+$, $CD4^+$, and $CD8^+$. There exists distinct correlation between the extent of T lymphocyte damages and severity of the disease.

2.6.4 Test of SARS-Specific Antibodies

The method recommended by WHO for test of serum SARS-CoV antibodies is enzyme-linked immunosorbent assay (ELISA). Upon test of the SARS-CoV-specific antibodies in the infected patients, including IgG, IgM, or total antibody, seroconversion or increase by 4 times and above of any serum antibody in progress phase and recovery phase could serve as evidence for definite diagnosis.

2.6.5 PCR Test of SARS Virus

Polymerase chain reaction (PCR), a type of molecular biological test, could identify SARS virus genes from various specimens (blood, feces, respiratory tract secretions, tissue sections, etc.), that is, SARS virus RNA.

2.6.5.1 Positive Results

Presence of any of the following three circumstances could be SARS virus positive:

1. Clinical specimens from at least two different sites are tested positive (nasopharyngeal secretions and feces).
2. The same clinical specimens collected by at least 2 days apart are tested positive (two or more specimens of nasopharyngeal excretions).
3. The same clinical specimen is tested positive by two different methods or in different laboratories.
4. Repeated PCR examination indicated positive.

2.7 Clinical Diagnosis

2.7.1 SARS Diagnosis and Treatment Regimens

2.7.1.1 Basis of Diagnosis

Epidemiologic History

1. The patient has a history of intimate contact with patients or is one of the infected populations or consolidated having infected others by definite evidences.
2. The patient had been to or lived in the areas with SARS patients and secondary infection epidemics.

Symptoms and Signs

The onset is acute and initial symptom is fever, with body temperature >38 °C, and occasionally accompanied by concurrent chillness. Patients may also suffer from headache, joint and muscular soreness, fatigue, and diarrhea, and generally there is no upper respiratory tract catarrhal symptom. Patients may have cough, mostly dry with scanty sputum, and chest dullness. Severe patients demonstrate accelerated respiration, shortness of breath, or obvious respiratory distress. Pulmonary signs are not obvious, and light moist rales may be audible or pulmonary consolidation observable.

Laboratory Examination

There is generally no increase of peripheral white blood cell count or decrease. Besides, the lymphocyte count is found generally declined.

Chest X-Ray Examination

Lungs present different degrees of patchy and plaque-shaped infiltration shadows or reticulate changes, which may progress rapidly into large patchy shadows. These commonly occur at multiple lobes or both sides, and absorption and dissipation of shadows are relatively slow. Pulmonary shadows and symptoms and signs may be inconsistent. If the test indicates negative, reexaminations shall be conducted after 1–2 days.

Effects of the Antibiotics Treatment

There are no remarkable responses to antibiotics.

2.7.1.2 Criteria for Clinical Diagnosis

Criteria for Diagnosis of Suspected Cases

Patients in compliance with any of the following three circumstances are diagnosed as suspected cases.

1. The patient has a history of intimate contact with patients, or is one of the infected population, or is confirmed having infecting other people by concrete evidences, who also manifest aforementioned clinical symptoms but not high white blood cell count by test of peripheral blood.
2. The patient has been to or lived in areas reported with infectious SARS patients and patients suffering from secondary infections 2 weeks before the disease onset, who also have abovementioned clinical symptoms and consistent pulmonary shadows on chest X-ray films with the abovementioned characteristics.
3. Despite the lack of epidemic data, the patient has abovementioned clinical manifestations and not high peripheral white blood cell count, as well as pulmonary shadows on chest X-ray that accord with abovementioned characteristics.

In other words, the patient conform to the aforementioned 1 (1)+2+3 or 1 (2) +2+4 or 2+3+4.

Criteria for Diagnosis of Clinically Diagnosed Cases

In case of any of the three following circumstances, the patient could be clinically diagnosed with SARS.

1. The patient has a history of intimate contact with patients, or is one of the infected population, or is confirmed having infecting other people by concrete evidences, who also manifest aforementioned clinical symptoms and pulmonary shadows on chest X-ray image.
2. The patient has been to or lived in areas reported with infectious SARS patients and patients suffering from secondary infections 2 weeks before the disease onset, who also have abovementioned clinical symptoms, not high peripheral blood white cell count and pulmonary shadows on chest X-ray films.
3. The patient has been to or lived in areas reported with infectious SARS patients and patients suffering from secondary infections 2 weeks before the disease onset, who also have abovementioned clinical symptoms, pulmonary shadows on chest X-ray films, and no obvious response to anti-infectious treatment.

In other words, the patient conform to aforementioned 1 (1)+2+4 or 1 (2) +2+3+4 or 1 (2)+2+4+5.

2.7.2 Clinical Classification and Staging

2.7.2.1 Criteria for Classification of Clinically Diagnosed Cases

Light Type

The conditions are mild without pulmonary fibrosis and other sequela. The prognosis is good.

Common Type

Patients have typical clinical manifestations of the early phase, progression phase, and recovery phase. The onset is acute, and the first symptom is fever, with body temperature generally >38 °C. Besides, the patients have no obvious respiratory distress or hypoxemia. Some patients are auscultated with slight moist rales or observed with pulmonary consolidation. The prognosis is good without sequelae.

Severe Type

Severe type accounts for about 30 %. It is same with the common type in clinical process but presents severe conditions and rapid progression. Some cases may progress to acute pulmonary injury or ARDS, rapidly incurring respiratory failure or even death. The diagnosis could be reached in case of any of the following three circumstances:

1. Dyspnea adult respiratory frequency is ≥30 times /min, accompanied by one of the following conditions:
   The chest imaging shows that the total surface of multilobar lesions or foci occupies more than 1/3 of the two lungs on orthotopic imaging.
   Conditions progress, with the focal area increased by over 50 % within 48 h or accounting for over 1/4 of the two lungs on orthotopic imaging.
2. Obvious hypoxemia is detected, with the oxygenation index lower than 300 mmHg.
3. Shock or multi-organic dysfunction syndrome occurs.

Miscellaneous

There are still some atypical cases of this disease.

2.7.2.2 Criteria for Staging of Clinically Diagnosed Cases

Early Phase

This generally refers to the first 1–7 days. The onset is acute and initial symptom is fever. Half of the patients are accompanied by the nonspecific systemic symptoms such as chillness, headache, and joint and muscular soreness.

Progression Phase

This phase spans the day 8–14 of the disease course. Infectious toxic symptoms such as fever, fatigue, muscular soreness continue to exist or even aggravate. Patient's body temperature rises, possibly to 39 °C or higher in a short time, and the high fever is persistent. Lung lesions demonstrate progressive exacerbation. A few patients (10–15 %) may develop ARDS, which is life threatening.

Recovery Phase

It mostly takes place at day 15–21 of disease course. Most patients have good prognosis after recovery for about 2 weeks. Some severe patients could gradually recover within 2–3 months after discharge.

2.8 Imaging Techniques and Protection

2.8.1 Chest Imaging Techniques of SARS

2.8.1.1 Conventional Chest X-Ray Examinations

These mainly encompass standing chest X-ray and bedside chest X-ray, which are economic and effective examination methods and first optional examination for preliminary diagnosis and reexamination. Mobile X-ray bedside imaging should be applied for patients under observation and inpatients. As lung disease of SARS patients progress rapidly, chest X-ray reexamination within a short period could help observe changes of conditions, commonly once every 1–2 days at the early phase and progression phase. Regular chest X-ray also need to be conducted during recovery phase so as to ascertain absorption and dissipation of lesions, residual foci, and pulmonary interstitial fibrosis.

2.8.1.2 Chest CT Scan

For SARS patients, CT scan generally is not a preferred method and, if necessary, could be conducted under strict disinfected quarantine. If the foci could not be absorbed for a long term in SARS recovery phase or patients still have symptoms but normal chest presentations, CT scan need to be carried out for further observation as it can better visualize the subtle pulmonary interstitial changes, such as lung interlobular septum thickening, intralobular septum thickening, subpleural linear shadow, and small ground-glass-density lesion and regional and segmental bronchiectasis, and therefore is helpful for clinical diagnosis of pulmonary interstitial fibrosis. Thin-layer CT scan or HRCT scan can better visualize intrapulmonary low-density small lesions, thus contributory to early diagnosis of pulmonary interstitial fibrosis. CT examination could also aid identification of other concurrent lung lesions.

2.8.2 Protection and Quarantine of Department of Radiology

Medical staff in the room of imaging examination and department of radiology shall prevent infections in strict compliance with SARS disinfection and prevention requirements and meanwhile conscientiously implement X-ray protection.

2.8.2.1 Protection Requirements of Photographs at Bedside or Fever Clinic

1. Ward shall be equipped with bedside X-ray machine; Imaging for all SARS inpatients shall be conducted in wards and patients shall wear masks.
2. The personal protection for imaging technician should be subject to the level-two protection requirements and, when necessary (imaging for critically ill patients), to level-three protection requirements.
3. X-ray film magazine should be put into the isolation bag before imaging (one isolation bag for each person).
4. The imaging technicians should sterilize their hands before return to the radiological department and then remove protective clothing, gloves, and protective glasses at the designated place. They should wash hands thoroughly, gargle, take a shower, and change clean working clothes before work.

2.8.2.2 Disinfection and Protection of Department of Radiology

1. The department must strengthen interior ventilation and air disinfection . Ultraviolet irradiation may be assumed at night, 2–3 times per day, 30 minutes per time, and peracetic acid spray conducted 2 times per day.
2. Rigorous isolation measures: all subjects must wear masks. The operation staff must wear protective masks, gloves, and gowns, with masks changed every 4 h and gowns replaced in time, and should use disposal bed sheet and shoe covers, and dispose of and replace them timely after the examination.
3. SARS examination zone should be separated from conventional patient examination zone and examination staff shall be fixed. If feasible, special chest X-ray examination room and X-ray machines may be set up in the isolation zone to avoid cross-infections.

2.8.2.3 Protective Technical Requirements for CT Scan

1. The protective measures for subjects and operation staff are similar to those required about isolation protection in radiological department.
2. All the subjects must wear masks and, for examination in CT room, shall minimize the stay time as much as possible.
3. After the patient leaves, the environment and articles which may be polluted by patients shall be given terminal disinfection.
4. The department must enhance interior ventilation and air disinfection and, in addition to use of chemical disinfectant spray, may also initiate long-term ultraviolet irradiation at night for disinfection.
5. A pathway specific for SARS patients should be established.

2.9 Chest X-ray Diagnosis

2.9.1 Pathological Basis of Chest Imaging Manifestations

The imaging manifestations of SARS are closely related to its pathological changes. Besides edema, inflammatory cell infiltration and other nonspecific inflammatory changes, the more prominent pulmonary pathological feature of SARS is abundant exfoliation of epithelial cells, inducing obvious thickening and damage of alveolar septum, as well as significant organization of effusions inside alveolar cavities. All the three changes of inflammation in early phase (degeneration, exudation, hyperplasia) are observable. The mechanism of acute lung injury induced by SARS may be ascribed to SARS coronavirus direct attack of alveolar epithelia and alveolar capillary epithelia or (and) indirect damage via lymphocyte, macrophage and effector cells, and lymphokine, cytokine, and inflammatory mediator released by them. This suggests that besides viral direct infection, immune reactions are also involved in lung injury.

In severe lung injury, pulmonary interstitial and pulmonary parenchymal air cavity changes detected by autopsy pathology, especially pulmonary air cavity not completely filled by lesion or filled but coexistent with unfilled alveoli, are visualized as ground-glass-density shadows on X-ray and CT. Varying degrees of residual lung cavity present with different densities of ground-glass shadows on thin-layer CT or high-resolution CT (HRCT). Complete filling of the alveolar space leads to pulmonary consolidation shadows.

Once pulmonary edema and alveolar hyaline membrane are formed, patients clinically manifest decreased lung compliance, progressive dyspnea, and intractable hypoxemia. It is such rapid pathological changes of SARS that give rise to characteristic presentations by chest X-ray examination, including rapid progression of lesions, diverse morphological states, and wide range, often spanning several segments and lobes. Therefore, dynamic observation of chest image holds great significance for diagnosis of SARS.

2.9.2 Basic Imaging Manifestations of SARS

2.9.2.1 Ground-Glass-Density Shadows

Ground-glass-density shadows are pathologically the result of lesions mainly at pulmonary interstitium and alveoli, with pulmonary interstitial lesions frequently complicated by alveolitis. Ground-glass-density shadows incurred by alveolar consolidation are attributable to partial filling of alveoli or coexistence of filling and unfilled alveoli. Such shadows on X-ray and CT can be determined if the density of lesions is lower than that of blood vessels, and blood vessel presentations are observable inside. The density of lesions lower than that of pulmonary hila on X-ray could also help identify ground-glass-density shadows.

2.9.2.2 Pulmonary Consolidation Shadows

Pulmonary consolidation shadows are pathologically due to filling of alveoli by pathological tissues, which is frequently complicated with lung interstitial lesions. Pulmonary consolidation could be confirmed if the lesions are found with higher density than vascular shadows and without vascular shadows inside but with air bronchogram on X-ray and CT. It could also be determined if the lesions present higher density than pulmonary hila or similar density to mediastinum. The lesions are solitary or multiple in small patches, and some lesions are distributed along lung lobes and segments.

2.9.3 Chest X-Ray Manifestations of SARS

2.9.3.1 Early Phase of Onset

96 % of SARS patients may develop subsequently solitary and multiple small patchy shadows within seven days of onset, with relatively low density, blurry borders, and irregular shapes, predominantly solitary. Occasionally, the pulmonary textures around lesions are revealed increased and thickened and mainly distributed at peripheral area, more commonly at bilateral inferior lungs. Since chest X-ray can poorly visualize relatively small lesions and at sometimes posteroanterior X-ray can hardly display lesions overlapping with heart shadows, orthotopic chest imaging should be conducted at the same time (Fig. 2.9).

2.9.3.2 Progression Phase

The conditions of most patients become worse within 14 days after onset. The small patchy shadows in the early phase may progress into large patchy, multiple, or diffusive lesions. The lesions may spread from unilateral lung to both lungs and from one lung field to several fields. Severe patients may demonstrate obvious changes 1–2 days after onset.

Lesions present mainly as ground-glass-density shadows or coexist with lung consolidation shadows. The center of some shadows with high density indicates consolidation, and relatively low-density peripheral area suggests ground-glass

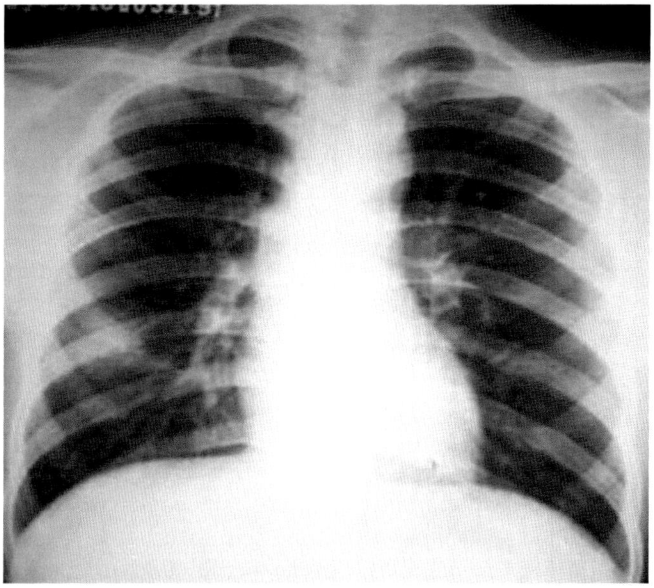

Fig. 2.9 The 18-year-old male patient diagnosed with SARS. The specific segment RT-PCR of SRS virus is positive. On day 5 of onset, the right inferior lung field was observed with patchy ill-demarcated shadows of increased density

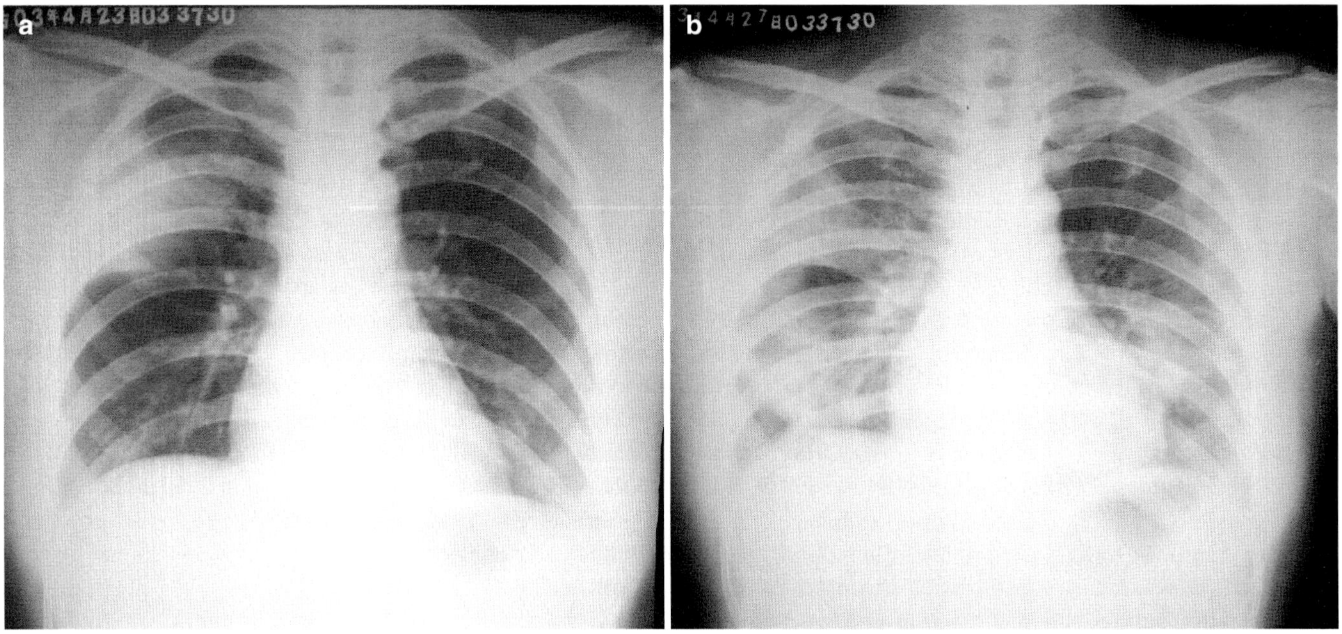

Fig. 2.10 (**a**, **b**) The 37-year-old female patient was examined with positive SARS antibody and diagnosed with SARS. (**a**) On the 11th day after onset, the right upper lung field was detected with large ill-defined patchy shadows. (**b**) On day 14 after onset, the right middle and inferior lung field and left middle and inferior lung field were seen with large patchy strip blurry shadows. Compared with afore imaging, the foci demonstrated obvious progression

density which may be complicated with thickening and increase of pulmonary textures. Severe patients may develop "white lung."

Some cases may have pneumothorax, pneumomediastinum, and subcutaneous emphysema after the use of ventilator.

A small part of lesions adjacent to the pleura may be complicated with local pleural thickening or revealed with mild tentiform adhesion. Pleural changes may reside after absorption of intrapulmonary lesions. Complication of slight pleural effusions may also be observable (Fig. 2.10).

2.9.3.3 Recovery Phase

The lesions of SARS patients begin to be absorbed in 15–30 days, which can be completely absorbed for majority patients. A few patients may show pulmonary fibrosis or pulmonary interstitial hyperplasia, with apparent pulmonary interstitial hyperplasia occurring 30–40 days after the onset. The intrapulmonary patchy shadows present with shrinkage and increase of density to gradually form high-density cord-like and honeycomb-shaped shadows in lungs. Severe pulmonary interstitial proliferation could dwindle the lung volume and make the mediastinum shift to the affected side. The imaging may reveal local irregular high-density plaque and cord-shaped shadows. Occurrence of intrapulmonary honeycomb-shaped shadows and tractional bronchiectasis is the characteristic of pulmonary interstitial fibrosis (Fig. 2.11).

2.9.4 Section Four Dynamic Changes of Chest X-Ray Manifestations

As rapid change is an important feature of SARS chest X-ray manifestations, dynamic X-ray studies and observations could provide evidences for SARS definite diagnosis. Therefore, observation of the disease dynamic change is critical to SARS chest X-ray, which is a major difference from X-ray examinations of other pneumonia. In the early phase and progression phase of SARS, lung foci may undergo remarkable changes within a short time (24 h at the shortest), such as expansion and dissemination, which are characterized by changes in shape, extent, and site of the foci. This suggests that clinical physicians shall conduct chest orthotopic imaging once every 24–48 h after the SARS patients are hospitalized so as to ascertain the disease changes.

Imaging dynamic changes are associated with multiple factors, such as age, original underlying disease, treatment method, and efficacy. The lesions are generally absorbed 14 days after onset but possibly on day 7 in some mild patients. The focal shadows may become smaller with the density gradually decreased. One characteristic dynamic change of SARS is migrating change of lesions in some patients, suggesting that the foci firstly occur at the unilateral inferior lung field and then spread to contralateral and/or superior and middle lung field. Patients with worse lesions may manifest wider imaging extent and new foci, and severe patients may develop "white lung." ARDS is a key cause leading to death of patients (Fig. 2.12).

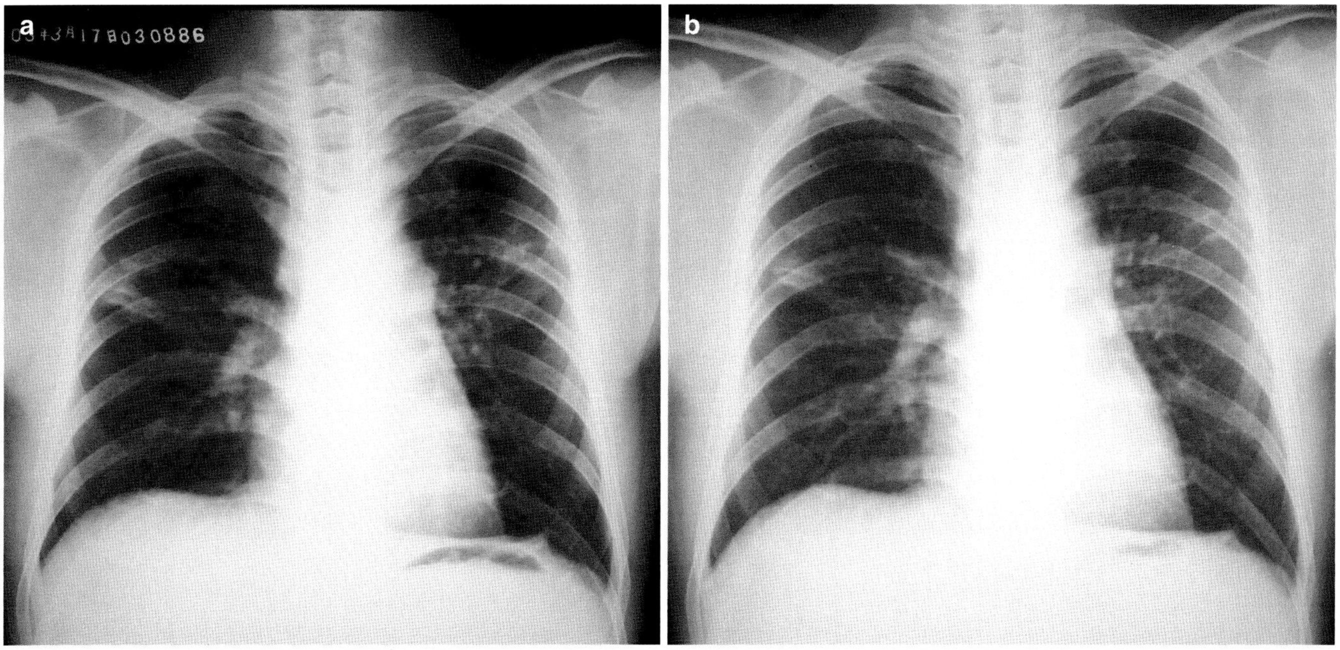

Fig. 2.11 (**a**, **b**) The male patient aged 34 years old was tested positive for specific segment RT-PCR of SARS virus RNA and was diagnosed with SARS. (**a**) 31 days after onset, both the middle and superior lung fields were detected with patchy and strip shadows as well as spotted shadows. (**b**) 38 days after onset, the foci at both superior lung fields presented with absorption and improvement, but a few linear shadows

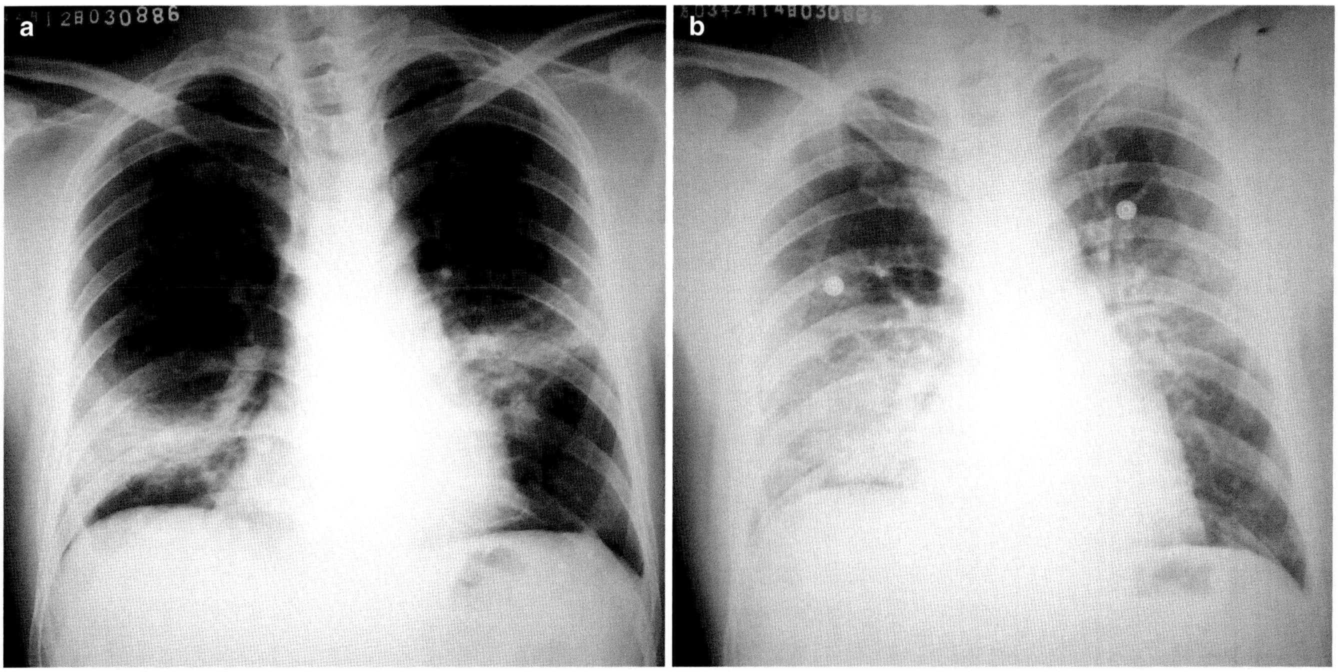

Fig. 2.12 (**a**–**e**) The male patient aged 34 years old was confirmed with SARS. (**a**). 4 days after onset (February 12, 2003), right inferior lung and left middle lung field was detected with large patchy and strip shadows, which had inhomogeneous density and blurry borders. (**b**) 6 days after onset, the foci at both lung fields expanded obviously to inferior lung field, which presented light-density patchy and strip shadows with migrating changes. (**c**) 10 days after onset, partial foci at both lung fields were absorbed and improved and became lighter in density, with absorption of right inferior lung field foci more obvious. (**d**) On day 13 of onset, foci at right inferior lung field were absorbed and improved and both superior lung fields were observed with ill-defined patches and strips of increased density. (**e**) On day 26 of onset, the blurry patchy and strip shadows on both superior lung fields were visualized with lighter density and slight shrinkage

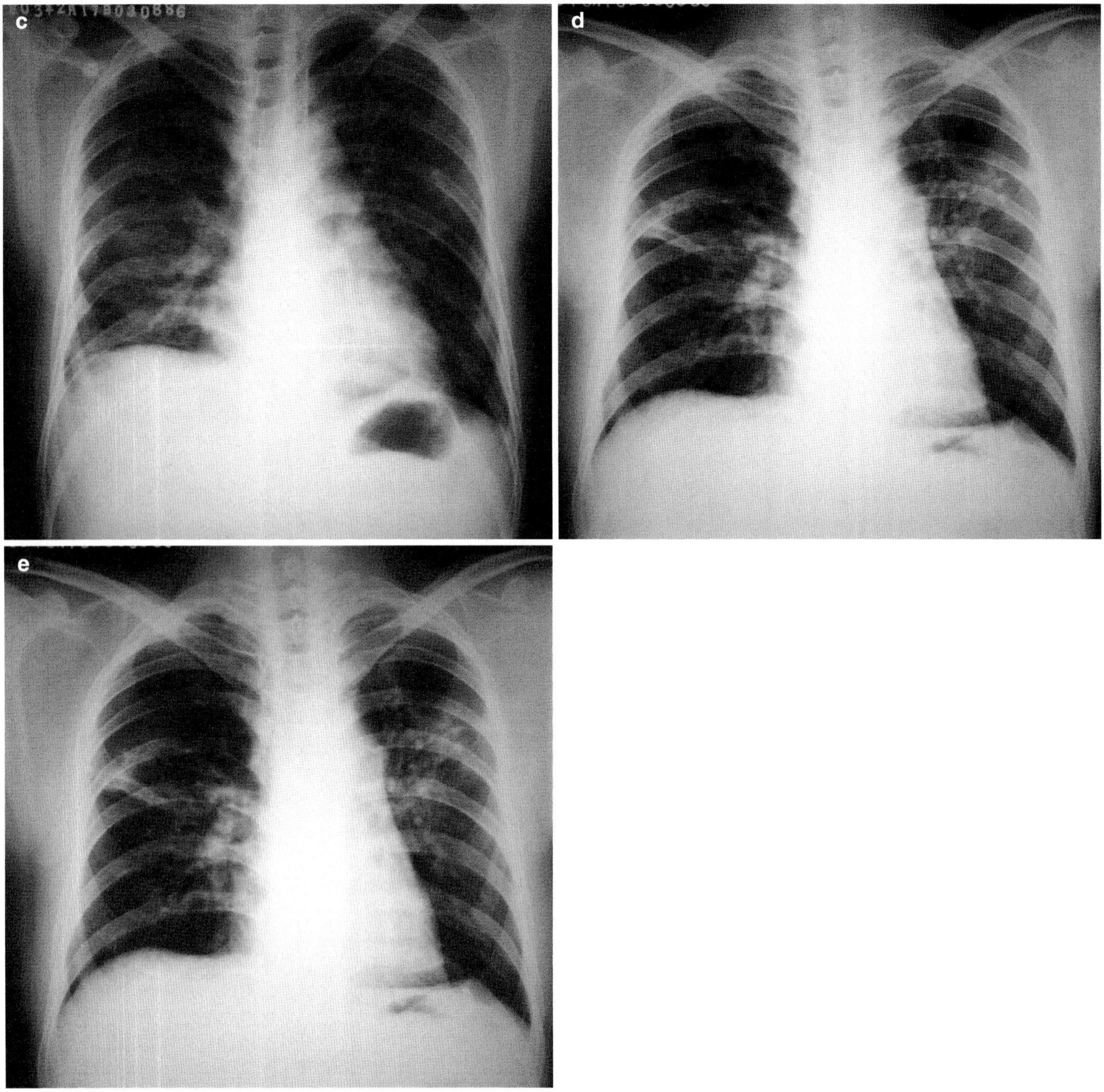

Fig. 2.12 (continued)

2.10 Chest CT Diagnosis

2.10.1 CT Manifestations of SARS

Lung imaging examination is an important basis for SARS diagnosis, and continual imaging examination could visualize the dynamic change characteristics of the disease.

2.10.1.1 Initial Phase

After SARS infection, chest abnormal changes frequently occur on day 1–7. In initial phase, focal shadows are frequently seen, which might be unilateral but dominantly bilateral. CT reveals small patchy ground-glass-density shadows, some of which are quasi-circular. Lesions present as solitary small patchy lung consolidation and multiple small patchy or relatively large patchy shadows. Large foci may appear as

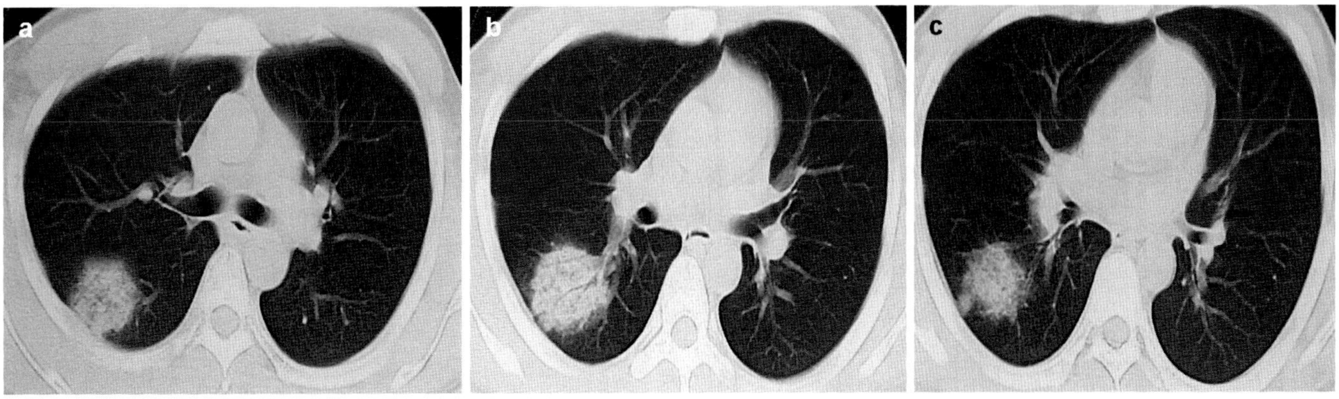

Fig. 2.13 (a–c) The male patient aged 25 years old was diagnosed with SARS (right inferior lung segment pneumonia). On day 6 of onset (March 28, 2003), CT plain scan lung window indicated patchy shadows of increased density at the posterior segment of right superior lobe, which had relatively clear borders

ground-glass-density shadows and concurrent lung consolidation shadows, with relatively higher-density vascular shadows observable in the former. Besides, some foci are found with increased vascular shadows at the periphery. In addition, lesions are unveiled frequently at the bilateral lung inferior fields and lung margins (Fig. 2.13).

2.10.1.2 Progression Phase

Lesions in majority patients may progress and worsen within 14 days after onset. The small patchy shadows in early phase could expand into large patchy, multiple, or diffusive lesions within 3–7 days. Besides, lesions extend from unilateral lung to bilateral lungs, from one lung field to multiple lung fields. Most patients could develop the severest infiltration of lungs on day 8–14, namely, peak phase or "critical" phase. CT presentations are still predominated by ground-glass-density shadows, which may be complicated by pulmonary consolidation. Lesions are commonly multiple and in diffusive distribution at both lungs, and lesions of varying shapes may coexist, with quasi-circular foci relatively common. Some cases appear with ground-glass-density shadows all the time from onset to absorption of lesions.

When ground-glass-density shadows are complicated by pulmonary consolidation, the large patchy, small patchy, or quasi-circular ground-glass-density shadows could be observed with pulmonary consolidation shadows of relatively high density. Ground-glass density and pulmonary consolidation may also occur at different parts of the lung and could be visualized on the same layer or different layers of CT. For lesions typical of pulmonary consolidation, pulmonary consolidation appears as plaque-shaped high-density shadows or consolidation signs at lung lobes and segments. In addition, lesions are frequently recorded at lung lobe segment of the inferior lobe and outer band of lung field (Fig. 2.14).

2.10.1.3 Recovery Phase

Lesions usually begin to be absorbed 2–3 weeks after onset, with the shadow shrunk and density gradually reduced and absorbed. Although the clinical symptoms of some patients improve and disappear, light ground-glass-density shadows could still be seen in lungs on CT. It may prolong a relatively long time. During the absorption of intrapulmonary lesions, there is also concurrent pulmonary interstitial proliferation, which begins to be absorbed under dynamic observation. Some lesions may develop into pulmonary interstitial fibrosis, characterized by lobular septum, intralobular septum, interstitial thickening, and subpleural curvature imaging signs as well as regional irregular high-density plaque and cord-like presentations. Occurrence of intrapulmonary honeycomb manifestations and tractional bronchiectasis signifies pulmonary interstitial fibrosis (Fig. 2.15).

2.11 Imaging Diagnosis of Complications

SARS complication is an important factor affecting prognosis, which should be given enormous attentions. During SARS treatment, antiviral drugs are administered as well as glucocorticoids and broad-spectrum antibiotics. Some patients may still need airway positive pressure ventilation, tracheotomy, and tracheal intubation. Reasonable use of such measures is of great significance for improving the treatment rate and lowering mortality of SARS patients. However, to be noted, such treatment drugs and methods may incur adverse reactions and cause complications. SARS complications already detected encompass pulmonary secondary infection, mediastinal and subcutaneous emphysema, pneumothorax, bone aseptic necrosis, empyema, brain secondary infection, and pulmonary interstitial

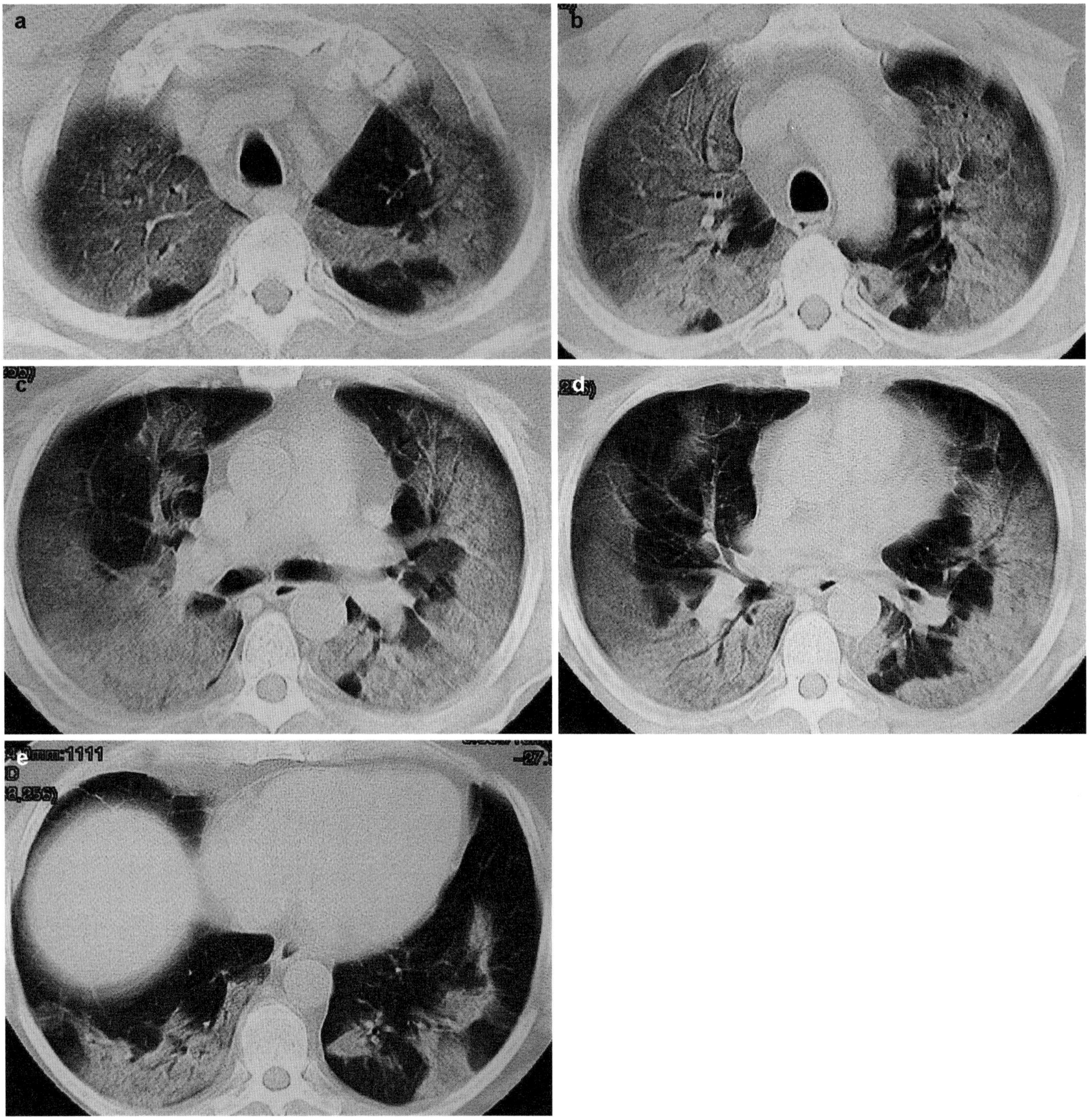

Fig. 2.14 (**a–e**) The male patient aged 52 years old was tested positive for the specific segment RT-PCR of SARS virus RNA. On day 4 of onset (April 2, 2003), chest CT plain scan revealed extensive large patchy ground-glass blurry shadows at bilateral superior, middle and inferior lung fields, and consolidation and air bronchogram at different layers

fibrosis. Such complications or sequela changes are also mainly identified by imaging examinations. Familiarity about SARS imaging manifestations and knowledge about complication imaging presentations could elevate SARS diagnostic level, therefore increasing cure rate and decreasing mortality.

2.11.1 Imaging Diagnosis of Pulmonary Interstitial Fibrosis

2.11.1.1 Pathogenesis and Clinical Data

In the early phase, SARS manifests bronchiolar and peripheral interstitial pneumonia, which could further progress into

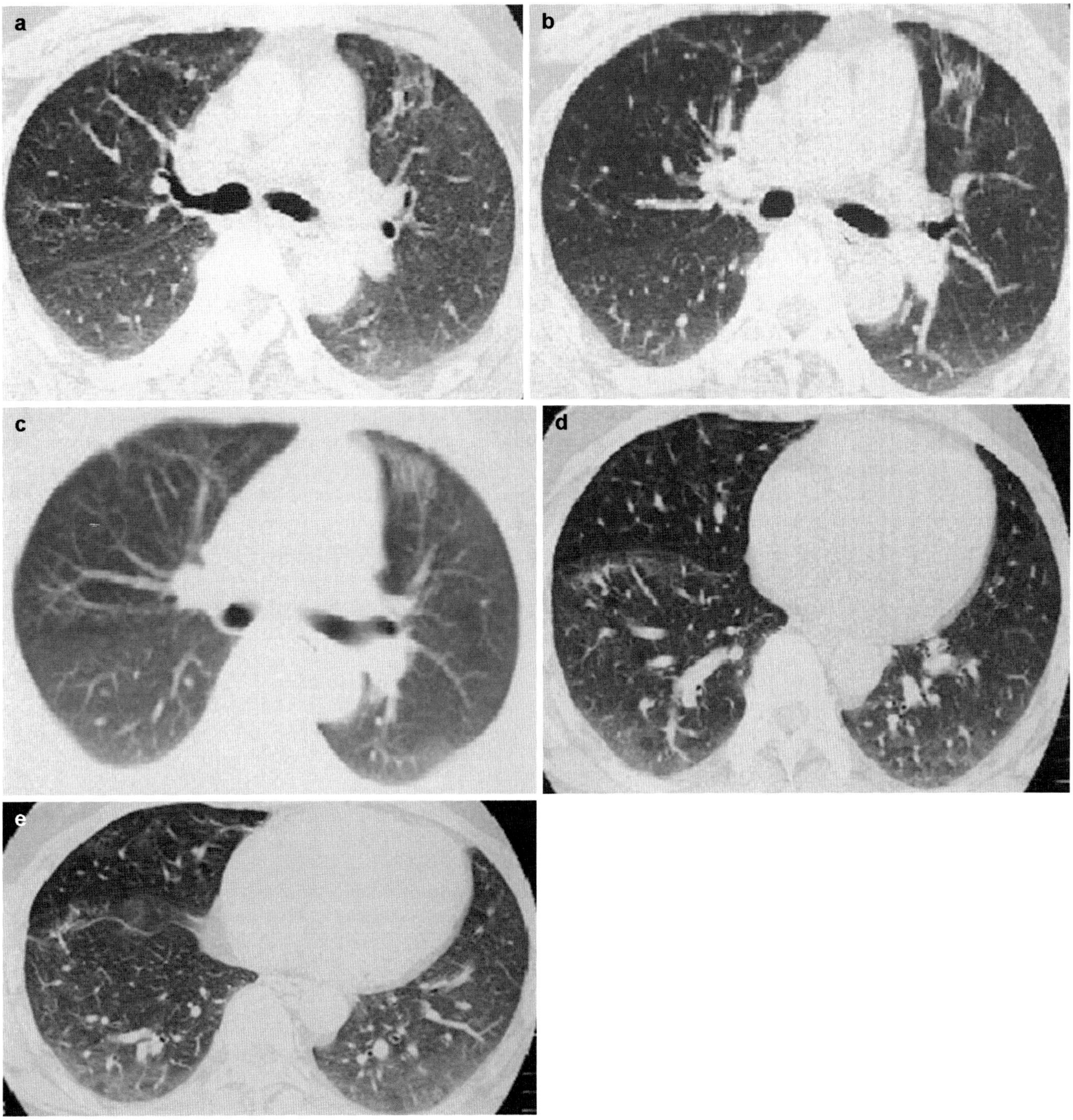

Fig. 2.15 (**a–e**) The male patient aged 44 years old was confirmed with SARS. On day 82 of onset (April 16, 2003), chest CT plain scan revealed cord-like shadows and ground-glass-density shadows at the left lung superior segment ligule and right lung inferior lobe antero-basal segment. Right lung middle and inferior lobe was detected with lobular septum thickening and subpleural curvature shadows

alveolar consolidation, with interstitial lesions present persistently and mostly reversible. In the recovery phase, only some cases develop into pulmonary interstitial proliferation and then cause fibrotic changes. Pulmonary interstitial proliferation and fibrosis degree and outcome are associated with the extent of pulmonary involvement in peak phase, occurrence of complications, and treatment. Generally, if lesions on chest image are light in peak phase, there will be fewer pulmonary changes left in recovery phase. Contrarily, patients with diffusive lung interstitial thickening in recovery phase are often those suffering from relatively severe pulmonary injury in peak phase and involvement of the great mass of lungs, particularly patients with recurrent conditions, protracted course, and concurrent infections. Researches demonstrate that 7–8 % of SARS patients have pulmonary fibrosis of varying degrees and male patients display relatively more obvious pulmonary impairment than female patients. Primary manifestations are lung dysfunction, such as decrease of pulmonary diffusion capacity, lung capacity impairment, and change of total lung capacity particularly residual volume.

2.11.1.2 Imaging Manifestations

Generally obvious pulmonary interstitial proliferation occurs at about 30–50 days after onset, which presents firstly lobular septum and intralobular thickening and subpleural curvature shadows. Then there is the shrinkage of intrapulmonary patchy shadows with increase of density and gradual formation of high-density cord and honeycomb shadows inside lungs. Severe pulmonary interstitial proliferation could diminish lung volume and compel the mediastinum to affected side. Besides, pulmonary interstitial proliferation could occur extensively inside lungs, predominated by lobular septum, intralobular interstitial thickening, and subpleural curvature shadows, as well as irregular high-density plaque and cord-like shadows at some regions. Honeycomb-shaped shadows and tractional bronchiectasis are signs of pulmonary interstitial fibrosis. CT reveals cord, reticulate, and honeycomb-shaped shadows, and HRCT could better visualize the subtle abnormal changes of pulmonary interstitium, such as lobular septum thickening, intralobular interstitial thickening, subpleural curvature shadows, and honeycomb-shaped shadows. Whether the cord-like and reticulate changes visualized by CT are completely absorbed or induce persistent fibrosis still entails long-term follow-up observation (Fig. 2.16).

2.11.2 Aseptic Necrosis of Femoral Head

2.11.2.1 Pathogenesis and Clinical Data

Numerous SARS patients develop osteonecrosis after recovery, which mostly appears as femoral head necrosis and also possibly necrosis of the ankle joint, knee joint, and shoulder joint. Scans of bilateral hips and knees of 82 SARS patients in rehabilitation phase disclosed that 51 patients (62 %) suffered from osseous abnormality, of which bone ischemia accounts for 17 % and implication of three sites for 20 %. Its pathogenesis still remains not completely ascertained, and it may be ascribed to improper use of hormones and injury of sclerotin from SARS viruses, bacterial embolism, lipid embolism, or multiple mixed factors. The primary pathological change of aseptic necrosis of femoral head is degenerative alteration due to femoral head blood circulation disturbance, mainly characterized by limping and pain. The lower limb of the affected side is relatively shorter and presents with light flexion and adduction, as well as with slightly limited abduction and intorsion.

2.11.2.2 Imaging Manifestations of Aseptic Necrosis of Femoral Head

Initial X-ray examinations suggest that the involved femoral head has normal appearance but inhomogeneous density, with spotted osteoporosis. Gradually ensue the increase of density as a result of osteonecrosis, which meanwhile is interspersed with some transparent shadows. Femoral head may become flat, fragmented, and irregular in contour from pressures. Typical femoral head necrosis appears in the shape of wedge, with the base toward articular surface and the top toward metaphysis. Since lesions are dominantly confined at the anterosuperior area of femoral head, lateral imaging of hip joints could clearly reproduce the extent of lesions. The necrotic area is encircled by a ring of transparent band. Hip articular cavity may become wider and irregular due to flattening of the femur. Sometimes, there may be complication of dislocation. The fragments of femoral head may be shed off into the joint, giving rise to joint mouse.

Normal femoral head is located at the acetabular center in the transverse CT image and may appear in the shape of sphere or hook on different layers, with delicate high-density bone cortex at the periphery. The high-density trabeculae inside femoral head are arranged in stelliform formation from the center continually to bone cortex, named as "stelliform sign." CT manifestations of aseptic necrosis of femoral head can be divided into early and advanced phase. In the early phase, the stelliform sign formed by the trabeculae of femoral head is deformed or absent, presenting spotted and patchy shadows of increased density inside femoral head and fasciculate changes or mutual fusion at its periphery. In the advanced phase, femoral head become ruptured and out of shape, and absorption of sclerotin between bone fragments appears as irregular low-density area, with stelliform sign disappeared.

MRI manifestations of aseptic necrosis of femoral head include: necrotic areas of femoral head of early cases have no repair reactions or mechanic collapse and still maintain normal lipid signals of medullary bones. However, low-signal margins incurred by sclerosis reactions could be seen at the periphery of foci. The T1 high signals of normal femoral head on T1-weighted image are detected with black linear low signals (representing demarcation between normal and ischemic bone tissues). On T2-weighted image, a high-signal line is visible at the medial low-signal sclerotic reaction line, thus forming the typical double-line sign. The double-line sign could reflect congestion and inflammation of granula-

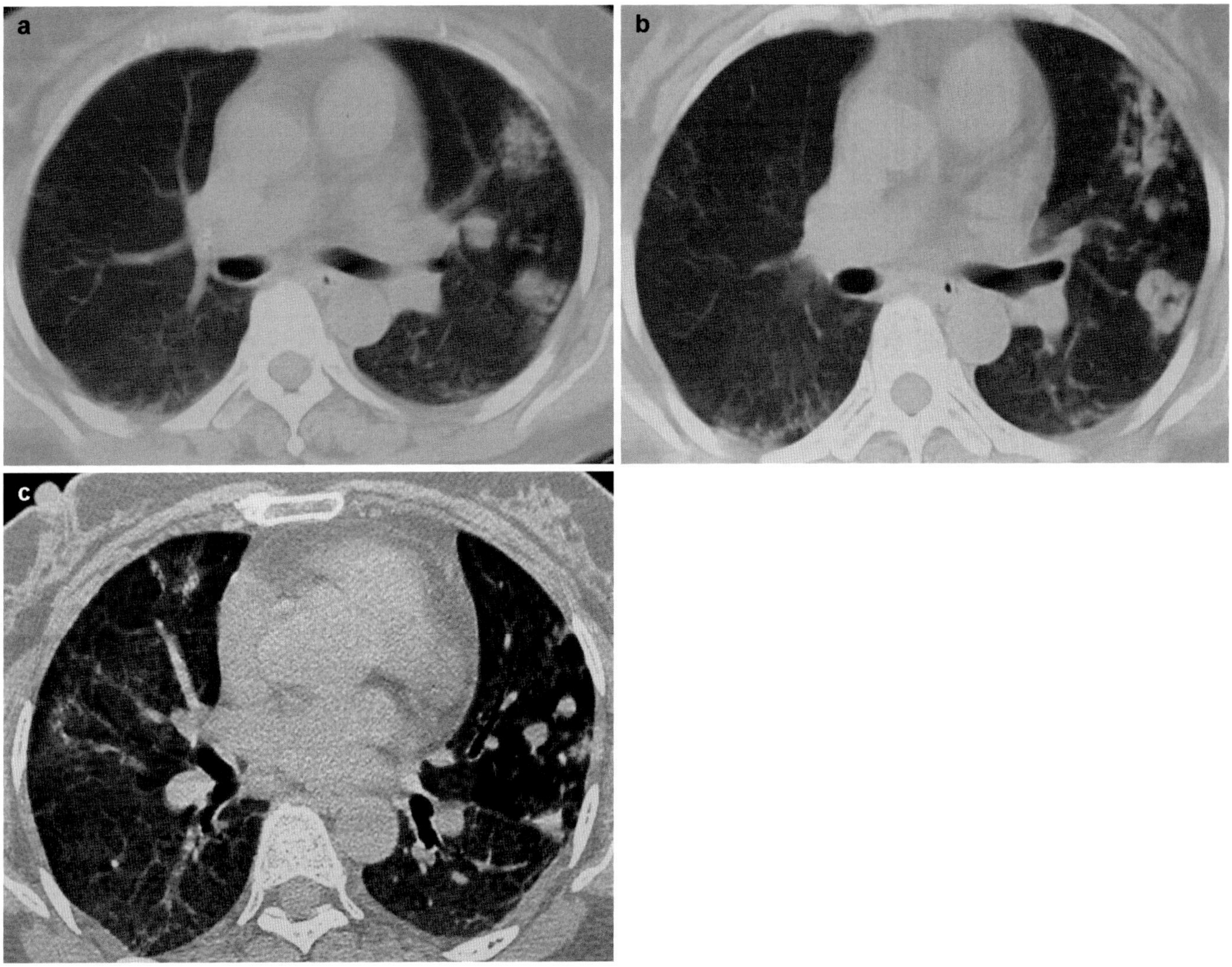

Fig. 2.16 (**a–c**) The female patient aged 54 years old was detected with SARS complicated by pulmonary interstitial fibrosis. On February 20, 2003, the patient had continuous fever, cough without sputum but accompanied with shortness of breath. The patient was hospitalized on March 4, 2003, and cured and discharged on May 15, 2003. On July 21, 2003, CT revealed scattered plaque shadows of increased density, subpleural curvature shadows, and other pulmonary interstitial fibrosis presentations at both lung fields

tion tissues and proves specific to aseptic necrosis of femoral head. Severe inflammation, congestion, fibrosis, and sclerosis could greatly deplete the amount of lipids of femoral head, which presents liquid-like signals on MRI, low signals on T1-weighted image, and high signals on T2-weighted images. Advanced cases are typical of fibrosis and sclerosis, and the affected area present with fibrotic MRI features, that is, low signals on T1- and T2-weighted and proton density-weighted imaging. Complication with effusions in hip joints appears as T1 low signals and T2 high signals.

Based on MRI presentations, aseptic necrosis of femoral head could be classified into four phases: phase I is characterized by homogenous or inhomogeneous low-signal areas adjacent to the joint above the femoral head on T1-weighted imaging; phase II is visualized with wedge-shaped low-signal bands; phase III presents with sequestrum crescent sign and cortex collapse; phase IV manifests joint degeneration and joint space narrowing besides presentations of phase III. In light of the aforementioned MR staging criteria, SARS cases complicated by aseptic necrosis of femoral head already reported are mostly in phase II.

Additionally, aseptic necrosis after use of hormones, besides most frequently involvement of the femoral head, could also implicate other joints, such as the knee joint, elbow joint, ankle joint, and acetabulum. Therefore, if necessary, MR examinations of other joints shall be conducted to ascertain the extent and degree of lesions. If SARS patients complain of pain at both hip joints and limited movement, CT scan or MRI examination of both hip joints is recommended to conclude definite diagnosis. X-ray plain scan is not sensitive to early bone ischemic necrosis, which therefore is not preferred (Fig. 2.17 and 2.18).

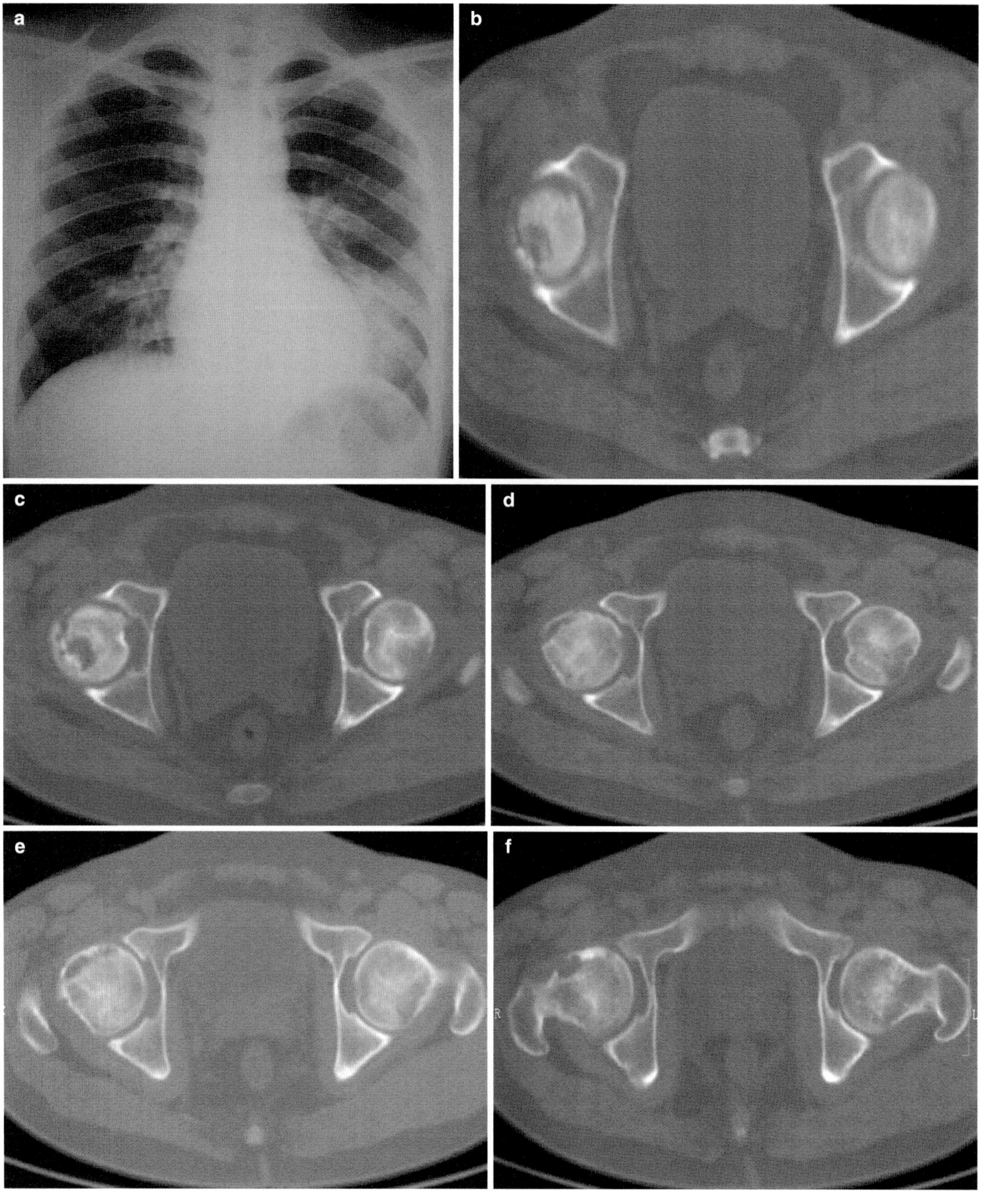

Fig. 2.17 (**a–f**) The male patient aged 28 years old was examined with SARS and concurrent ischemic necrosis of right femoral head. Methylprednisolone 1880 mg was administered. (**a**). Early chest imaging demonstrated band or patchy blurry shadows in the left inferior lung field. (**b–f**). 33 months after onset, CT visualized irregular low-density damaged area at the right femoral head and neck

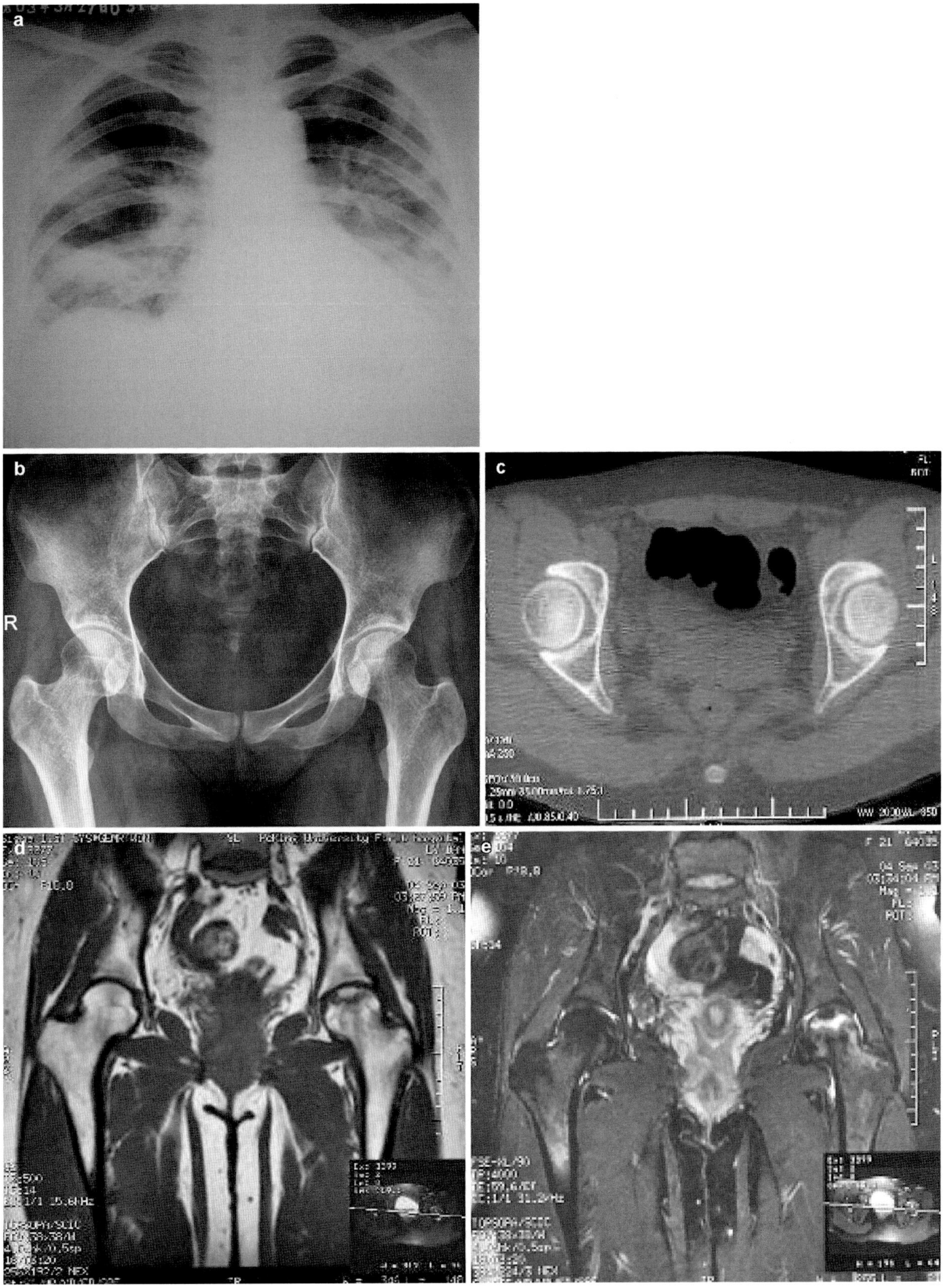

Fig. 2.18 (**a**–**e**) The female patient aged 40 years old was confirmed with SARS complicated by left femoral head ischemic necrosis. Methylprednisolone 4180 mg was given. (**a**) On day 15 after onset, both middle and inferior lung fields were seen with large patchy irregular color shadows of increased density. (**b**) On day 32 after onset, X-ray plain scan indicated bilateral femoral heads free of obvious abnormalities in shape and density. (**c**) On day 40 after onset, axial CT scan suggested bilateral femoral heads without obvious abnormalities in shape and density. (**d**) On day 185 after onset, MRI T1WI revealed left femoral head with linear T1 low signals. (**e**) On day 185 after onset, MRI T2WI visualized left femoral head with wedged-shaped T2 high signals

Further Reading

1. Huang WJ, Xu H, Li ZB, et al. The first case of severe acute respiratory syndrome in Heyuan City, Guangdong Province. Chin J Tuberc Respir Dis. 2003;26(11):736–7.
2. Shuyun X, Guang Z, Jie L, et al. Analyses on one case of severe acute respiratory syndrome "super transmitter" and chain of transmission. Chin J Epidemiol. 2003;24:449–53.
3. Ksiazek TG, Erdman D, Goldsmith CS, et al. A novel coronavirus associated with severe acute respiratory syndrome. N Engl J Med. 2003;348(20):1953–66.
4. Peiris JS, Lais ST, Poon LL, et al. Coronavirus as a possible cause of severe acute respiratory syndrome. Lancet. 2003;361(9366): 1319–25.
5. Drosten C, Gunther S, Preiser W, et al. Identification of a novel coronavirus in patients with severe acute respiratory syndrome. N Engl J Med. 2003;348(20):1967–76.
6. Poutanen SM, Low DE, Henry B, et al. Identification of severe acute respiratory syndrome in Canada. N Engl J Med. 2003; 348(20):1995–2005.
7. Tsang KW, Ho PL, Ooi GC, et al. A cluster of cases of severe acute respiratory syndrome in Hong Kong. N Engl J Med. 2003; 348(20):1977–85.
8. Rota PA, Oberste MS, Monroe SS, et al. Characterization of a novel coronavirus associated with severe acute respiratory syndrome. Science. 2003;300(5624):1394–9.
9. Marra MA, Jones SJ, Astell CR, et al. The genome sequence of the SARS-associated coronavirus. Science. 2003;300(5624): 1399–404.
10. Boping Z, Xinchun C, Huosheng W, et al. Identification and molecular cloning and sequence analysis of a novel coronavirus from patients with SARS by RT PCR. Chin J Exp Clin Virol. 2003;5:137–40.
11. Fouchier RA, Kuiken T, Schutten M, et al. Aetiology: Koch's postulates fulfilled for SARS virus. Nature. 2003;423(6937):240.
12. Brown EG, Tetro JA. Comparative analysis of the SARS coronavirus genome: a good start to a long journey. Lancet. 2003;361(9371):1756–7.
13. LIU YN, FAN BX, FANG XQ, et al. The quantitative detection of anti-coronavirus antibody titer in medical personnel closely contacted with severe acute respiratory syndrome patients. Chin J Tuberc Respir Dis. 2003;26(10):583.
14. YIN CB, ZHANG FC, TANG XP, et al. Measurement of subsets of blood T lymphocyte in 93 patients with severe acute respiratory syndrome and its clinical significance. Chin J Tuberc Respir Dis. 2003;26(6):343.
15. Guan Y, Zheng BJ, He YQ. Isolation and characterization of viruses related to the SARS coronavirus from animals in southern China. Science. 2003;302(5643):276–8.
16. Krokhin O, Li Y, Andonov A, et al. Mass Spectrometric Characterization of Proteins from the SARS virus: a preliminary Report. Mol Cell Proteomics. 2003;2(5):346–56.
17. Yan CG, Xie Q, Lu ZM. Research advance in origin of severe acute respiratory syndrome virus. Chin J Infect Dis. 2003;21(4): 297–300.
18. Zheng-lun XIAO, Yi-min LI, Rong-chang CHENG, et al. Severe acute respiratory syndrome in 78 patients:a retrospective study. Chin J Tuberc Respir Dis. 2003;6:334–8.
19. Booth CM, Makutas LM, Tomlinson GA, et al. Clinical features and short-term outcomes of 144 patients with SARS in the greater Toronto area. JAMA. 2003;289(21):2801–9.
20. Donnelly CA, Ghani AC, Leung GM, et al. Epidemiological determinants of spread of causal agent of severe acute respiratory syndrome in Hong Kong. Lancet. 2003;361(9371):1761–6.
21. Yang WZ, Wang HZ, Zhang J, et al. Preliminary analysis of the infectious atypical pneumonia and its prevention and control measures. Chin J Epidemiol. 2003;24(6):432–3.
22. Zhong-zhi LI, Kun-ling SHEN, Xin-miao WEI, et al. Clinical analysis of 18 pediatric cases with severe respiratory syndrome. Chin J Pediatr. 2003;41(8):574–7.
23. Yong gang LI, Fu sheng WANG, WANG M, et al. Association of disease progression with dynamic alterations of clinical immunological and virology factors in patients with severe acute respiratory syndrome. Chin J Infect Dis. 2003;21(4):241–5.
24. Yang-bo TANG, Yi-zhou TAN, Xiao-ping TANG, et al. Detection and analysis of antibody of severe acute respiratory syndrome associated coronavirus. Chin J Infect Dis. 2003;21(3):172–5.
25. Poon LL, Chan KH, et al. Early diagnosis of SARS Coronavirus infection by real time RT-PCR. J Clin Virol. 2003;28(3):233–8.
26. Zhou BP, Tang XP, Lu PX, (eds). SARS. People Health Publishing House, Beijing; 2003. pp. 52–78
27. Jing min Z, Guang de Z, Yan ling S, et al. Clinical pathology and pathogenesis of severe acute respiratory syndrome. Chin J Exp Clin Virol. 2003;17:217–21.
28. Yan-qing DING, Hui-jun WANG, Hong SHEN, et al. Study on etiology and pathology of severe acute respiratory syndrome. Chin J Pathol. 2003;32(3):195–200.
29. Zhen-wei L, Li-jie Z, Xin M, et al. A clinicopathological study on 3 cases of severe acute respiratory syndrome. Chin J Pathol. 2003;32:201–4.
30. Riguan L, Xiaodong F, Zhuo-cai W, et al. Pathological and ultramicrostructural changes of tissues in a patient with severe acute respiratory syndrome. Chin J Pathol. 2003;32:201–4.
31. Nicholls JM, Poon LL, Lee KC, et al. Lung pathology of fatal severe acute respiratory syndrome. Lancet. 2003;361(9371):1773–8.
32. Li W, Moore MJ, Vasilieva N, et al. Angiotensin-converting enzyme 2 is a functional receptor for the SARS coronavirus. Nature. 2003; 426(6965):450–4.
33. Peiris JS, Chu CM, Cheng VC, et al. Clinical progression and viral load in a community outbreak of coronavirus-associated SARS pneumonia: a prospective study. Lancet. 2003;361(9371): 1767–72.
34. Collin AR. In vitro detection of apoptosis in monocytes/macrophages infected with human coronavirus. Clin Diagn Lab Immunol. 2002;9(6):1392–5.
35. Wong RS, Wu A, To KF, et al. Haematological manifestations in patients with severe acute respiratory syndrome. BMJ. 2003; 326(7403):1358–62.
36. Graham RL, Sparks JS, Eckerle LD, et al. SARS coronavirus replicase proteins in pathogenesis. Virus Res. 2008;133(1):88–100.
37. So LK, Lau AC, Yam LY, et al. Development of a standard treatment protocol for severe acute respiratory syndrome. Lancet. 2003;361(9369):1615–7.
38. Totura AL, Baric RS. SARS coronavirus pathogenesis: host innate immune responses and viral antagonism of interferon. Curr Opin Virol. 2012;2(3):264–75.
39. Xiao-qing LIU, Si-bei CHEN, Guo-qing HE, et al. Management of critical severe acute respiratory syndrome and risk factors for death. Chin J Tuberc Respir Dis. 2003;26(6):329–33.
40. LU PX, ZHOU BP, HU YW, et al. Clinical and chest X-ray characteristics of 5 cases with severe acute respiratory syndrome in children in Shenzhen area. Chin J Pediatr. 2003;41(9):645–7.
41. Jang TN, Yeh DY, Shen SH, et al. Severe acute respiratory syndrome in Taiwan: analysis of epidemiological characteristics in 29 cases. J Infect. 2004;48(1):23–31.
42. Xue-xiang J, Xiao-ying W, Jiang-xi X. MRI in the Following up of the Osteonecrosis in SARS Patients. Chin J Med Imag Technol. 2003;10(10):1279–80.

43. Tang X, Yin C, Zhang F, et al. Measurement of subgroups of peripheral blood T lymphocytes in patients with severe acute respiratory syndrome and its clinical significance. Chin Med J (Engl). 2003;116(6):827–30.
44. Xinwei W, Gang C, Biao D, et al. Establishment of fluorescent PCR Method for Detection of SARS coronavirus and the clinical trial. Chin J Lab Med. 2003;26:300–2.
45. Zhang QF, Cui JM, Huang XJ, et al. Morphology and morphogenesis of severe acute respiratory syndrome (SARS) associated virus. Sheng Wu Hua Xue Yu Sheng Wu Wu Li Xue Bao (Shanghai). 2003;35(6):587–91.
46. Enserink M. Albert Osterhaus profile. The virus collector. Science. 2003;300(5623):1228–9.
47. Shi Y, Yi Y, Li P, et al. Diagnosis of severe acute respiratory syndrome (SARS) by detection of SARS coronavirus nucleocapsid antibodies in an antigen-capturing enzyme-linked immunosorbent assay. J Clin Microbiol. 2003;41(12):5781–2.
48. Ng ML, Tan SH, See EE, et al. Proliferative growth of SARS coronavirus in Vero E6 cells. J Gen Virol. 2003;84(Pt 12):3291–303.
49. puxuan L, boping Z, xinchun C. Chest X-ray imaging of patients with SARS. Chin Med J. 2003;116(7):972–5.
50. Pu-xuan* LU, Bo-ping ZHOU, Ming-yuan YUAN, et al. Investigation of chest X-ray manifestations of severe acute respiratory syndrome. Chin J Radiol. 2003;37(8):682–5.
51. Puxuan LU, Boping ZHOU, Gendong YANG, et al. Clinical characteristics and chest X-ray manifestations in SARS. J Emerg Med. 2003;12(7):437–9.
52. Wei* WANG, Da-qing MA, Da-wei ZHAO, et al. CT appearances and dynamic changes in severe acute respiratory syndrome. Chin J Radiol. 2003;37(8):686–9.
53. Da-wei* ZHAO, Da-qing MA, Wei WANG, et al. Early X-ray and CT manifestations of SARS. Chin J Radiol. 2003;37(7):143–5.
54. Grinblat L, Shulman H, Glickman A, et al. Severe acute respiratory syndrome: radiographic review of 40 probable cases in Toronto Canada. Radiology. 2003;228(3):802–9.
55. Antonio GE, Wong KT, Hui DS, et al. Thin-section CT in patients with severe acute respiratory syndrome following hospital discharge: preliminary experience. Radiology. 2003;228(3):810–5.
56. Brecher CW, Aviram G, Boiselle PM. CT and radiography of bacterial respiratory Infections in AIDS patients. AJR. Am J Roentgenol. 2003;180(5):1203–9.
57. Wong KT, Antonio GE, Hui DS, et al. Thin-section CT of severe acute respiratory syndrome: evaluation of 73 patients exposed to or with the disease. Radiology. 2003;228(2):395–400.
58. Muller NL, Ooi GC, Khong PK, et al. Severe acute respiratory syndrome: radiographic and CT findings. AJR Am J Roentgenol. 2003;181(1):3–8.
59. Antonio GE, Wong KT, Hui DS, et al. Imaging of severe acute respiratory syndrome in Hong Kong. AJR Am J Roentgenol. 2003;181(1):11–7.
60. Pu-xuan LU, Bo-ping ZHOU, Ming-yuan YUAN, et al. Chest CT manifestations of severe acute respiratory syndrome. Chin J CT MRI. 2003;1(1):35–7.
61. Puxuan LU, Boping ZHOU, Xiaolong GONG, et al. Chest roentgenographic features of severe acute respiratory syndrome. J Clin Radiol. 2003;22(6):449–54.
62. LU PX, YANG GL, YU WY, et al. Imaging follow-up of SARS patients complicated with pulmonary fibrosis. Chin J Med Imag Technol. 2004;20(12):1901–3.
63. Yang GL, Hu YW, Yao HY, et al. X-ray contrast study of severe and ordinary SARS patients complicated with pulmonary fibrosis and femoral head necrosis. Chin J Infect Dis. 2005;23(2):136–8.
64. Rigetu Z. Overview and outlook of treatment of SARS patients. Chin J Pediatr. 2003;42(6):403–4.
65. Hon KL, Leung CW, Cheng WT, et al. Clinical presentations and outcome of severe acute respiratory syndrome in children. Lancet. 2003;361(9370):1701–3.
66. Lipsitch M, Cohen T, Cooper B, et al. Transmission dynamics and control of severe acute respiratory syndrome. Science. 2003; 300(5627):1966–70.

Human Avian Influenza A H5N1, H7N9, H10N8 and H5N6 Virus Infection

3

Pu-Xuan Lu, Yuan Jing, Le Xiao-Hua, Bo-Ping Zhou, Shi Yu-Xin, Zhang Zhi-Yong, Zhou Yu-Shen, Deng Ying-Ying, Ran Xian-Gui, Ge Yang, He Jian, Lin Jia-Fu, Zeng Qing-Si, Li Jing-Jing, Yan De-Min, and Huang Xiang-Rong

3.1 Overview

Yuan Jing

3.1.1 Definition of Human Avian Influenza

Avian influenza is an infectious disease induced by avian influenza viruses in poultry, commonly called genuine fowl plague or European fowl plague.

Human avian influenza is an acute respiratory tract infection caused by some strains of subtypes of avian flu viruses. At present, the subtypes of avian influenza virus confirmed able to infect human beings are H5N1, H7N9, H10N8, H5N6, H7N2, H7N3, H7N7, and H9N2. Among these, human avian influenza H5N1 is severe with a high mortality, which is designated as highly pathogenic avian influenza (HPAI). Since February 2013, 3 cases of human H7N9 avian influenza have been detected in Shanghai City, Anhui province, and Jiangsu province with two dead, which was the first report in the world.

3.1.2 Discovery of Human Avian Influenza

In 1878, a severe disease was firstly reported in Italy among chickens, called fowl plague. In 1901, it was confirmed to be caused by viruses, which were identified as influenza A virus in 1955. In 1981, such disease was formally named avian influenza on the first international avian influenza conference.

3.1.2.1 Discovery of Human Avian Flu Subtype H5N1

On May 5, 1997, H5N1 human avian influenza was firstly found in Hong Kong of China in a 3-year-old child, who died from Reye syndrome and multiple organ failure 10 days after onset of the disease. On May 9, 1997, the US CDC and Rotterdam state influenza center of WHO laboratory isolated the H5N1 AIV strain from the bronchial secretions of this 3-year-old boy, which was named "A/HongKong/157/97." This body is the first case of human infected with highly pathogenic avian influenza H5N1 virus. In December, there were in total 18 cases of human avian influenza confirmed in Hong Kong, China with 6 cases deceased. By December 31, 2014, 667 cases of highly pathogenic human avian influenza H5N1 were documented around the globe, including 393 deaths with the mortality at 58.92 %.

Pu-Xuan Lu (✉)
Department of Radiology, Shenzhen Third People's Hospital
Guangdong, Shenzhen, China
e-mail: lupuxuan@126.com

Yuan Jing • Bo-Ping Zhou
Department of Infection, Shenzhen Third People's Hospital
Guangdong, Shenzhen, China
e-mail: 13500054798@139.com; zhoubp@hotmail.com

Le Xiao-Hua • Li Jing-Jing • Yan De-Min • Huang Xiang-Rong
The Shenzhen No.3 People's Hospital, Guangdong College, Shenzhen, China

Shi Yu-Xin • Zhang Zhi-Yong
The Shanghai Public Health Clinical Center, Shanghai, China

Zhou Yu-Shen
China's Military Academy of Medical Sciences, Microbial Institute of Epidemic, Guangzhou, China

Deng Ying-Ying
Shenzhen Yantian Hospital, Shenzhen, China

Ran Xian-Gui • Ge Yang
The Second People's Hospital of Fuyang City in Anhui Province, Fuyang, China

He Jian
The First Hospital of Nanchang, Nanchang, China

Lin Jia-Fu
Affiliated Hospital of North Sichuan Medical College, Nanchong, China

Zeng Qing-Si
The First Affiliated Hospital of Guangzhou Medical University, Guangzhou, China

P.-X. Lu, B.-P. Zhou (eds.), *Diagnostic Imaging of Emerging Infectious Diseases*, DOI 10.1007/978-94-017-7363-8_3

3.1.2.2 Discovery of Human Avian Influenza H7N9

Since February 2013, 3 cases were confirmed with avian influenza H7N9 successively in Shanghai, Anhui, and Jiangsu provinces, with 2 cases dead. Besides, this is firstly reported human avian influenza H7N9 in the world. By December 31, 2014, there were in total 451 cases of human avian influenza H7N9 in China, of which 174 cases passed away, with the mortality up to 38.58 %.

3.1.2.3 Discovery of Human Avian Influenza H10N8

On December 6, 2013, 1 case with human avian influenza H10N8 complicated with severe pneumonia was reported in Jiangxi province, China, which was the first around the world. Thereafter, 2 cases of human avian influenza H10N8 were respectively reported on January 25, 2014, and February 13, 2014, in Nanchang Jiangxi province. Of the three cases, 2 cases passed away.

3.1.2.4 Discovery of Human Avian Influenza H5N6

On May 6, 2014, the throat swab of one severe pneumonia case was detected positive for H5N6 avian influenza virus nucleic acid in Sichuan province of China, which was confirmed as avian influenza virus H5N6 via further tests by China CDC. This patient had a history of contact with fowl dead from diseases and was clinically diagnosed with acute severe pneumonia, but passed away due to unresponsive to emergent treatment. This was the global first case. On December 23, 2014, the second human avian influenza H5N6 was found in Guangdong province of China. This male patient was aged 58 years old. Further re-examination by CDC on December 22, 2014, revealed that the avian influenza A H5N6 nucleic acid was positive. This patient is now receiving treatment at the intensive care unit.

3.2 Etiology

Yuan Jing

3.2.1 Morphological Structure and Physiochemical Nature of the Virus

3.2.1.1 Morphological Structure

H5N1 is a segmented negative single-stranded RNA virus belonging to *Influenzavirus A* genus, *Orthomyxoviridae* family of *Mononegavirales* order. The typical shape of avian influenza virus under electric microscope is spherical in a diameter of 80–120 nm and has a capsid in helical symmetry as well as envelope. The initially isolated strains may appear like filament in a diameter of about 20 nm and length of 300–3000 nm. The hemagglutinin protuberance is a homotrimer composed of 3 non-covalently bound protein molecules, and the neural aminase presents with homotetramer made up by head and stem like a mushroom.

The structures of the virus are subsequently envelope, matrix protein, and viral core from inside to outside. The surface glycoprotein club-shaped hemagglutinin (HA) and neural aminase (NA) are embedded into the lipid bilayer of the viral envelope together with ion channel protein. Matrix protein binds to the inner surface of viral envelope and associates with the helical ribonucleoprotein of the viral core to form a layer of membrane-like structure to protect the viral core. RNP comprises nucleocapsid protein (NP), three polymerases (PB1, PB2, PA), and eight viral RNA segments.

3.2.1.2 Physicochemical Properties of the Virus

Similar to human influenza virus, avian influenza virus is sensitive to diethyl ether, chloroform, and acetone and other organic solvents as well as heat and ultraviolet rays. It could be deactivated after exposure to sunlight for 40–48 h and frequently used disinfectants such as sodium hypochlorite, phenolic compounds, quarternary ammonium disinfectants, aquae formalin, and other aldehydes, and iodine compounds could rapidly destroy the infectivity of the viruses. Under general conditions, influenza viruses could survive for 30 days under 0 °C, under 22 °C for 4 days, and under 56 °C for 3 h. Besides, it could be deactivated after half an hour under 60 °C and killed after merely 1 min under over 100 °C. However, under natural conditions, viruses in feces possess tremendous resistance due to protection from organics.

3.2.2 Pathogenicity of the Virus

HA on the envelope of influenza virus, as an attachment protein, could combine with the sialic acid residues of host cell receptors at the top of the globular head, which is key to the viral infection. However, influenza virus could only recognize specific sialic acid molecules on host cell membranes. Neu5Acα2-6Gal binding on the membrane of human respiratory tract mucous cells is key to infection of humans by avian influenza virus. Hyaluronic acid (HA) of the virus combines with host cell receptors and by pinocytosis mediated by such receptors and then enters coated pits which further internalizes HA into coated vesicle. Then the coated vesicle with viruses generates endosome which combines with lysosome to form endosomic lysosome. The acidic pH value inside endosome lysosome changes HA structure and decreases the aggregation force of trimer to expose segment N of HA and fuse with plasma membrane. Besides, the low pH value activates M2 ion channel and facilitates H+ to enter virion, thus decreasing pH value inside the virus. Therefore, the direct interaction between M1 and NP is damaged to free RNP, thus resulting in uncoating of the virus. Thereafter, the genome of the virus is released into the cell plasma and again transported to the nucleus. Both the transcription and replication of the influenza virus RNA segments take place in the host cell nuclei, and RNP must enter the cell nuclei.

3.3 Epidemiology

Yuan Jing

It has been proved that the avian influenza subtypes able to infect humans are H5N1, H7N9, H10N8, H5N6, H9N2, H7N7, H7N2, and H7N3, of which H5N1 presents with relatively strong infectiveness and causes severe conditions and high mortality. Besides, in 2013, patients infected with H7N9 avian influenza also manifested relatively severe conditions and high mortality.

3.3.1 Sources of Infection

Avian influenza viruses have been confirmed widely distributed in many poultry (including the turkeys, chicken, guinea fowl, pigeons, geese, and ducks) and wild fowl (including wild ducks, swans, and various kinds of sea birds) with diseases induced by avian influenza viruses in domesticated chicken and turkey most severe. Besides, there exists silent infection in domesticated poultry which could prolong several months.

The poultry infected by avian influenza or carrying avian influenza virus such as chicken, ducks, geese, and pigeons, particularly chicken, serve to be the important source of infection. The secretions and excretions, feathers, tissue organs, and fowl eggs may also carry viruses.

The influenza A virus could also be seen in humans, horses, pigs, monkeys, domestic cats, rats, tigers, and American leopards, and occasionally in ferret-polecat, seal, whales, and other mammals. In 1970, Kundin found H3N2 subtype antibodies in pigs and isolated similar virus.

Whether human could spread infection needs to be further consolidated, and whether patients with human avian influenza are source of infection has not been determined. Besides, human avian influenza H5N1 and H7N9 are also reported in individual interpersonal infection case.

3.3.2 Route of Transmission

Avian influenza viruses is mainly disseminated through the feces and excretions of infected poultry, contaminated drinks, drinking water, egg holders, chicken embryos, gas-soluble gels, poultry eggs, transportation tools, and other channels. This virus could spread the infection through human respiratory tract, digestive tract, gas-soluble gel, as well as skin damages and eye conjunctiva, particularly respiratory tract and digestive tract. Direct contact with infected poultry or indirect contact with viral pollutants is also regarded as the main route of infection; viral secretions, feces, and any subjects contaminated by poultry corpses could also transmit the epidemic; direct contact with the viral strains could also spread this disease.

3.3.3 Susceptible Population

Considering human avian influenza cases already detected, patients of any case could be infected irrespective of gender.

3.3.4 Epidemiological Characteristics

3.3.4.1 Season of Epidemic

There could be epidemic in all the four seasons, but mainly in the alternate season between winter and spring as well as between autumn and winter, so frequently upon sudden attack of cold current and drastic change of temperature. Generally, human avian influenza is seldom reported in summer but could also occur sporadically such as the first case of avian influenza H5N1 in Shenzhen of China in June. The newly emerging human avian influenza H7N9 in 2013 in China also mainly occurred in February to March.

3.3.4.2 Area Distribution Characteristics of Avian Influenza

Human avian influenza develops mainly in the vast village areas in various countries in the world. In China, the highly pathogenic human avian influenza epidemic is mostly documented in rural areas and surrounding areas of provincial capitals. Meanwhile intimate contact with dead poultry and their secretions and excretions provide main conduit for dissemination of human avian influenza.

3.3.4.3 Human Population Distribution Characteristics

Among patients with human avian influenza, children and the young people occupy a relatively high proportion, and the ratio between the male and female is at 7: 14, with the latter remarkably higher than the before. Besides, farmers and rural students or children take a large proportion. However, for avian influenza H7N9, the middle old-aged account for a relatively high proportion.

3.4 Pathogenesis and Pathological Changes

3.4.1 Pathogenesis

Influenza virus belongs to influenza virus genus of orthomyxovirus family and is an enveloped, negative single-branded and segmented RNA virus. Influenza virus falls into type A, type B, and type C in light of the antigen of nucleoprotein (NP). Influenza virus type A could be further divided into subtypes according to the antigen difference of hemagglutinin (HA) and neuraminidase (NA) embedded in the lipid bilayer outer membrane. Avian influenza virus (AIV) of different types or subtypes demonstrates varying pathogenicity due to the difference in viral genome structure and sequence expressing protein polypeptide. Some mutant viruses could even surmount genus and order barriers to infect humans, such as H5N1, H7N7, H9N2, and H7N9, among which H5N1 or H7N9 infection could induce severe conditions and high mortality.

HA on the outer membrane of influenza virus type A plays critical roles in the pathogenesis of AIV. HA, as the main component of envelope spike, is key to viral attachment and transmembrane process and could stimulate generation of neutralizing antibody and cellular immunity to ward off viral infection and disease. In the course of infection, HA, could be hydrolyzed into peptide chain HA1 and HA2, with the former able to combine with host cell receptors and the latter as a critical subunit to mediate fusion of the virus and host cell membranes. Therefore, the influenza virus could integrate with host cell receptors mediated by HA1 and fuse with cell membrane mediated by HA2 to promote release of ribonucleoprotein (RNP).

Another important component of highly pathogenic AIV infecting human body cells may be NS1 protein, which could inhibit interferon (IFN) and tumor necrosis factor-alpha (TNF-α). Fas signal pathway may mediate cell apoptosis related to influenza virus infections. The inflammatory reaction factors may mediate the systematic inflammatory reaction syndrome in severe patients, acute respiratory distress syndrome, and multiple organ failure, while corticosteroids may delay or decrease such reactions, suggesting that immune injury may participate in pathogenesis of human avian influenza.

3.4.2 Pathological Changes

Highly pathogenic human avian influenza is induced by human avian influenza virus H5N1 and H7N9 characteristic of acute respiratory system lesions and with high mortality. In light of domestic and foreign literature reports, its main pathological changes could be summarized as severe lung disease, toxic changes, and secondary infections of immune organs and other viscera. Main causes of death include (1) progressive respiratory failure incurred by pulmonary diffusive alveolar injury; (2) complication with multi-organ damages such as liver, kidneys, and heart; and (3) immunosuppression and secondary infections.

3.4.2.1 Lungs

Naked-Eye Observation

Lung tissues are revealed swollen and heavier, with the left lung up to 770–2250 g and right lung 785–800 g (both lungs 1550–1950 g). Both lungs present with dark red color and distinct consolidation, particularly at the lower lobes of the lungs. There may be slight adhesions between the lungs and parietal pleura. Lung sections demonstrate notable congestion and edema as well as exudation of light red bubbly blood-stained fluids. Trachea and bronchi are viewed with congestion at mucosa and light red bubbly secretions inside the lumen. The pleural cavity is observed with slight light yellow effusions.

Examination Under Light Microscope

Early phase: It manifests diffuse alveolar injury at both lungs, typical of acute disseminated exudative disease. The alveolar spaces are full of pinkish exudates and inflammatory cells of varying amount, including mainly lymphocytes, monocytes, plasma cells, and macrophages as well as a few neutrophilic granulocytes. The alveolar spaces could also be seen with exfoliated, degenerated, and necrotic alveolar epithelial cells. Part of the alveolar spaces are found with bleeding and fibrin as well as hyaloid membrane. Alveolar type II epithelial proliferation is also observable. No inclusion bodies are observed in megakaryocytes and nucleus or plasma. Part of the alveolar septum become lightly thicker with vascular dilatation, congestion, and inflammatory cell (type similar to that inside alveolar space) infiltration but without intravascular fibrinous thrombi. Middle phase (disease course over 10 days): it presents changes of proliferation phase. Diffuse alveolar damages and alveolar epithelial reactive proliferation are seen but cellular changes related to virus absent. Alveolar space is seen with fibrinous exudation, bleeding, formation, and mechanization of hyaloid membrane. Interstitium is detected with vascular congestion, reactive fibroblast proliferation, and light lymphocyte infiltration. Part lung tissues are found with fungal infections. Advanced phase (disease course over 3 weeks): it presents changes of fibrosis. Part alveolar epithelium is revealed with necrosis and exfoliation as well as reactive proliferation (Figs. 3.1 and 3.2) but without viral inclusion body in epithelial cells. Alveolar spaces are observed with effusion of plasma fluid, fibrin, red cells, and neutrophilic granulocytes, formation of hyaloid membrane, organization of squamous epithelia, and mechanization of exudates (Fig. 3.3). Part alveoli are detected with collapse or compensatory emphysema. Pulmonary interstitium is seen with fibrosis and occasional presence of lymphocytes, plasma cells, and reactive hemophagocytes. Pulmonary interstitial capillaries are viewed with transparent emboli and DIC as well as occasionally obliteration (Fig. 3.4). Pulmonary bleeding and secondary infection could also be seen.

3.4.2.2 Immune Organs

Lymph Nodes

Lymphocytes decrease and scatters and lymph sinus is found dilated and with focal necrosis. Histiocytes proliferate

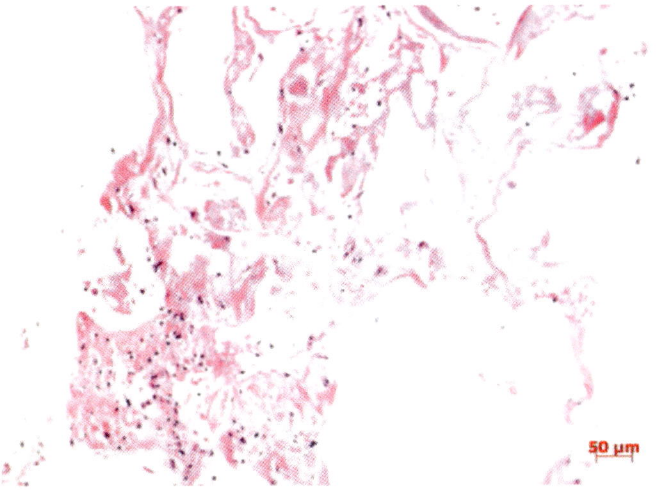

Fig. 3.1 Degeneration and necrosis of lung tissues and light lymphocyte infiltration HE staining

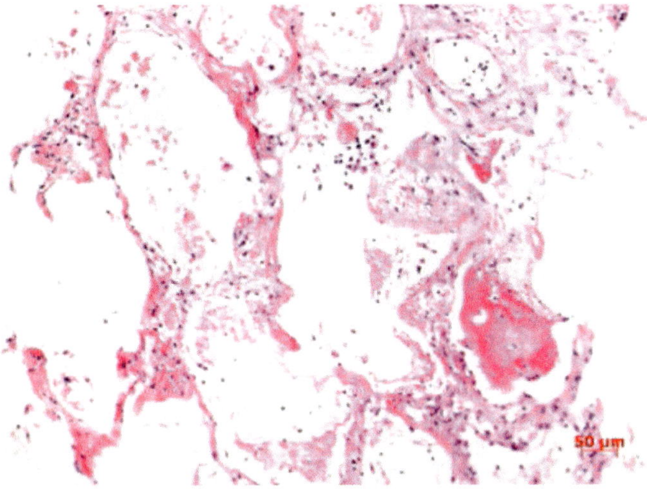

Fig. 3.3 Exfoliation of alveolar epithelia, and presence of reddish liquid, fibrin and slight amount of lymphocytes in pulmonary alveolar spaces. HE staining

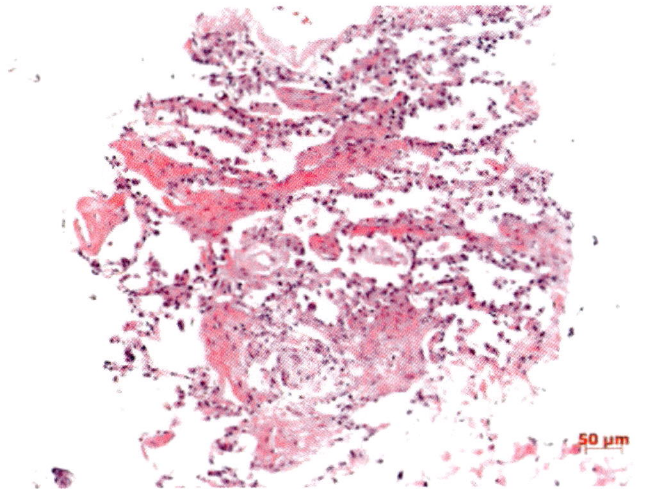

Fig. 3.2 Reactive proliferation of alveolar epithelium and fibrosis of pulmonary interstitium HE staining

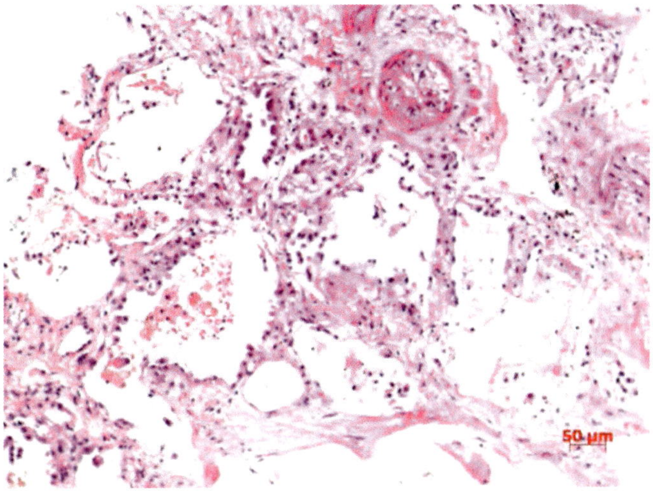

Fig. 3.4 Proliferation of lung epithelial cells, with partial exfoliations, and vascular occlusion HE staining

accompanied by phenomenon of phagocytosis of the hemophagocytes and lymphocytes.

Spleen

The spleen presents with mild enlargement, smooth surface, and dark red color. Microscopy suggests extravasated blood, edema, atrophy of white marrow, and enlargement of red marrow. Peripheral to the white marrow is atypical lymphocytes. Part spleen sinuses are seen with slight inflammatory cell infiltration and histiocytosis accompanied by hemophagocytosis.

Bone Marrow

Bone marrow tissues are revealed with reactive histiocytosis and hemophagocytosis.

3.4.2.3 Other Main Organs

Cerebrum, Cerebellum, and Spinal Cord

The brain is unveiled with extravasated blood at the surface blood vessels and slight widening of gyrus. Microscopy visualizes wider spaces between the cerebrum, cerebellum, and spinal nerve cells and small blood vessels, as well as extravagated blood in blood vessels.

Heart

Cardiac chambers are found with dark-brown blood clots. Microscopy indicates degeneration of cardiocyte vacuole and cardiocytes with swelling and loss of striated patterns as well as partial pyknosis. Interstitium manifests light edema and extravagated blood in blood vessels.

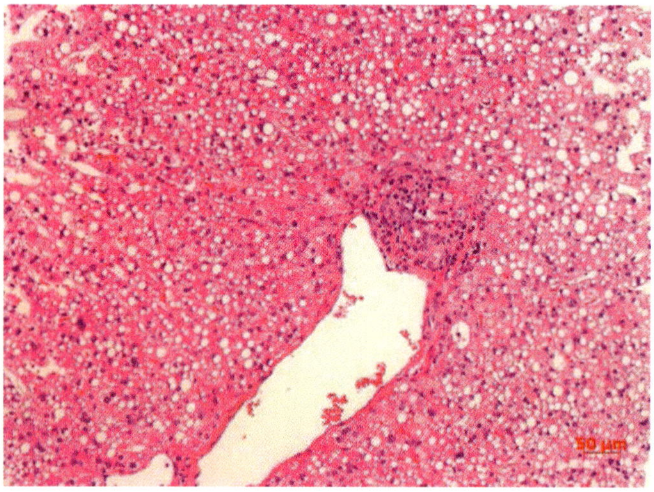

Fig. 3.5 Presence of lipid droplets at liver cellular plasma and slight lymphocyte infiltration at the portal area HE staining

Liver

The surface of the liver is smooth, grayish red, and with homogeneous section. The liver lobule presents normal structure, with slight hydropic degeneration and fat degeneration (Fig. 3.5) at liver cells and central necrosis. Interstitium is unveiled with light extravagated blood and part portal area with light lymphocyte infiltration.

Kidney

The kidney becomes swollen and the renal capsule is easily to be separated. The cortex and medulla are well demarcated with slight blood stasis at the latter. Under the microscope, multiple glomerular capillaries are seen with dilatation and blood stasis, and the renal tubules with necrosis. The blood vessels of renal interstitium are revealed with extravagated blood and thrombosis.

3.5 Laboratory Examination

Yuan Jing

3.5.1 Blood Routine Examination

Patients with human avian influenza are characterized by decrease of the peripheral blood WBC count, particularly decrease of lymphocytes, which meanwhile is closely related with the occurrence of ARDS and mortality rate.

3.5.2 Blood Biochemical Examination

Creatine kinase, lactate dehydrogenase, aspartate aminotransferase, and alanine aminotransferase are mostly found elevated and so are C-reactive protein and myoglobin.

3.5.3 Virus Antibody and Virus Nucleic Acid Test

3.5.3.1 Immunofluorescence Test

Influenza viruses infect mainly the epithelial cells of respiratory tract. Positive experiment suggests that this patient or cultured subject has influenza virus and could directly conclude infection of the corresponding type or subtype of influenza virus. This experiment is superior in specificity and sensitivity, which are 5–10 times higher than direct immunofluorescence assay.

3.5.3.2 Colloidal Gold Test

The sample extract from the test kit is mixed with any clinical specimen to separate virus antigens, which are then dropped on the test membrane already adsorbed with alkaline phosphatase-labeled anti-influenza virus A nucleoprotein monoclonal antibody and substrate liquid. The thorough reaction between the antigen and antibody could develop color under the catalysis of enzymes.

This method is applicable to quantitative measurement of influenza virus A and B in nasal suction liquid, nasal scrubbing liquid, and laryngopharyngeal scrubbing liquid specimens.

3.5.3.3 Enzyme-Linked Immunosorbent Assay (ELISA)

Competitive block method is adopted to test H5 antibodies in the serum specimen. The coating monoclonal antibodies on the microwell plate of the agent kit are added with serum specimen and antigen reaction liquid, which forms "coating monoclonal antibody-antigen specimen antibody" complex. Then enzyme-marked antibodies are added. If the serum specimen could distinctly inhibit the combination of enzyme-marked antibodies with antigens, it suggests the presence of avian influenza H5 antibodies.

1. Cutoff value: The Cutoff value = average negative control OD × 0.5
2. Positive judgment: Sample OD value <Cutoff value indicates positive, and otherwise negative. Rise of serum H5 antibodies by four or above times in the early stage of onset and stage of recovery could serve as evidence for definitive diagnosis.

3.5.3.4 Nucleic Acid Test

Polymerase chain reaction (PCR), as a molecular biological assay, could test avian influenza virus nucleic acid in various specimens (blood, feces and excretion, respiratory secretions, and tissue secretions).

3.5.3.5 Virus Isolation

Chicken-embryo culture is a common method of viral culture which is simple to operate and easy to manage. It is very sensitive to orthomyxovirus, paramyxovirus, Poxvirus, and herpes virus and could be used to separate afore viruses from patient samples. The frequently used method for influenza virus is double chicken embryo allantoic cavity and amniotic cavity inoculation. If the chicken embryo dies after 24 h or HA test is positive, it indicates presence of viral infection and CF, IF, EIA, HI, and NT shall be conducted further for differentiation.

In case of diagnosis of suspected cases, both the titer of serum-neutralizing antibody in the acute and recovery periods shall be tested, which could establish diagnosis if the serum antibody level in latter is higher than that the former (≥4). In children, particularly those below 3 years old, the titer of serum influenza virus antibody increasing by two times holds diagnostic value.

3.6 Clinical Diagnosis

Yuan Jing

3.6.1 Diagnostic Criteria

The diagnosis of human avian influenza could be derived based on epidemiological history, clinical manifestation, and laboratory examination results. If the epidemiological history is not clear, diagnosis of human avian influenza H5N1, H7N9, H10N8, and H5N6 could be reached according to clinical manifestations, supplementary examinations, and laboratory test results, particularly separation of avian influenza H5N1, H7N9, H10N8, and H5N6 from patient respiratory tract secretions; avian influenza virus H5N1, H7N9, H10N8, and H5N6 nucleic acid test positive; or avian influenza virus H5N1, H7N9, H10N8, and H5N6 specific antibody level in double serum samples 4 times or above higher by dynamic test.

3.6.2 Severe Human Influenza Diagnostic Criteria

The presence of any of the following five items could conclude diagnosis of severe human avian influenza:

1. Dyspnea: The adult respiratory rate under resting state is ≥30 times/min concurrently with either following circumstance: (i) chest imaging suggests that multilobar lesions or foci occupy over 1/3 of the total area of both lungs on orthotopic film and (ii) conditions progress with lesions increasing by over 50 % and accounting for over 1/4 of total area of both lungs on orthotopic film within 40 h.
2. Distinct hypoxemia: Oxygen inhalation at 3–5 L/min, arterial partial pressure of oxygen (PaO2) <70 mmHg (1 mmHg = 0.133 kPa), or pulse blood oxygen saturation (SpO2) <93 %, or already diagnosed as acute lung injury (ALI) or acute respiratory distress syndrome (ARDS). If the oxygenation index is below 300 mmHg (1 mmHg = 0.133 kPa), it could be diagnosed as ALI; and if the oxygenation index is below 200 mmHg, it could be diagnosed as ARDS.
3. Occurrence of shock or multiple organ dysfunction syndrome (MODS).
4. Occurrence of viral encephalitis.
5. Infected children manifest Reye syndrome.

3.7 Chest Imaging Diagnosis

For imaging examination of human avian influenza virus pneumonia, CT possesses distinct advantages, which could contribute to accurate determination of the degree, extent, and site of lung injury and identify the meticulous dynamic changes of lesions via the high resolution of tissue density and adjustment of window breath and position to obtain more information about lesions than chest X-ray, therefore offering evidence for clinical diagnosis and treatment. Lung interstitial fibrosis is an important complication of this disease, and high-recognition CT (HRCT) can better visualize the subtle changes of pulmonary interstitial fibrosis, such as pulmonary lobular septum thickening, and subpleural curvature shadow, which could aid efficacy evaluation and prognosis estimation.

3.7.1 Chest Manifestations of Human Avian Influenza Virus Pneumonia

3.7.1.1 Early Phase of Onset

The incubation phase of patients with human avian influenza H5N1, H7N9, H10N8, and H5N6 is commonly 1–7 days, mostly 2–4 days, but may last 8 days in a few patients. After the incubation ensues, the early phase of the onset which generally prolongs 1–4 days. The initial symptom is fever with body temperature >38°C, and over half of the patients are accompanied with influenza-like symptoms such as chilliness, headache, soreness of joints and muscles, fatigue, dry and nonproductive cough, as well as chest pain. Chest X-ray or CT inspections may be manifested as (1) lobular septum thickening and acinar nodular shadows; (2) solitary or multiple patchy ground-glass shadows in the lungs and lesions mostly located at unilateral inferior lung lobe; and (3) patchy pulmonary consolidation shadows with air bronchogram in between or ground-glass shadows at the periphery or other long lobes (Figs. 3.3, 3.4, 3.5, and 3.6).

3.7.1.2 Progression Phase

The lesions aggravate within 14 days after the onset in most patients. The patchy shadows of the early phase progress into large patchy, multiple, or diffusive lesions in 3–7 days. The lesions may extend from unilateral to bilateral lungs and from single lung lobe to multiple lobes. In progression phase, severe patients manifest multilobar lesions or lesions advancing by over 50 % within 48 h (Fig. 3.7).

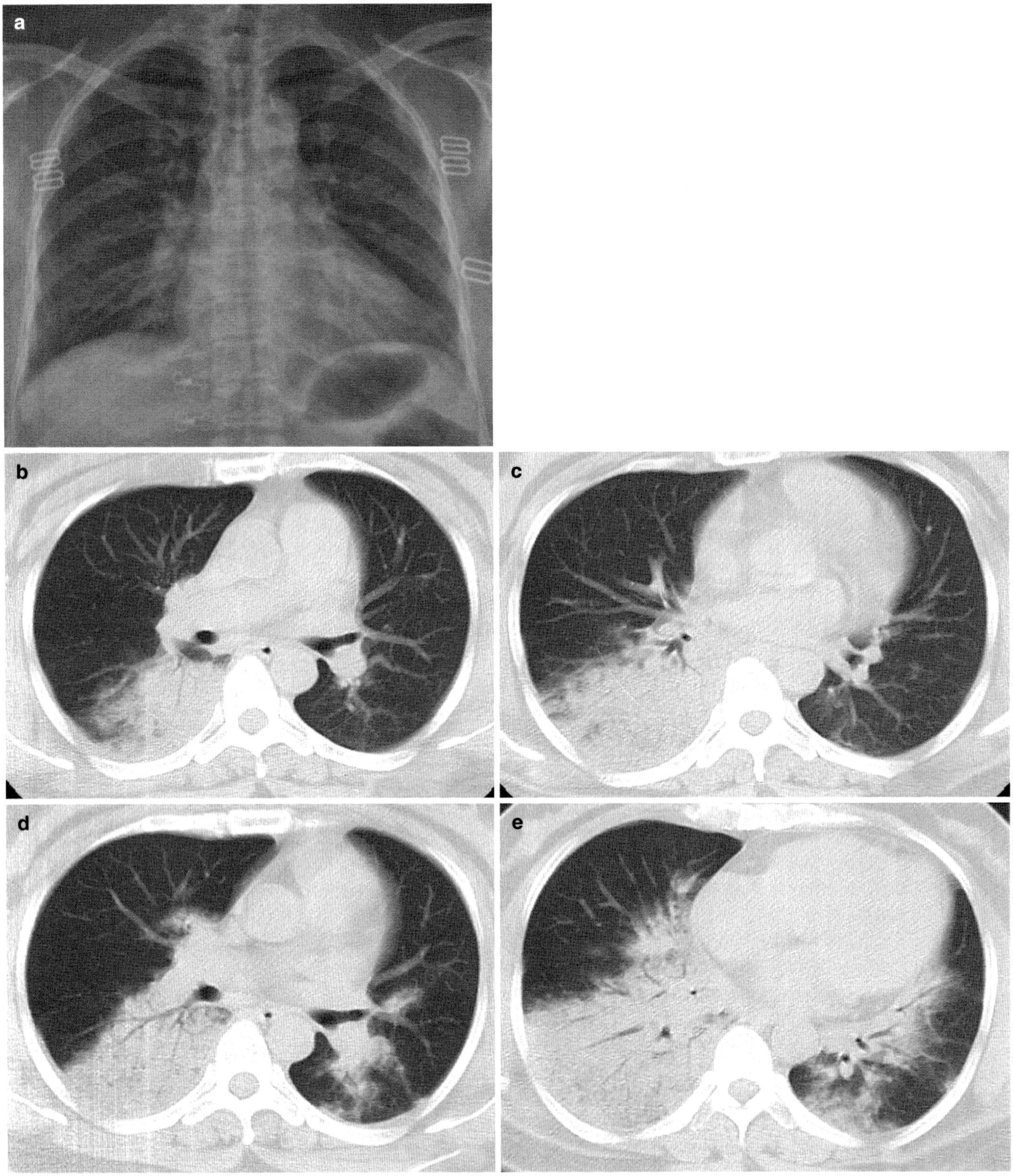

Fig. 3.6 (**a**–**e**) The female patient aged 39 years old is infected with avian influenza virus H7N9 pneumonia. (**a**) On 2nd day after onset, chest X-ray plain films of both lungs did not detect distinct abnormalities. (**b**, **c**) On 4th day after onset, chest CT scan visualized large patchy consolidation shadow at posterior basal segment of right lung inferior lobe, with air bronchogram in between. (**d**, **e**) On 6th day after onset, chest CT scanning revealed that the large patchy consolidation shadow at the right lung inferior lobe progressed notably and the basal segments of right lung middle lobe and left lung inferior lobe were observed with scattering plaque or large patchy consolidation shadows and ground-glass shadows at the periphery

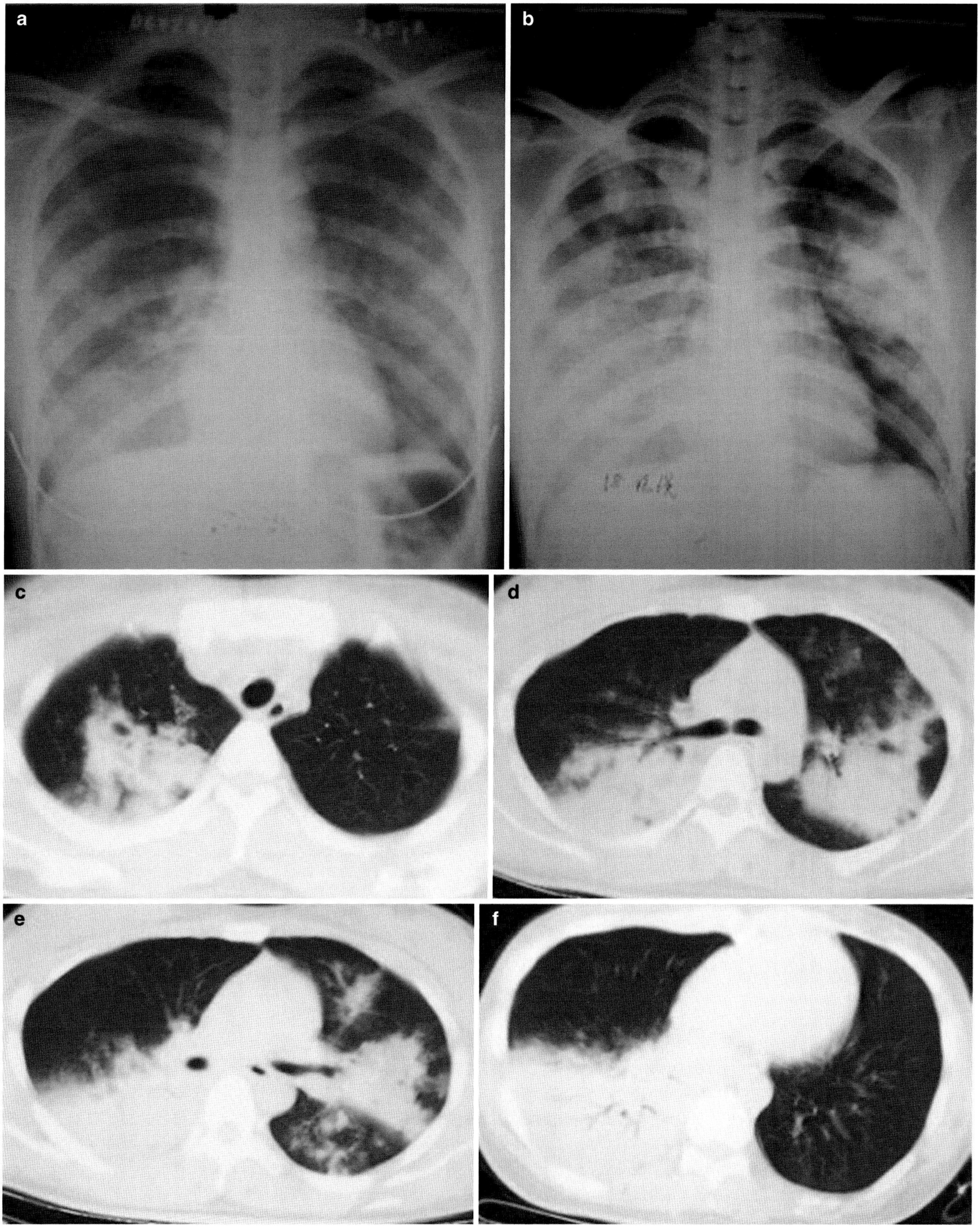

Fig. 3.7 (**a–f**) The female patient aged 26 years old was infected with avian influenza H5N1. (**a**) On the 6th day of the onset of the disease. Chest X-ray revealed large patchy ground-glass shadows at both middle and inferior lung fields and consolidation shadows at the right inferior lung. (**b**) On the 7th day of the onset of the disease. Chest X-ray unveiled rapid development of lesions, with the foci at both lungs enlarging distinctly. Extensive consolidation shadows were seen in both lung fields. (**c–f**) On the 7th day after onset of the disease. The CT lung window showed: The middle and inferior right lung lobe manifested large patchy consolidation shadows, with air bronchogram inside. The left lung was visualized with large patchy consolidation shadows and patchy ground-glass shadows

Chest Imaging Presentations

1. Most frequently seen is large patchy consolidation shadows at the lungs, with air bronchogram inside; plaque-shaped consolidation shadows could also be seen, with foci distributed at lung lobes or lung segments or quasi-circular consolidation shadows of varying sizes observable (Figs. 3.3, 3.4, 3.5, 3.6, 3.7, and 3.8).
2. Lung consolidation shadows and ground-glass dense shadows appear concurrently, predominantly consolidation (Figs. 3.3, 3.4, 3.5, 3.6, 3.7, 3.8, and 3.9).
3. In severe cases, both lungs develop disseminated infiltration foci and ground-glass shadows observable at the anterolateral large patchy lung consolidation shadows, presenting ARDS changes (Figs. 3.3, 3.4, 3.5, 3.6, 3.7, 3.8, 3.9, and 3.10).

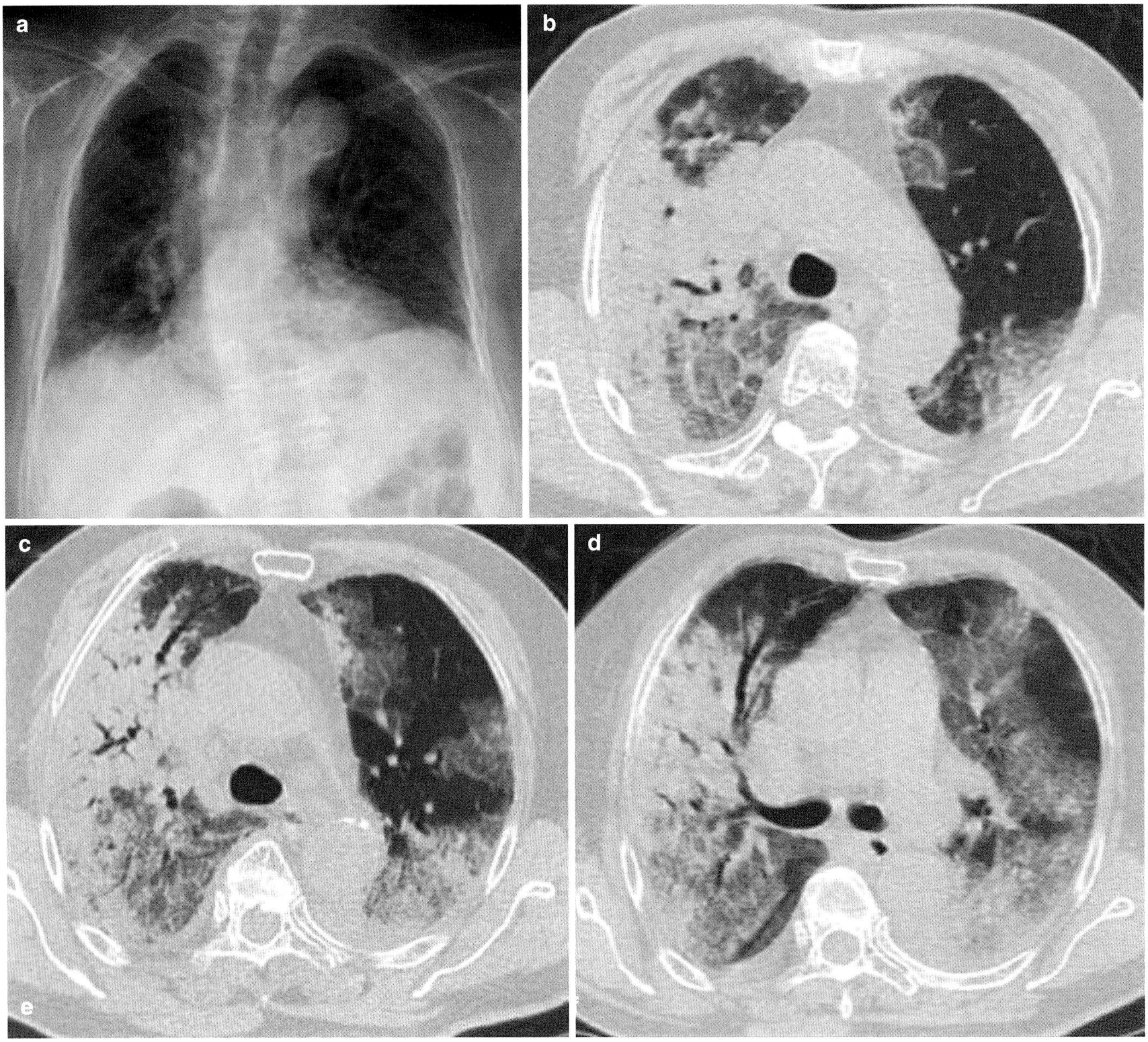

Fig. 3.8 (**a–e**) The female patient aged 82 years old was infected with avian influenza H7N9 pneumonia. (**a**) On the 4th day of the onset of the disease, chest X-ray visualized thickening of lung textures at both inferior lungs, but no distinct consolidation shadows inside the lungs. (**b–e**) On the 6th day of the onset of the disease, chest CT lung window viewed extensive ground-glass shadows and consolidation shadows at both lungs, with mainly consolidation shadows at the right lung lobes and air bronchogram observable. The left inferior lung was found with consolidation and left superior lung with mainly ground-glass shadows. (**f**) On the 6th day of the onset of the disease, chest CT longitudinal window indicated consolidation shadows at both lungs accompanied by slight effusions in the right thoracic cavity

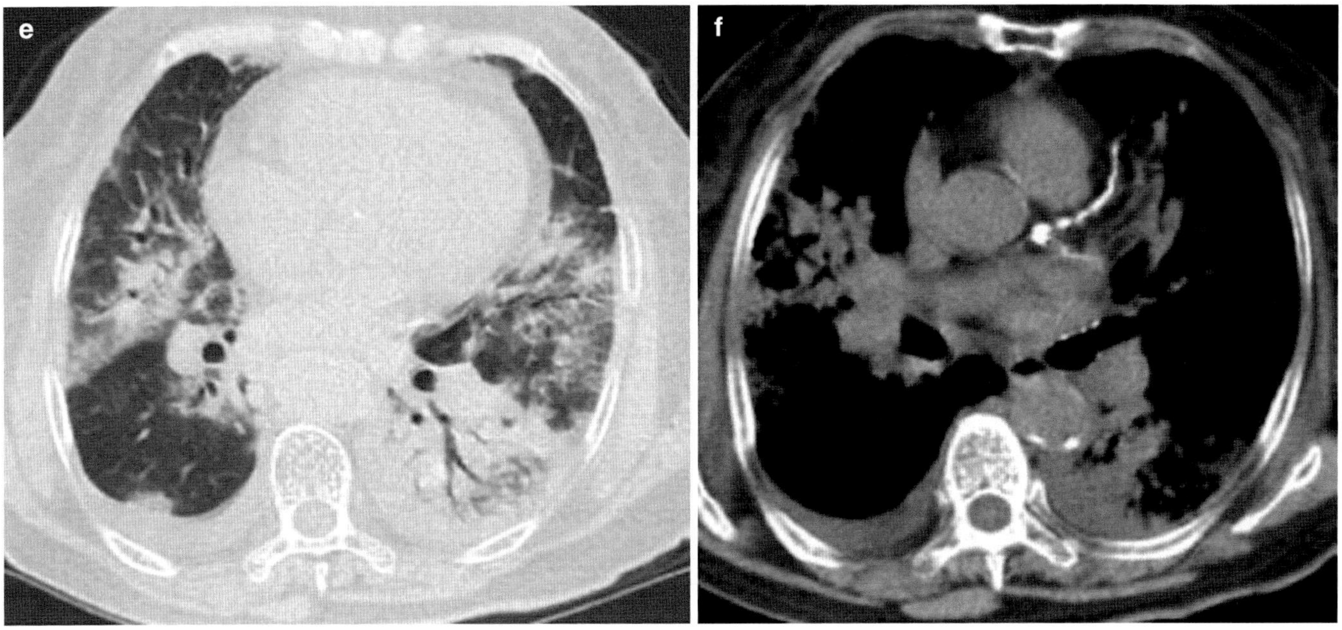

Fig. 3.8 (continued)

4. Pleural effusion is relatively common, particularly in patients with severe pneumonia. The absorption of pleural effusion and lung foci are synchronous generally.

3.7.1.3 Phase of Recovery

After effective treatment in progression phase, the conditions of patients with human avian influenza pneumonia are under control and foci begin to be absorbed. The majority foci of patients with human avian influenza virus pneumonia free of secondary infections are completely absorbed within 30 days, while the lungs of part of the patients may present with fibrosis or proliferation of lung interstitium. For a few severe patients, the foci absorption is relatively slow, and absorption of lung shadows still takes a relatively long time, even years, resulting in interstitial fibrosis. Imaging presentations in the phase of recovery: (1) The large patchy pulmonary consolidation shadows are gradually absorbed and become smaller and light in color, and the consolidation pulmonary tissues gradually swell. Imaging presentations are characterized by plaque-shaped and striped consolidation shadows. (2) Ground-glass-density shadows shrink gradually or are completely absorbed. (3) Pulmonary interstitium presents with fibrosis typical of lobular septum thickening, subpleural curvature shadows, paraseptal emphysema, paramediastinal pulmonary bulla, and bronchiolar dilation (Figs. 3.3, 3.4, 3.5, 3.6, 3.7, 3.8, 3.9, 3.10, and 3.11). (4) The pleura shows limited thickening and adhesion. (5) Pulmonary air sacs are observable during absorption of lesions, which might be induced by pulmonary parenchymal necrosis and formation of valves and could be absorbed after treatment (Figs. 3.3, 3.4, 3.5, 3.6, 3.7, 3.8, 3.9, 3.10, 3.11, and 3.12).

3.7.1.4 Characteristics of the Dynamic Changes of Human Avian Influenza Virus Pneumonia

The characteristic dynamic changes of human avian influenza virus pneumonia are as follows: ① The foci present with rapid dynamic changes, and the foci in severe pneumonia cases could disseminate to multiple lobes and segments within 48 h. ② Lesions in the early phase and progression phase mainly manifest as consolidation shadows and ground-glass shadows. ③ Absorption of the foci is slow. Some patients may present with lung interstitial fibrosis in the lungs several years after discharge (Figs. 3.3, 3.4, 3.5, 3.6, 3.7, 3.8, 3.9, 3.10, 3.11, 3.12, and 3.13). ④ During the course of absorption in recovery phase, the foci in the middle and upper lung lobe are absorbed at an earlier time than those in the dorsal inferior lung lobes and subpleura; and foci firstly formed in the early and progression phase are absorbed at a later time. On the contrary, foci that appear at a later time are absorbed more early. ⑤ Chest imaging changes and clinical symptoms and signs are inconsistent, that is a delay of imaging signs of absorption of pulmonary lesions from clinics (Figs. 3.3, 3.4, 3.5, 3.6, 3.7, 3.8, 3.9, 3.10, 3.11, 3.12, 3.13, and 3.14).

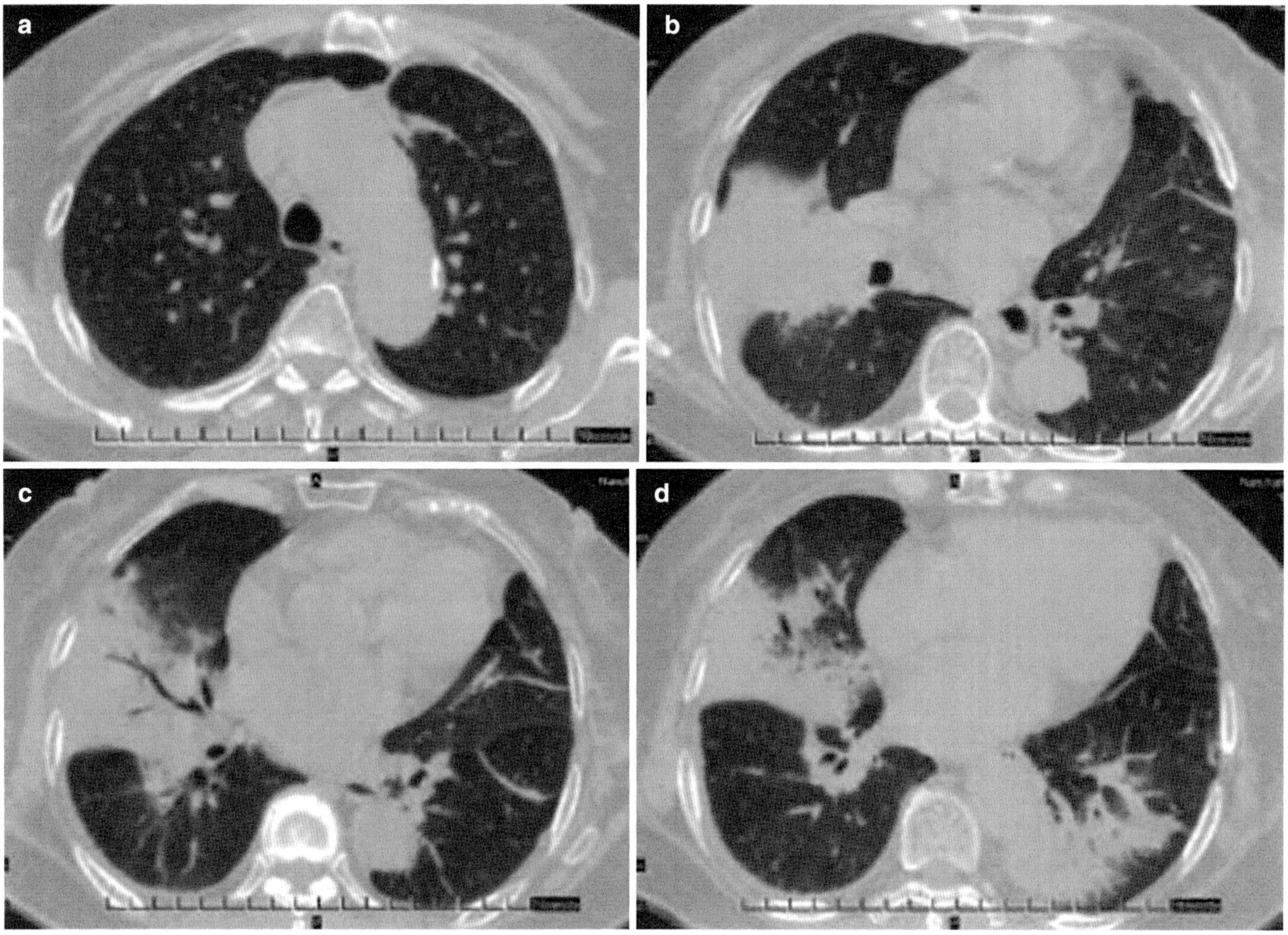

Fig. 3.9 (**a**–**d**) The female patient aged 73 years old was diagnosed with avian influenza H10N8 pneumonia and underwent chest CT on December 1, 2013 (on the 4th day of onset of the disease). (**a**) Beside the left superior lung aortic arc, patchy shadows of increased density were observed. (**b**) Right middle lung lobe was seen with large patchy consolidation shadows and left superior lung with patchy ground-glass-density shadows. (**c**) Right middle lung lobe was found with large patchy consolidation shadows, with air bronchogram in between, and left inferior lung with cord-shaped high-dense shadows. (**d**) Large patchy consolidation shadows were detected beside the right middle lung lobe and left lung lobe thoracic aortic arc

3.7.2 Imaging Differential Diagnosis of Human Avian Influenza Pneumonia

The imaging manifestations of human avian influenza pneumonia comprise disseminated lung consolidation shadows and ground-glass shadows, and intrapulmonary foci occur at an early time and last a long time. Pulmonary lesions present with rapid progression and could extend rapidly into large patchy and disseminated lesions in a short period. The density change of the lesions, or the mutual transformation between ground-glass change and consolidation density, is also very fast. Besides, imaging signs of acute respiratory distress syndrome may also appear in a short time. Due to the lack of specific diagnostic method of human avian influenza pneumonia, clinical diagnosis entails comprehensive analysis of several examination methods, including epidemiologic history, laboratory examination, chest imaging, and observation of the effects of antibiotics therapy.

The differential diagnosis of human avian influenza pneumonia depends on imaging manifestations combined with the patients' history and clinical and laboratory examinations. Clinically the disease must be differentiated from viral pneumonia such as H1N1 and SARS, mainly from the epidemiological history; laboratory examinations, clinical and imaging characteristics; as well as immune impairment. Their common imaging presentations are ground-glass shadows and pulmonary consolidation shadows, with lesions of rapid change and progression. However, human avian influenza pneumonia demonstrates the fastest progression of the foci and early lesions mainly at the both inferior lung lobes, but such characteristics are not obvious in the case of H1N1 and SARS.

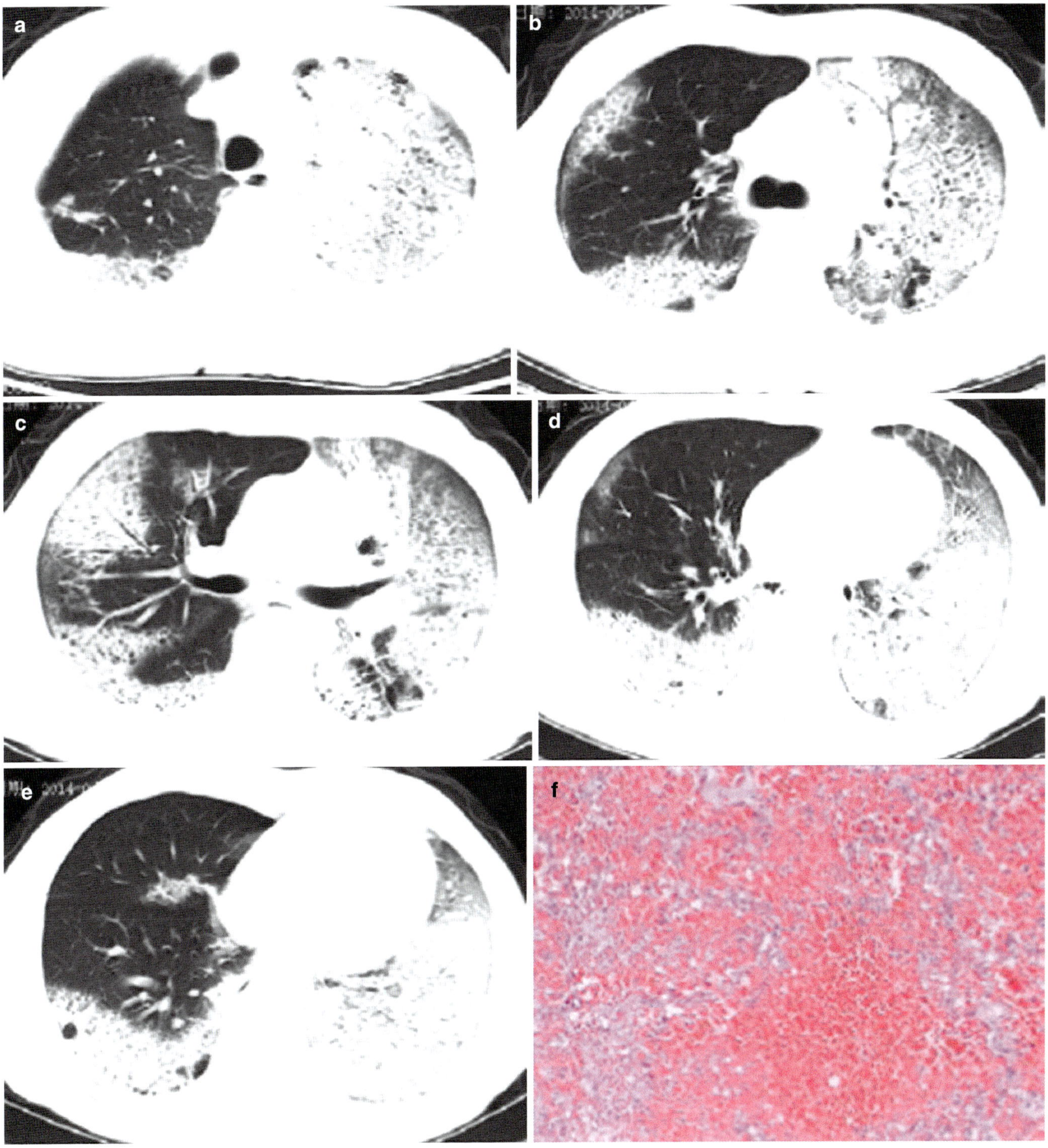

Fig. 3.10 (**a–g**) The 50-year-old male patient was confirmed with avian influenza H5N6 pneumonia and received chest CT on April 21, 2014 (the 8th day of onset). (**a**) The left superior lung was detected with large patchy high-density consolidation shadows and apicoposterior segment of right superior lung with patchy shadows at subpleural area. (**b**) The left superior lung was seen with large patchy high-density shadows with air bronchogram in between. The posterior basal segment of right inferior lung lobe and subpleural area of right superior lobe with high-density shadows. (**c**) The inferior layer of the protuberance was revealed with left lung consolidation shadows and right lung superior and middle lobes and the middle and lateral band of the posterior basal segment of right inferior lobe with patchy consolidation shadows. (**d**) For the venous layer of right inferior lung, left lung and right inferior lung were observable with large patchy consolidation shadows, and the subpleura of the right middle lung and right lingula with ground-glass shadows. (**e**) For the diaphragmatic layer, the subpleural area of posterior basal segment of right inferior lobe and left inferior lobe were seen with consolidation shadows, and the subpleural area of the posterior segment of right lung inferior lobe with multiple pulmonary bulla shadows. (**f**) Pulmonary interstitium and alveolar wall capillaries were unveiled with diffusive dilation and congestion accompanied with focal hemorrhage and part of the lung areas with obvious hemorrhage. (**g**) The alveolar cavities were filled with pinkish homogenous effusions, inflammatory cells, and fibrin

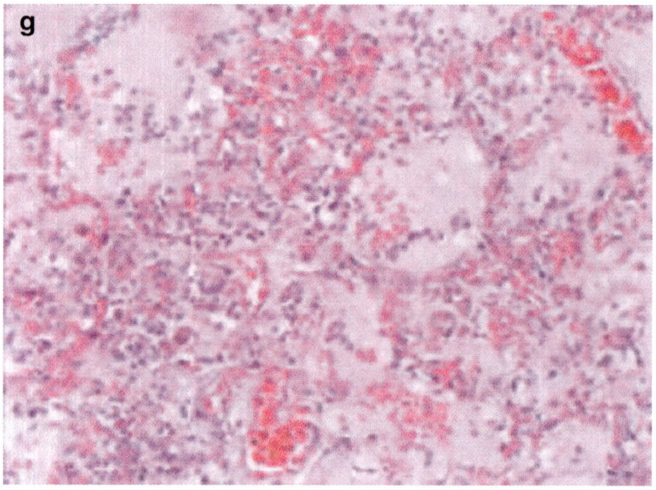

Fig. 3.10 (continued)

3.7.3 Imaging Manifestations of the Complications of Human Avian Influenza Pneumonia

Complication of human avian influenza pneumonia is an important factor affecting the prognosis, which should be highlighted. In the course of treatment of human avian influenza, antivirus drugs, glucocorticoid steroids, and broad-spectrum antibiotics are administered, and positive airway pressure or tracheal cannula may be applied in some patients. Reasonable use of such procedures is of great significance for raising the successful therapeutic rate of patients with human avian influenza pneumonia and lowering mortality rate. However, due to the decrease of the resistance of patients, the drugs and therapies themselves may induce side reactions t and incur corresponding complications. The primary complications of human avian influenza pneumonia encompass secondary lung

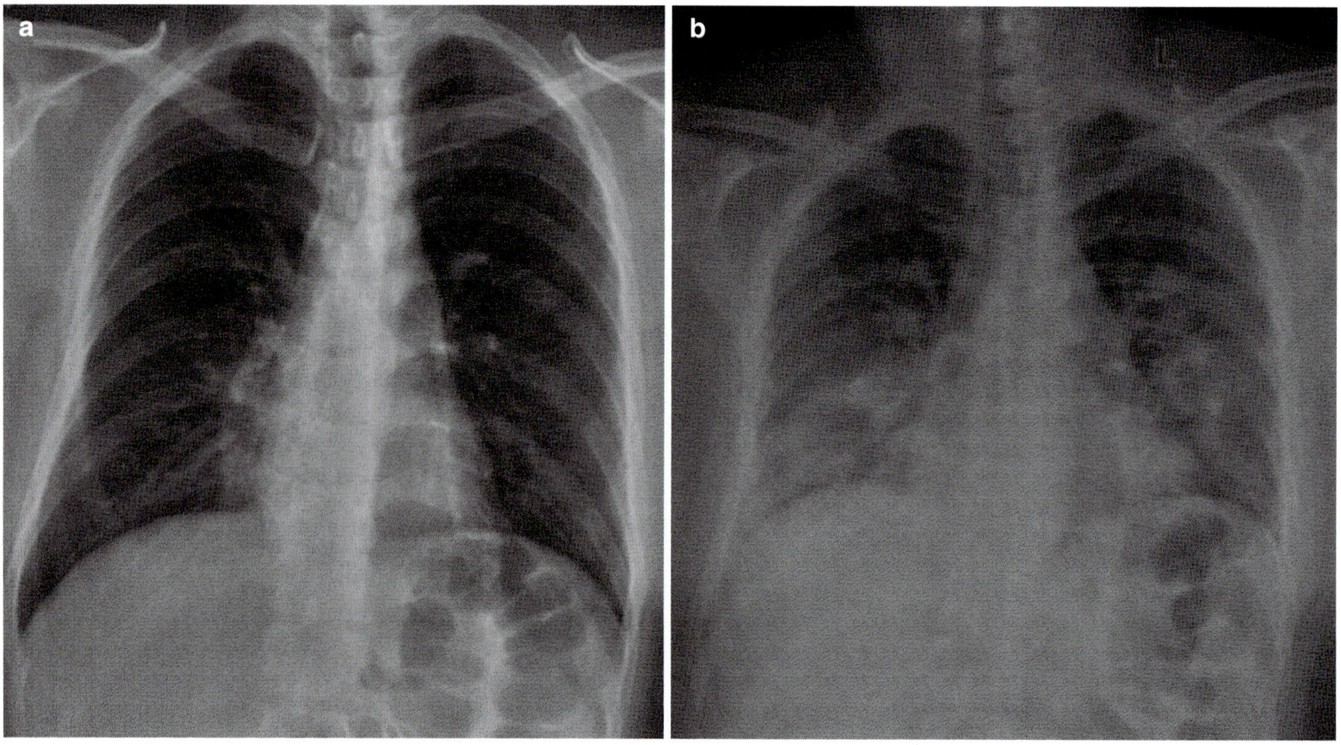

Fig. 3.11 (**a**–**n**) The 31-year-old male patient was confirmed with avian influenza H7N9 pneumonia. (**a**) On the third day after onset of the disease, chest X-ray shows patchy shadows of increased density at mesial margin of the right inferior lung field. (**b**) On the 5th day of the disease onset, chest X-ray visualized large patchy shadows of increased density in the middle and inferior lung fields of both lungs. (**c**–**e**) On the 5th day after the onset of the disease, chest CT demonstrated ground-glass shadows and consolidation shadows scattering at both lungs. Besides, among the consolidation shadows of the right lower lung, air bronchogram was visualized. (**f**–**h**) On the 8th day after the onset of the disease, chest CT revealed extensive ground-glass shadows and consolidation shadows, with the foci increased in number and progressing obviously. (**i**–**k**) On the 11th day after the onset of the disease, after effective treatment, chest CT re-examination disclosed a slight amount of ground-glass density shadows and cord-like and small patchy shadows, indicating entry into recovery phase. (**l**–**n**) On the 15th day after the onset of the disease, chest CT re-examination demonstrated cord-shaped and small patchy shadows, lobular septum thickening, subpleural curvature shadows, bronchiolar dilation, and pleural limited thickening and adhesion at both lungs

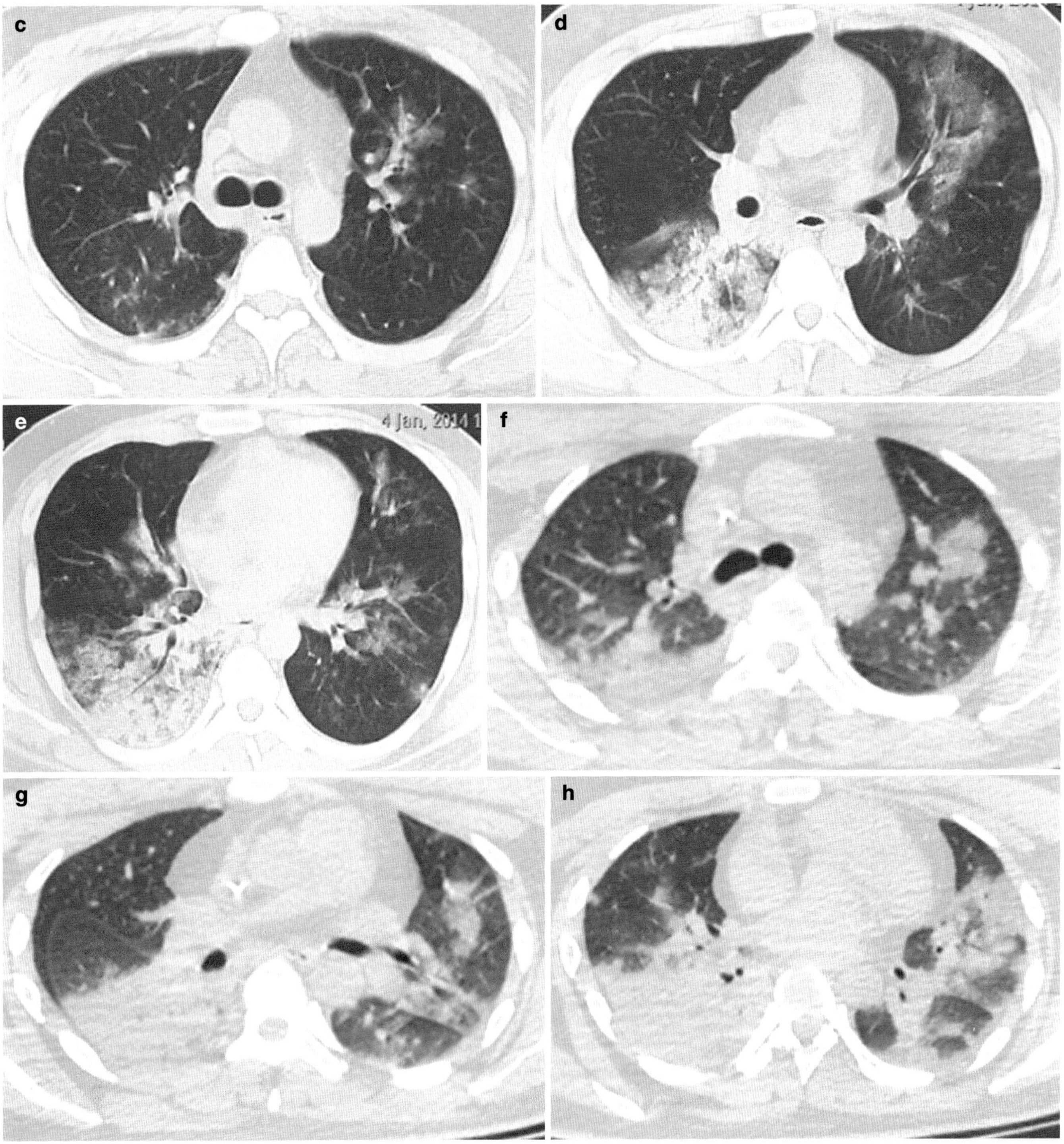

Fig. 3.11 (continued)

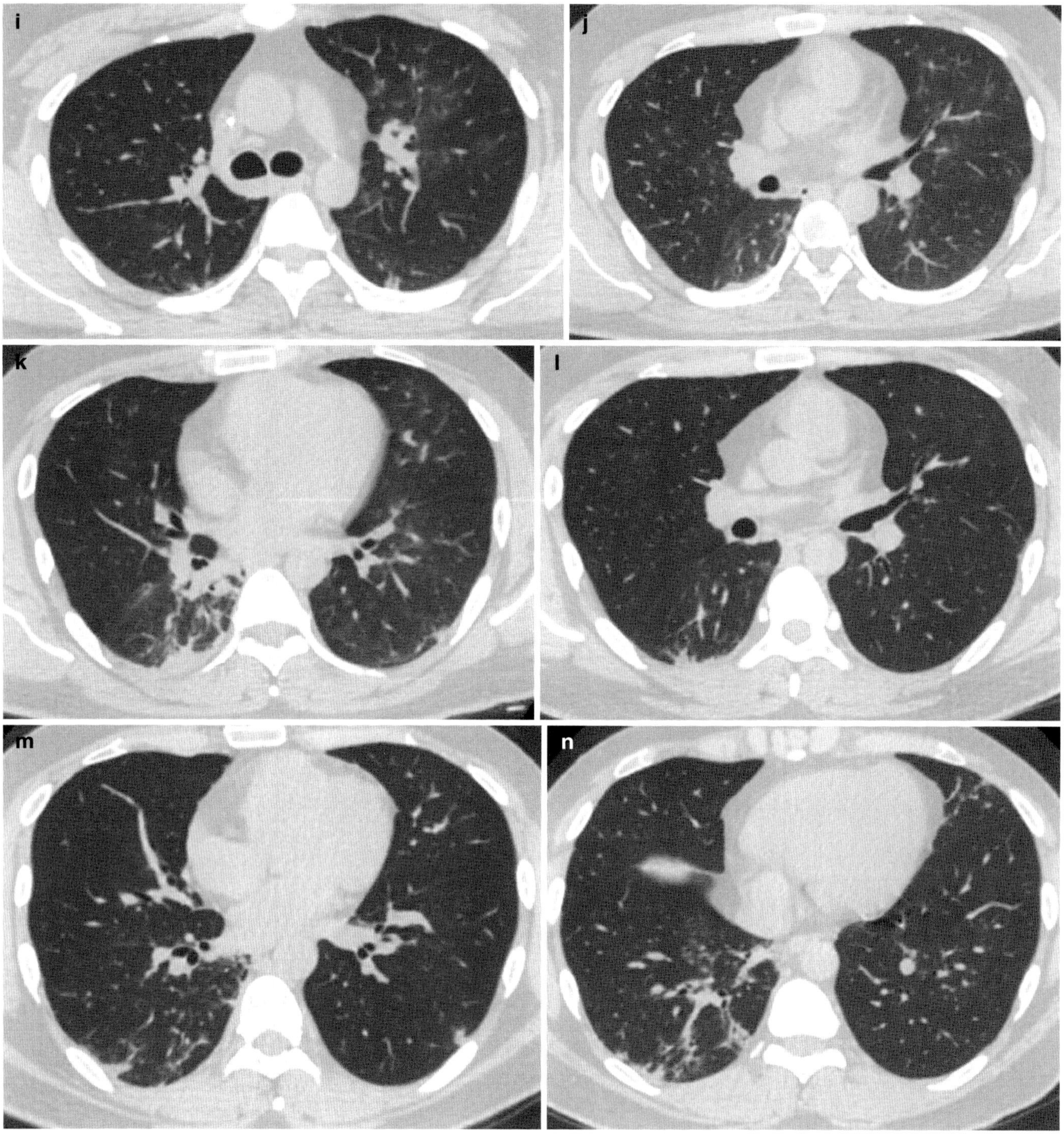

Fig. 3.11 (continued)

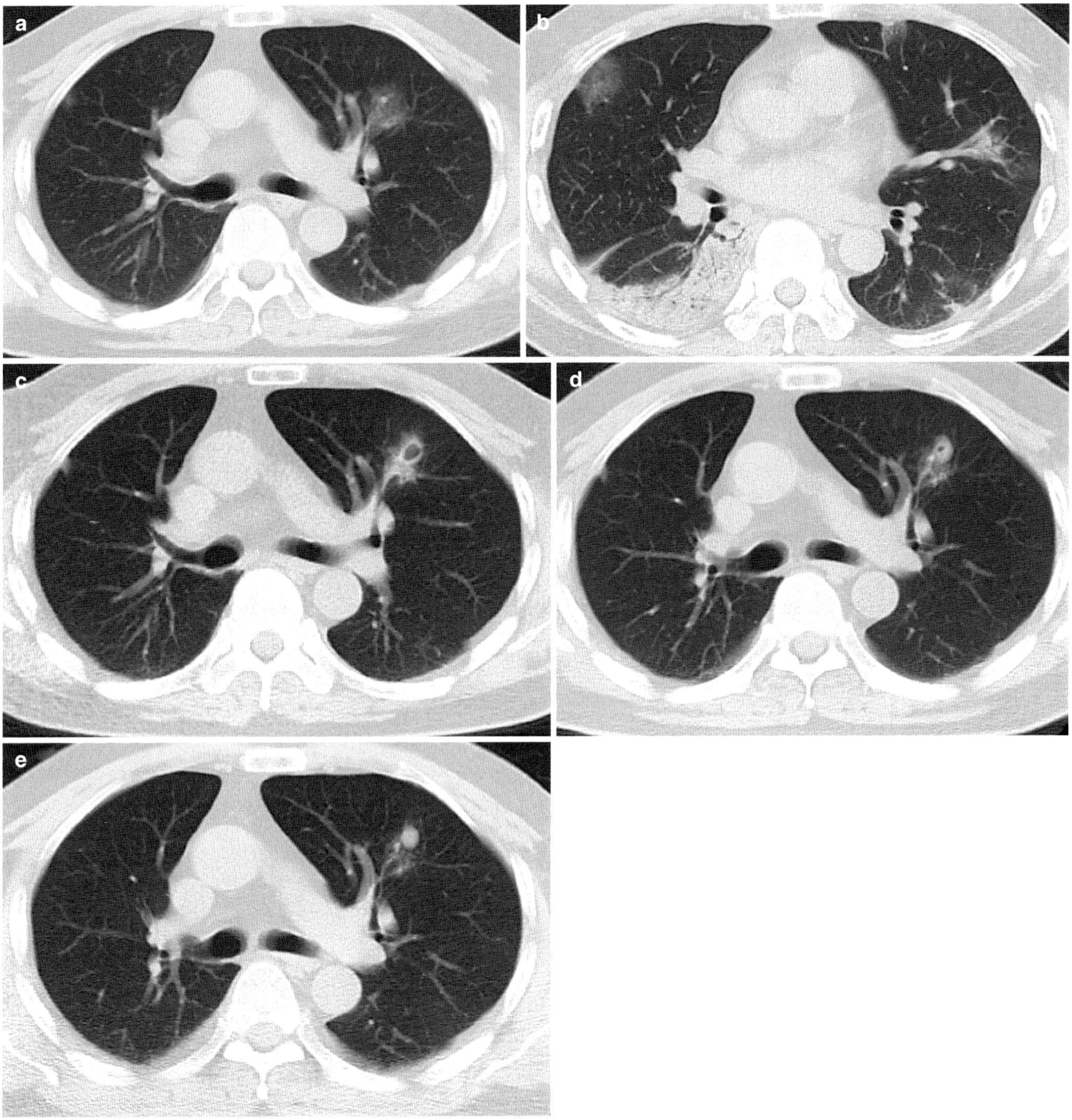

Fig. 3.12 (**a–e**) The male patient aged 56 years old was diagnosed with avian influenza H7N9 pneumonia. (**a**, **b**) On the 6th day after onset of the disease, chest CT scan demonstrated consolidation shadows and air bronchogram at the right inferior lung lobe and scattering patchy ground-glass shadows at the right middle lobe and subpleural area of the left lung. (**c**) On the 22nd day after the onset of the disease, chest CT showed absorption of the majority of right inferior lung consolidation shadows and presence of small lung air sacs at left superior lung with relatively clear inner wall. (**d**) On the 26th day after the onset, chest CT suggested absorption of small pulmonary air sacs at left superior lung. (**e**) On the 43th day after the onset of the disease, chest CT indicated basal absorption of small lung air sacs at left superior lung and presence of nodular shadows

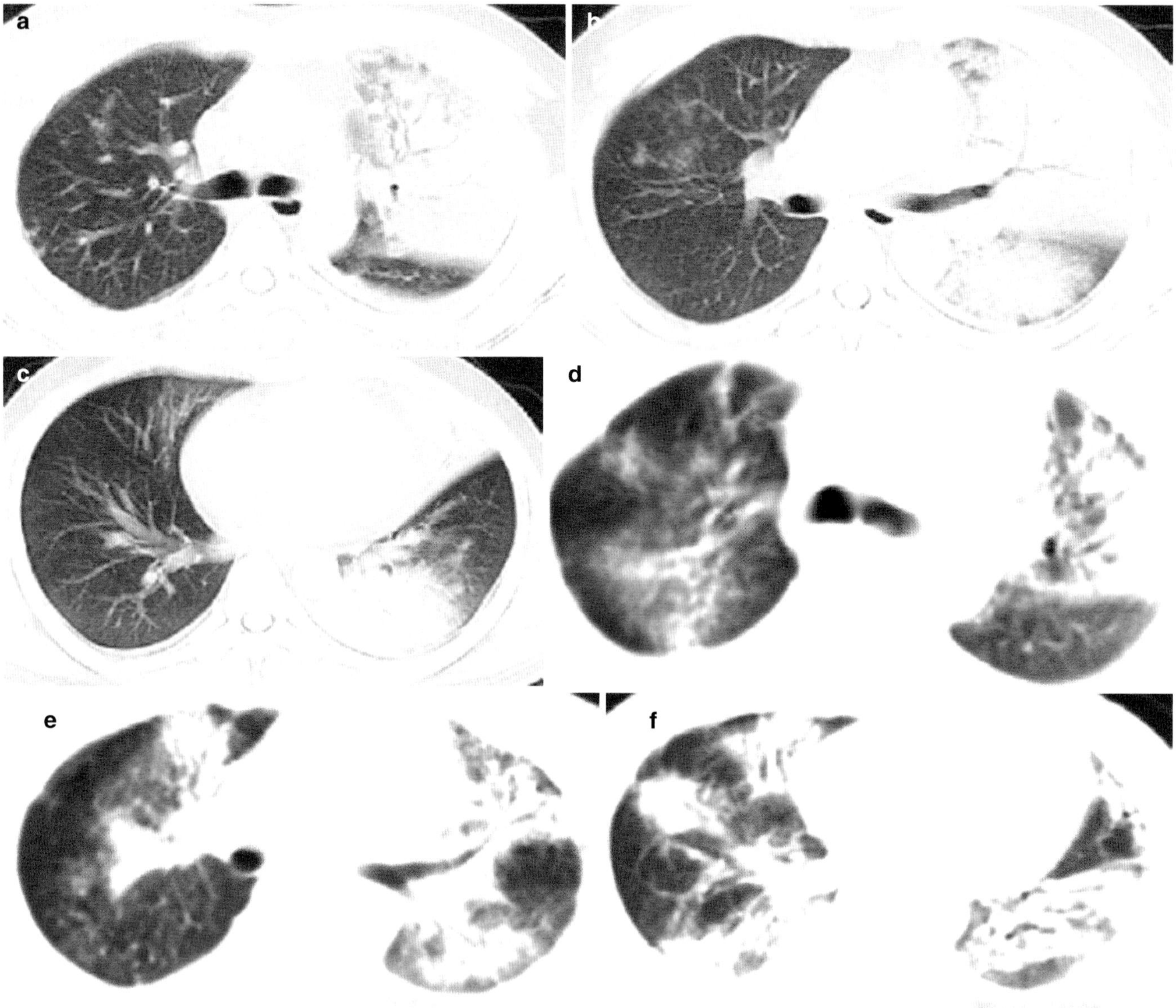

Fig. 3.13 (**a**–**u**) The male patient aged 31 years old was confirmed with human avian influenza subtype H5N1severe pneumonia complicated by ARDS. (**a**–**c**) On the 9th day after the onset of the disease, chest CT showed large patchy consolidation shadows at the left lung, with air bronchogram observable in between. The right lung was seen with scattered patchy ground-glass shadows. (**d**–**f**) On the 34th day after the onset of the disease, both lungs were found with extensive consolidation shadows and ground-glass shadows; the left lung presented mainly consolidation shadows and air bronchogram. There were shrinkage of left inferior lobe and aggregation of lung texture. (**g**–**i**) On the 96th day after the onset, both lungs were visualized with patchy inhomogeneous consolidation shadows and cord-like shadows, with patchy ground-glass shadows seen peripheral to consolidation shadows at both lungs. (**j**–**l**) On the 286th day after the onset of the disease, CT revealed that foci of both lungs were predominated by pulmonary interstitial changes such as fibrous cord-like and latticed shadows, with concurrent ground-glass shadows. Absorption of the foci slowed down distinctly. (**m**–**o**) 2 years after onset of the disease, CT unveiled fibrous strip and latticed shadows in both lungs, and patchy ground-glass shadows at the left superior lung and bilateral inferior lungs. Compared with the chest CT presentations 1 year before, the foci were slightly absorbed. (**p**–**s**) 39 months after the onset of the disease, chest CT suggested fibrous strip and latticed shadows at bilateral superior lungs as well as thickening of interlobular septum, paramediastinal emphysema, small consolidation shadow, and signs of bronchiectasis. The left superior and right inferior lung were detected with small patchy ground-glass shadows. (**t**–**u**) 5 years and 7 months after the onset of the disease, both lungs were visualized still with fibrous strip shadow, latticed shadow, and bronchiectasis signs, particularly at the right middle lobe and left superior lobe. Both lungs were found with small consolidation shadows and small patchy ground-glass shadows

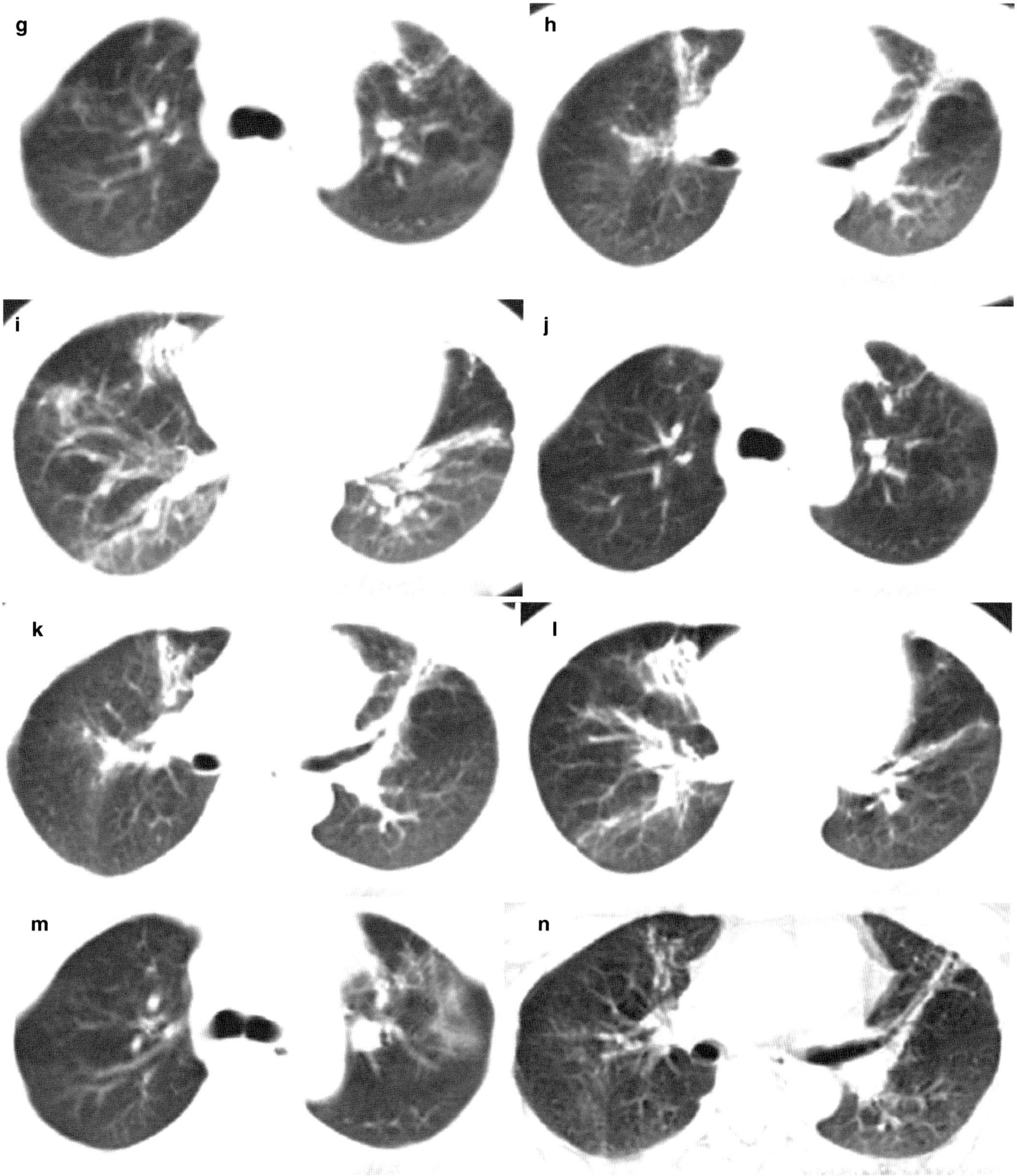

Fig. 3.13 (continued)

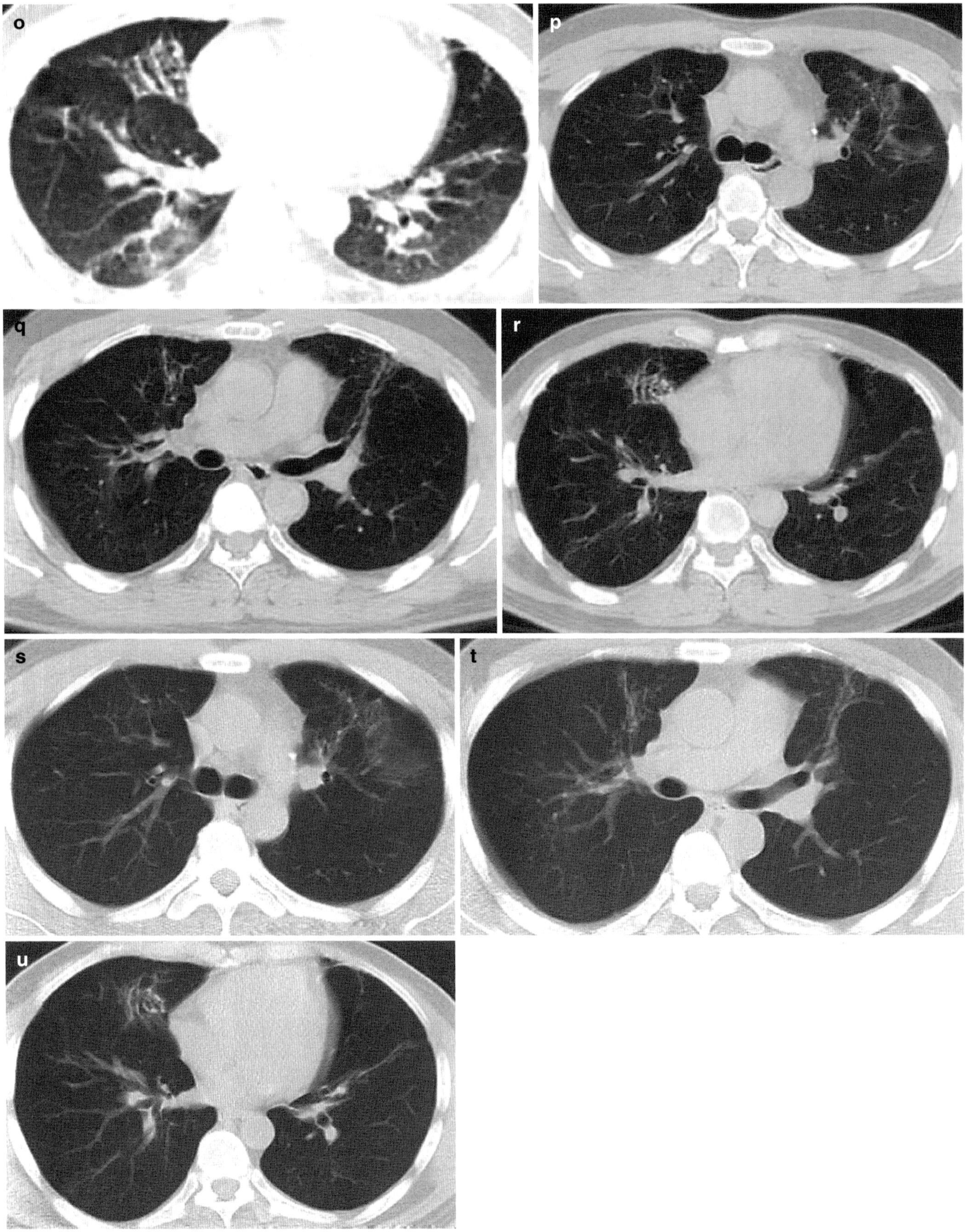

Fig. 3.13 (continued)

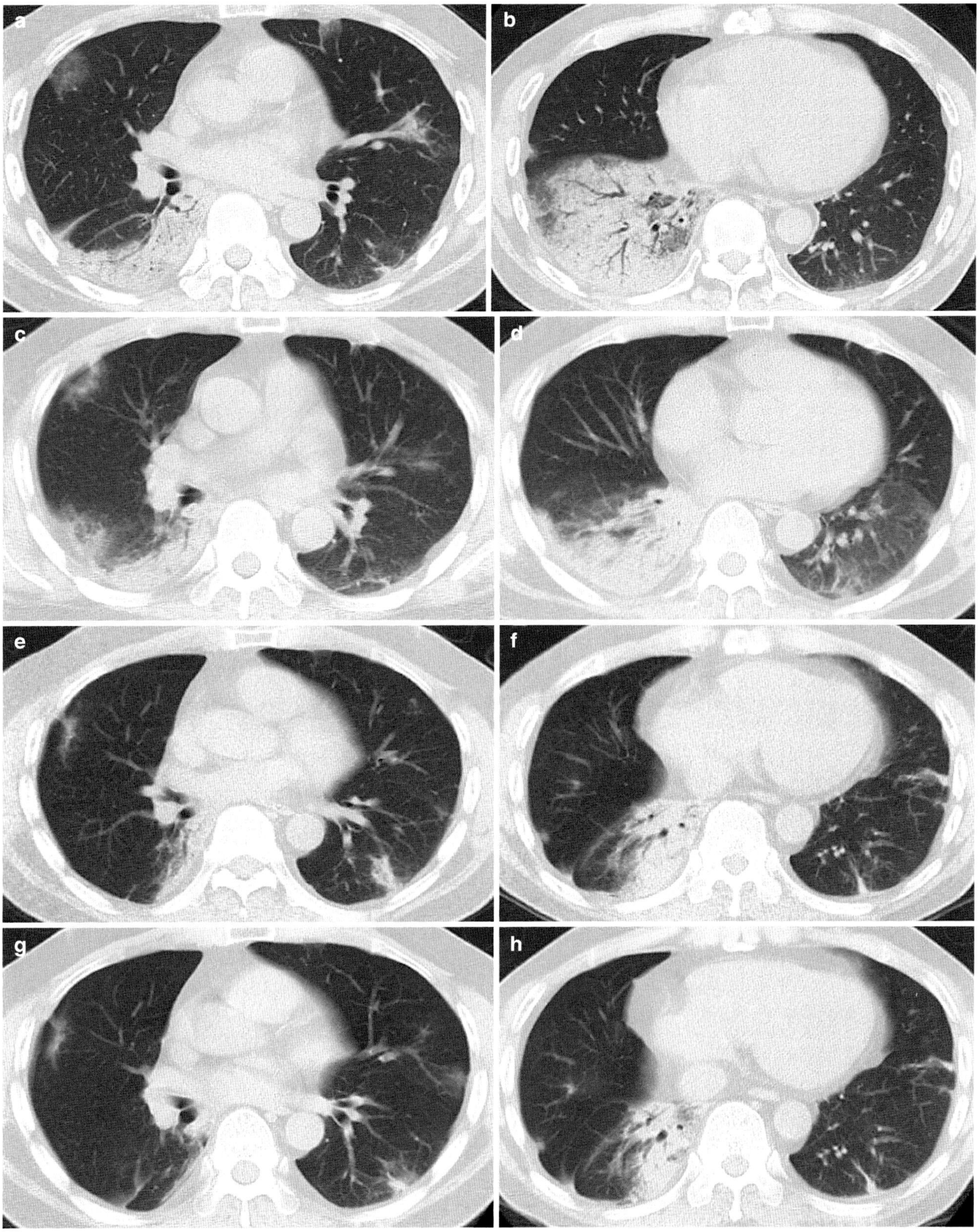

Fig. 3.14 (**a–h**) The 56-year-old male patient was detected with avian influenza H7N9 pneumonia. (**a**, **b**) On the 6th day after the onset of the disease, chest CT indicated large patchy consolidation shadows at right inferior lung lobe accompanied by air bronchogram. The right middle lobe and subpleural area of left lung were visualized with scattered patchy ground-glass shadows. (**c**, **d**) On the 13th day after the onset of the disease, chest CT suggested absorption of large patchy consolidation shadows at the right inferior lung lobe. The left inferior lung was found with ground-glass shadows. (**e**, **f**) On the 21st day after the onset of the disease, chest CT demonstrated obvious absorption of large patch of consolidation at right lung lobes. (**g**, **h**) On the 25th day after the onset of the disease, chest CT revealed fibrous strip shadows at the right lung lobes. The left lung and right superior lung presented with absorption of the patchy ground-glass shadows

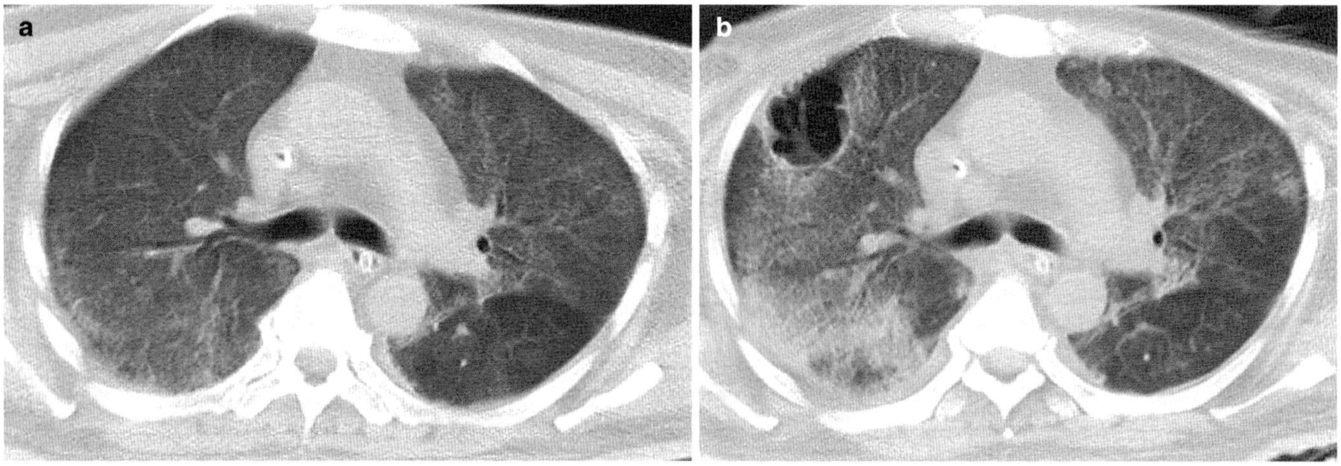

Fig. 3.15 (**a**, **b**) The male patient aged 48 years old was diagnosed with avian influenza H7N9 severe pneumonia accompanied by *Acinetobacter baumannii* infection. (**a**) On the 15th day after the onset of the disease, both lungs were revealed with ground-glass-density shadows and the original right inferior lung consolidation shadows were basically absorbed. Avian influenza virus H7N9 became negative. (**b**) On the 24th day after onset of the disease, the patient suffered from fever, and culture of deep sputum for two times showed *Acinetobacter baumannii*. CT visualized consolidation shadows at the right lung and small patchy consolidation shadow at the subpleural area of the left superior lung

infection, mediastinal and subcutaneous emphysema, pneumothorax, lung fibrosis, and nonbacterial necrosis of the head of the femur. These complications or sequelae are also discovered mainly by imaging. Knowledge about human avian influenza imaging presentations could help elevate the curative rate and decrease mortality of human avian influenza.

3.7.3.1 Lung Secondary Infections

Pathogenesis

Human avian influenza virus may attack the human immunity system directly and compromise immunity.

Large doses of glucocorticoids are administered during treatment which could undermine the immunity.

Some patients may still need such treatment as positive airway pressure or bronchial intubation and central venous indwelling catheter, which create conditions for secondary infection.

Meanwhile, abundant use of broad-spectrum antibiotics could disturb the normal bacterial flora. The most frequent and severe is a complication with *Acinetobacter baumannii* infection.

Clinical and Imaging Diagnosis of Complication of *Acinetobacter baumannii* Infection

Acinetobacter baumannii is highly capable of acquiring drug tolerance and clone dissemination, and *Acinetobacter baumannii* with multiple drug tolerance and broad drug tolerance is one of the most important pathogen of human avian influenza. *Acinetobacter baumannii* may induce nosocomial pneumonia, bloodstream infection, abdominal infection, central nervous system infection, urinary system infection, cutaneous soft tissue infection, and myelitis. The diagnosis may be concluded based on following evidences: (1) besides clinical symptoms, signs and imaging presentations consistent with pneumonia, new or sustained or aggravated lung exudates, infiltration, and consolidation are detected (Fig. 3.15). (2) Host factors including underlying disease, immune status, application of antibacterial medicines in early period, and duration of mechanical ventilation (3).

Sputum culture for over two times shows growth of pure *Acinetobacter baumannii* or dominant growth of *Acinetobacter baumannii*; or blood culture demonstrates with growth of *Acinetobacter baumannii*.

3.7.3.2 Mediastinal and Subcutaneous Emphysema

All patients with avian influenza suffer from different degrees of lung fibrosis and lung impairment, and the majority of patients need assisted respiration such as artificial assisted ventilation of the ventilator and tracheotomy intubation, which could heighten intrapulmonary pressure by different degrees. However, as patients with human avian influenza manifest varying degrees of inflammatory exudation from lung tissues, the occlusive fibrosis inside bronchioli may lead to rupture of alveolar elastic fibers, which may on one hand damage lung air exchange and on the other hand lower lung compliance. Under the condition of increased intrapulmonary pressure, pneumothorax and mediastinal and subcutaneous emphysema are more likely to occur.

Imaging presentations: CT suggests air-density linear shadows encircling the mediastinum and shift of the mediastinal pleura toward lung field. Air in the mediastinum escapes along the cervical fascial space to the neck and chest subcutaneous area, thus rendering subcutaneous gas-density imaging signs (Figs. 3.3, 3.4, 3.5, 3.6, 3.7, 3.8, 3.9, 3.10, 3.11, 3.12, 3.13, 3.14, 3.15, and 3.16).

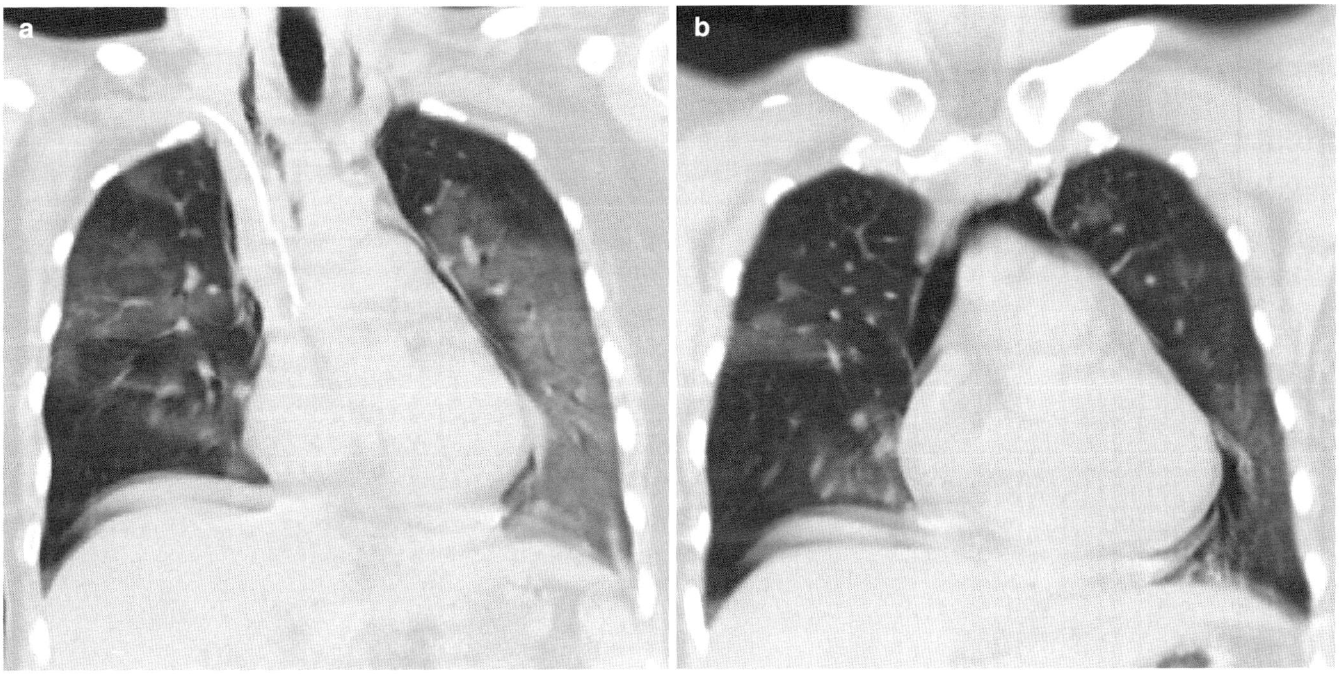

Fig. 3.16 (**a**, **b**) The 34-year-old male patient was diagnosed with avian influenza H7N9 severe pneumonia complicated with mediastinal pneumatosis. Coronal imaging visualized remarkable pneumatosis at the neck, mediastinum, and the periphery of the heart and large blood vessels

3.7.3.3 Lung Interstitial Fibrosis

Pathologic Basis of Clinical Imaging

In the early phase of onset, human avian influenza presents with bronchiolar and peripheral parenchymal or interstitial lesions, which may progress into alveolar parenchymal and interstitial lesions, mostly reversible. In the phase of recovery, some cases may advance into pulmonary interstitial proliferation and then into fibrosis. The degree and outcome of lung interstitial proliferation and fibrosis are related to the scope of lung involvement in the climax phase, presence of complications, as well as treatment.

Imaging Manifestations

The initial signs of lung interstitial proliferation are thickening of lobular septum and intralobular interstitium as well as subpleural curvature shadows. The intrapulmonary patchy become smaller and denser, and high-density cord and honeycomb-like shadows are gradually observable in the lungs. Severe lung interstitial proliferation could make the lungs shrink and mediastinum shift toward the affected side. Lung interstitial proliferation may exist extensively in the lungs, predominated by thickening of interlobular septum and interlobular interstitium as well as subpleural curvature imaging changes. It may also manifest local irregular high-density plaque and cord-shaped shadows. Intrapulmonary honeycomb-like imaging presentation and traction bronchiectasis are primary signs of lung interstitial fibrosis.

CT reveals cord-like, reticular, and honeycomb-shaped shadows. HRCT could better display the meticulous abnormal changes of pulmonary interstitium, such as thickening of lobular septum, intralobular interstitial thickening, subpleural curvation shadow, honeycomb-like shadow, paraseptal emphysema, as well as bronchiolar dilatation (Figs. 3.17 and 3.18).

3.7.3.4 Ischemic Necrosis of Femoral Head and Osteomyelitis

Pathogenesis

TAt present its pathogenesis still remains unclear and it might be associated with the inflammatory reaction and damage from use of hormones and human avian influenza combined with bacterial infection (such as *Acinetobacter baumannii* infection) or multiple mixed factors on sclerotin and blood vessels. Femoral head aseptic necrosis is typical of degenerative changes due to femoral head blood circulation disturbance, with limping and pain as main symptoms. The affected lower limb is slightly shorter and manifests mild flexion and adduction. The abduction and intorsion slightly limited.

Imaging Presentations of Aseptic Necrosis of the Femoral Head

In the early phase of femur head aseptic necrosis, CT demonstrates that the stellate sign formed by femoral trabeculae become deformed or disappeared, visualized as spot or patchy shadows with increased density in the femoral head and tuft-

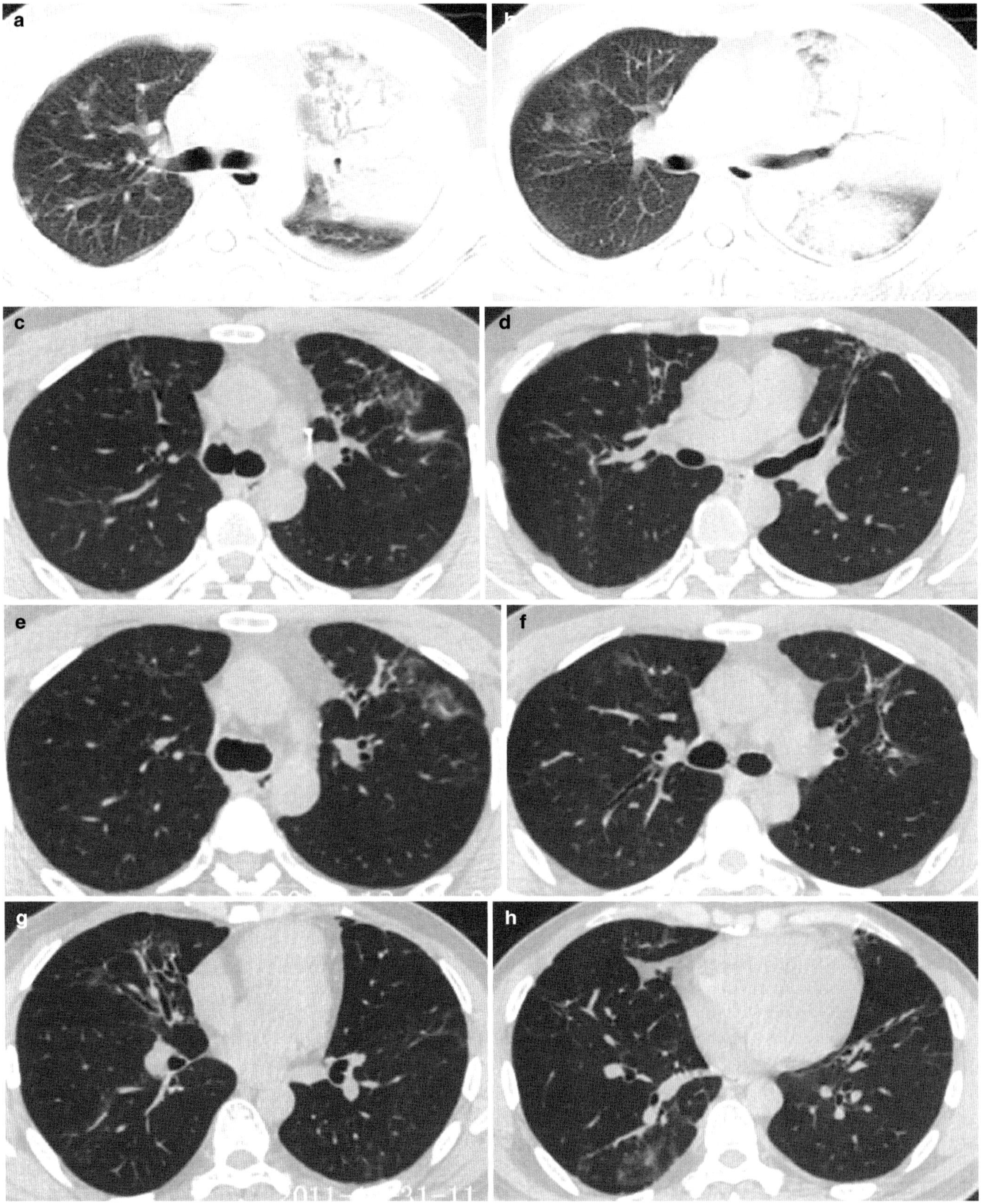

Fig. 3.17 (**a**–**j**) The male patient aged 34 years old was confirmed with human avian influenza H5N1 complicated by pulmonary interstitial fibrosis. (**a**, **b**) On the 9th day after the onset of disease, chest CT suggested large patchy consolidation shadows, with air bronchogram in between. The right lung was seen with scattered ground-glass shadows. (**c**, **d**) 5 years and 7 months after onset of the disease, chest CT follow-up revealed fibrous strip shadows and latticed shadows at both lungs as well as bronchiectasis. (**e**–**g**) The left lung ligule and right inferior lung middle lobe were detected with small patchy ground-glass shadows, fibrous strip shadows, and bronchiectasis. (**h**, **i**) The inferior lobes of both lungs were unveiled with strip consolidation shadows, small patchy ground-glass shadows, and paraseptal emphysema. (**j**) The coronal view of three-dimensional construction suggested a quasi-circular nodular shadow in a diameter of about 2 mm in left main bronchus

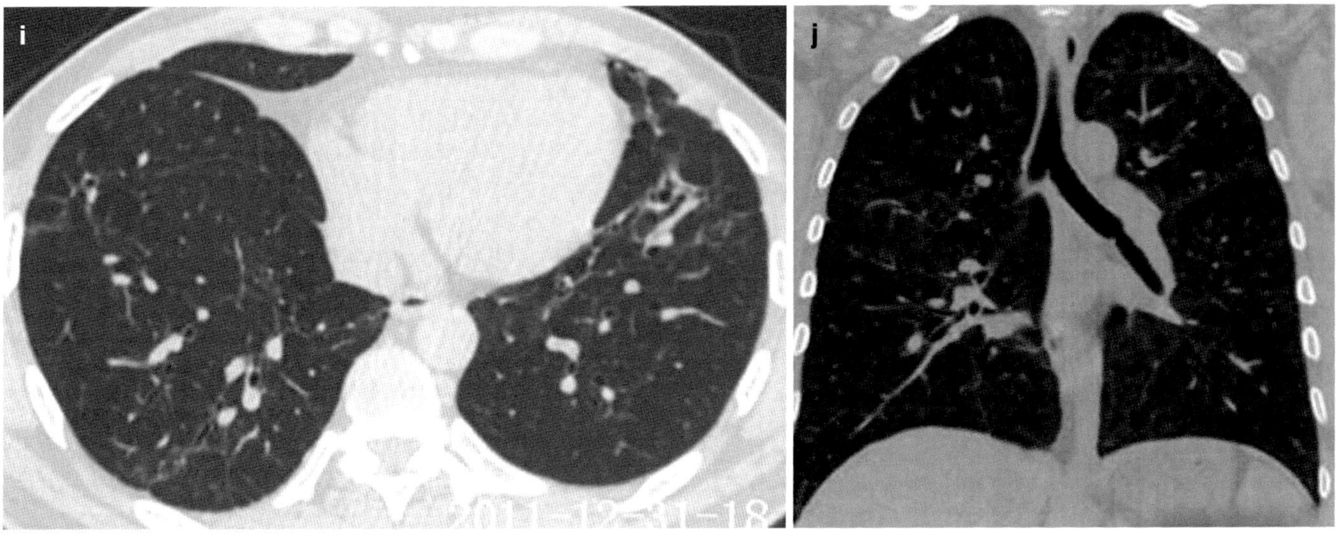

Fig. 3.17 (continued)

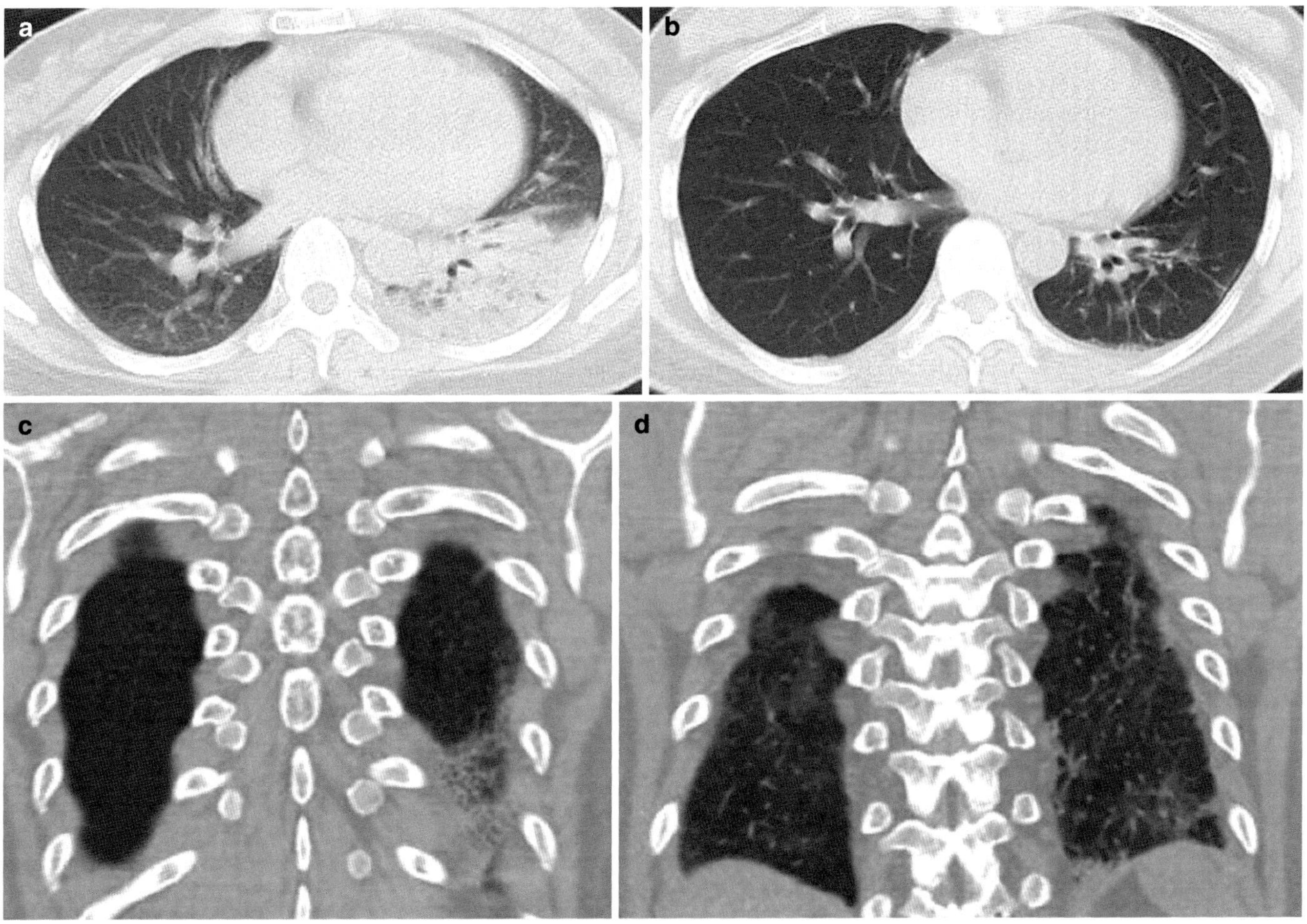

Fig. 3.18 (**a**–**e**) The female patient aged 43 years old was identified with avian influenza H7N9 severe pneumonia complicated by lung interstitial fibrosis. (**a**) On the 10th day after the onset of the disease, chest CT showed large patchy consolidation shadows at the right inferior lung. (**b**) On the 34th day after the onset of the disease, the transverse image of chest CT re-examination indicated fibrous strip shadows and subpleural curvature shadows. (**c**) Coronal view of three-dimensional reconstruction found mosaic sign at the left inferior lung. (**d**) Coronal view of three-dimensional reconstruction demonstrated extensive pulmonary interstitial proliferation at the dorsal sides of both lungs. (**e**) Coronal view of three-dimensional reconstruction unveiled emphysema at the right superior paramediastinum, and cord-like shadow at the right inferior lung; and bronchiectasis sign at the left inferior lung

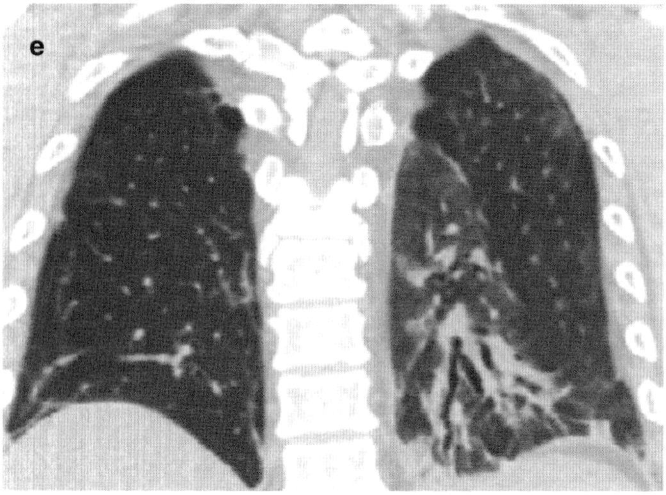

Fig. 3.18 (continued)

shaped change or mutual fusion at the periphery of stellate sign. In the advanced phase, the femur head becomes fragmented and deformed, and the absorption of sclerotin between fragmented bones presents irregular low-density area, with the stellate sign absent. Based on MRI presentations, aseptic necrosis of the femur head may be divided into the following four phases: Phase I shows homogenous or inhomogeneous low-signal areas adjacent to joints above the femur head on weighted T1 and T2 imaging; phase II manifests wedge-shaped mixed low-signal band; phase III is typical of sequestrum crescent sign and cortical collapse; phase IV manifests phase III signs accompanied by joint degeneration and joint space stenosis.

Besides, apart from the most common ischemic necrosis of the femoral head, osteomyelitis is also documented, mostly at the femur, which presents irregular low-signal area on T2 weighed imaging (Fig. 3.19).

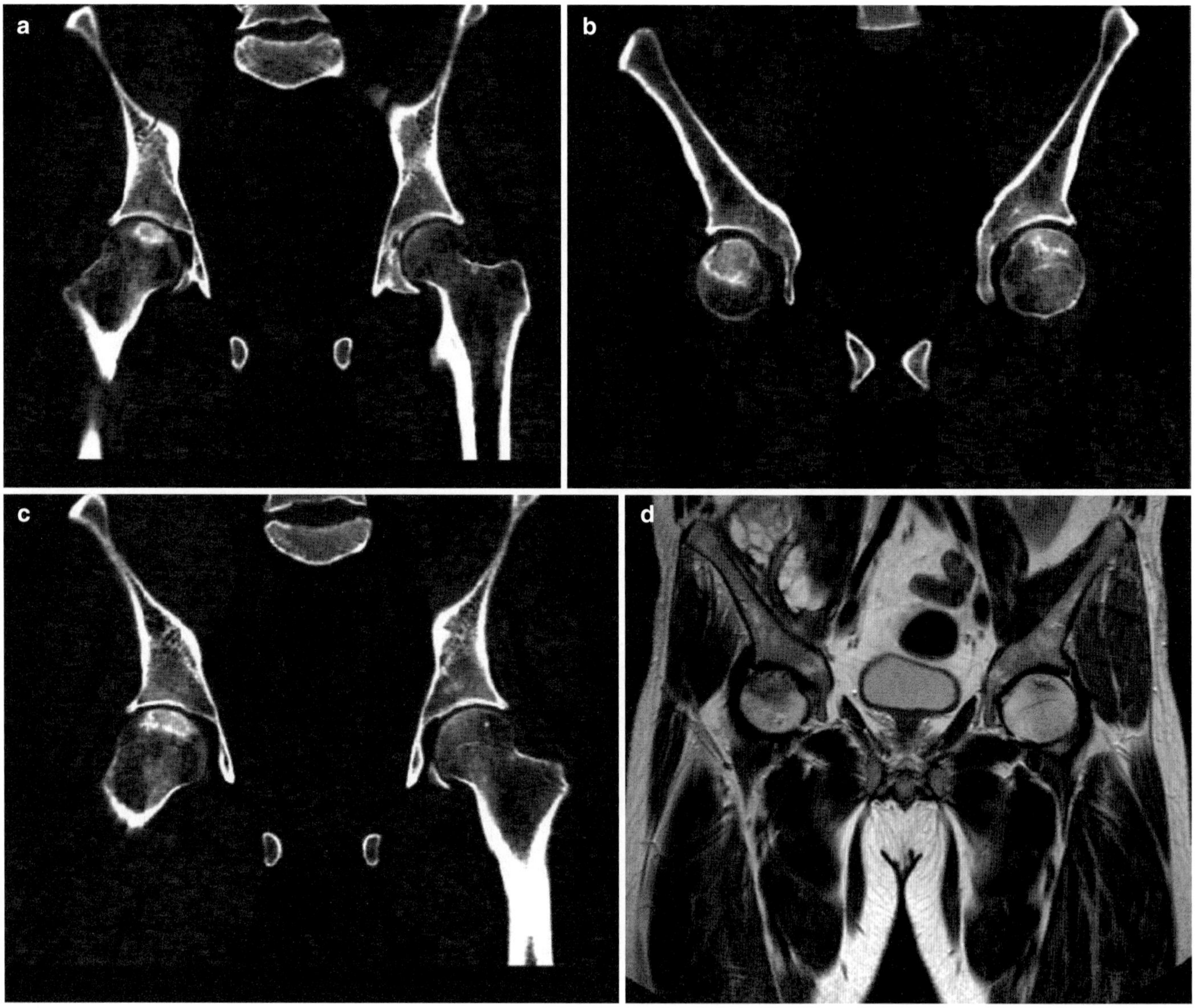

Fig. 3.19 (**a–g**) The 39-year-old male patient was detected with avian influenza H7N9 severe pneumonia accompanied by bilateral femur head ischemic necrosis and osteomyelitis of the middle and upper segment of the left and right femurs. (**a–c**) On the 27th day after onset of the disease, pelvic CT plain scan coronal view revealed patchy shadows of increased density at bilateral femur heads, prominently at the right femoral head. (**d–g**) On the 37th day after onset of the disease, pelvic MRI plain scan disclosed the bilateral femoral heads of irregular low signals on weighted T1 and T2 imaging, and the middle and upper segments of the left and right femur with irregular low signals on weighted T2 imaging

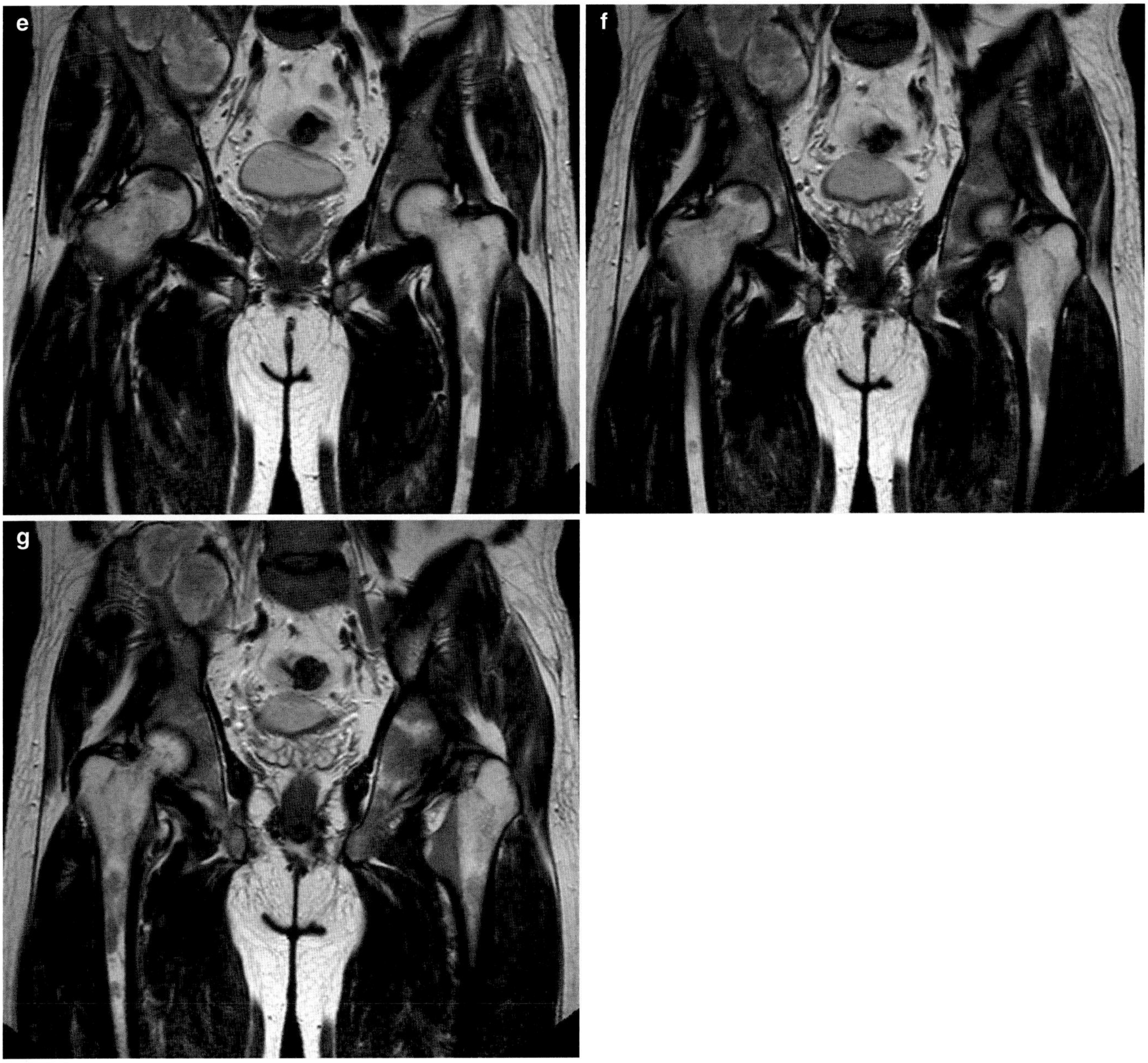

Fig. 3.19 (continued)

Further Reading

1. Luo RP, Zhu YM, Xu ZY, et al. Report of the first human case of H5N1 avian influenza pneumonia in China mainland. Chin J Pediatr. 2006;44(5):342–5.
2. Xu XY, Wang QY. Biology and epidemiology of human avian influenza. Nat Med J Chin. 2004;84(5):342–5.
3. Huang XR, Zeng Z, Lu PX, et al. Clinical Imaging Analysis of 12 cases of human avian influenza H7N9 pneumonia [J]. Chin J CT MRI. 2014;12(2):8–11.
4. Henter JI, Chow CB, Leung C, et al. Cytotoxic therapy for severe avian influenza A (H5N1) infection. Lancet. 2006;367(9513):870–3.
5. Ungchusak K, Auewarakul P, Dowell SF, et al. Probable person-to-person transmission of avian influenza A (H5N1). N Engl J Med. 2005;352(4):333–40.
6. Lin J, Zhang J, Dong X, et al. Safety and immunogenicity of an inactivated adjuvanted whole-virion influenza A(H5N1) vaccine: a phase I randomised controlled trial. Lancet. 2006;368(9540):991–7.
7. Oner AF, Bay A, Arslan S, et al. Avian influenza A (H5N1) infection in eastern Turkey in 2006. N Engl J Med. 2006;355(21):2179–85.
8. Obenauer JC, Denson J, Mehta PK, et al. Large-Scale Sequence analysis of avian influenza isolates. Science. 2006;311(5767):1576–80.
9. Li Q, Lan Y, Xu CL, et al. Study on a deceased pregnant patient with avian influenza (H5N1) [J]. Chin J Epidemiol. 2006;27(4):288–92.
10. Zhou BP, Yi-min LI, Lu PX. Human avian influenza. Peking: Science Press; 2007.
11. Yu HJ, Chen YX, Shu YL, et al. Investigation and confirmation of the first case of human avian influenza H5N1 in China mainland. Chin J Epidemiol. 2006;27(4):281–7.
12. Bai YQ, Xu G, Gong ZL, et al. Autopsy pathological analysis of human highly pathogenic avian influenza H5N1. Chin J Pathol. 2006;32:545–8.
13. Beigel JH, Farrar J, Han AM, et al. Avian influenza A (H5N1) infection in human. N Engl J Med. 2005;353(13):1374–85.

14. Zhang W*, Wen LY, Lu M, et al. Clinical characteristics of the first human highly pathogenic influenza H_5N_1 in Jiangxi Province. Chin J Tuberc Respir Dis. 2006;29(5):300–6.
15. Zeng Z, Lu PX, Zhou BP, et al. Imaging manifestations of human avian influenza H7N9 severe pneumonia. J Tuberc Lung Health. 2014;3(1):25–8.
16. Liang ZW, He DH, Weng WX, et al. Review and enlightenment of human avian influenza prevention and control in Hongkong. Chin J Tuberc Respir Dis. 2004;27(4):253–8.
17. Brown EG, Liu H, Kit LC, et al. Pattern of mutation in the genome of influenza A virus on adaptation to increased virulence in the mouse lung: identification of functional themes. Proc Natl Acad Sci U S A. 2001;98(12):6883–8.
18. Chen H, Deng G, Li Z, et al. The evolution of H5N1 influenza viruses in ducks in southern China. Proc Natl Acad Sci U S A. 2004;101(28):10452–7.
19. Cheung CY, Poon LL, Lau AS, et al. Induction of proinflammatory cytokines in human macrophages by influenza A (H5N1) viruses: a mechanism for the unusual severity of human disease? Lancet. 2002;60(9348):1831–7.
20. Chotpitayasunondh T, Ungchusak K, Hanshaoworakul W, et al. Human disease from influenza A (H5N1), Thailand, 2004. Emerg Infect Dis. 2005;11(2):201–9.
21. Shinya K, Hamm S, Hatta M, et al. PB2 amino acid at position 627 affects replicative efficiency, but not cell tropism, of Hong Kong H5N1 influenza A viruses in mice. Virology. 2004;320(2): 258–66.
22. Tran TH, Nguyen TL, Nguyen TD, et al. Avian influenza A (H5N1) in 10 patients in Vietnam. N Engl J Med. 2004;350(12):1179–88.
23. Carlson CM, Turpin EA, Moser LA, et al. Transforming growth factor-b: activation by neuraminidase and role in highly pathogenic H5N1 influenza pathogenesis. PLoS Pathog. 2010;6(10), e1001136.
24. Yuen KY, Wong SS. Human infection by avian influenza A H5N1. Hong Kong Med J. 2005;11(3):189–99.
25. De Jong MD, Bach VC, Phan TQ, et al. Fatal avian influenza A (H5N1) in a child presenting with diarrhea followed by coma. N Engl J Med. 2005;352(7):686–91.
26. Cai JP, Xiao R, Zhou XY. Biological characteristics and laboratory test of avian influenza virus. Chin J Lab Med. 2005;28(3):232–4.
27. Liu ST, Zhou BP, Yang DG, et al. Successful treatment of the first case of human H5N1 avian influenza in Shenzhen. Chin J Infect Dis. 2007;25(1):29–34.
28. Normile D. Avian influenza. Studies suggest why few humans catch the H5N1 virus. Science. 2006;311(5768):1692.
29. Doherty PC, Turner SJ, Webby RG, et al. Influenza and the challenge for immunology. Nat Immunol. 2006;7(5):449–55.
30. Pizza G, Amadori M, Ablashi D, et al. Cell mediated immunity to meet the avian influenza A (H5N1) challenge. Med Hypotheses. 2006;67(3):601–8.
31. Lu PX, Zhou BP, Zhu WK, et al. Imaging features of pneumonia caused by highly pathogenic H5N1 Subtype human avian influenza virus. Chin J Med ImagTechnol. 2007;23(4):532–5.
32. Lu PU, Deng YY. Epidemiological and imaging manifestations of human avian influenza. Chin Comp Med Imag. 2010;16(5):431–4.
33. Lu PX, Zhu WK, Ye RX, et al. CT manifestation and dynamic changes of grave pneumonia in adults caused by H5N1 subtype of human avian influenza virus. Chin J CT MRI. 2007;5(1):31–4.
34. Zhao DJ, Ma DQ. Imaging manifestations of human avian influenza. Chin J Radiol. 2006;40(3):319–21.
35. Puxuan L, Boping Z, et al. Radiological features of lung changes caused by avian influenza subtype A H5N 1 virus: report of two severe adult cases with regular follow -up. Chin Med J. 2010;123:100–4.
36. Tran TH, Nguyen TL, Nguyen TD, et al. Avian influenza A(H5N1) in 10 patients in Vietnam. N Engl J Med. 2004;35(12):1179–88.
37. Cheung CY, Poon LL, Lau AS, et al. Induction of proinflammatory cytokines in human macrophages by influenza A (H5N1) viruses: a mechanism for the unusual severity of human disease? Lancet. 2002;360(9348):1831–7.
38. Peiris JS, Yu WC, Leung CW, et al. Re-emergence of fatal human influenza A subtype H5N1 disease. Lancet. 2004;363(9409):617–9.
39. Lu PX, Zeng Z, Huang XR, et al. Imaging presentations and dynamic changes of severe pneumonia incurred by avian influenza H7N9. Radiol Pract. 2014;29(7):740–4.
40. Wang LQ, Shi YX, Zhang ZY, et al. Imaging preliminary observation of new recombinant avian influenza (H7N9) pneumonia. Chin J Radiol. 2013;47(6):505–8.
41. Qingle W, Zhiyong Z, Yuxin S, et al. Emerging H7N9 influenza A (Novel Reassortant Avian-Origin) pneumonia: radiologic findings [J]. Radiology. 2013;268(9):882–9.
42. Huang XH, Huang H, Lu PU, et al. CT presentations of human avian influenza H7N9 pneumonia and its correlation with viral load and CD4+ T cell. Radiol Pract. 2014;29(7):751–5.
43. Fu WJ, Hu MH, Liu XQ, et al. Retrospective analysis of one case of avian influenza H10N8 severe pneumonia in Jiangxi province. Chin J Public Health. 2014;30(6):818–9.
44. Chen HY, Yuan H, Gao RB, et al. Clinical and epidemiological characteristics of a fatal case of avian influenza A H10N8 virus infection: a descriptive study [J]. Lancet. 2014;383(9918):714–21.

Influenza A (H1N1)

4

Zeng Hong-Wu, Yuan Jing, Huang Wen-Xian, Li Hong-Jun, Pu-Xuan Lu, Le Xiao-Hua, Huang Hua, Mao Xiao-Ming, Zhou Lei, Hu Ya-Nan, Wang Hao-Peng, Zhang Qian-Qian, and Sha Ziling

In March 2009, an outbreak of human-infected swine influenza occurred in Mexico, with reports of deaths. Soon afterward, such cases were reported worldwide, namely, a pandemic outbreak. The prevailing disease is then defined as an acute respiratory infectious disease caused by swine-origin influenza A (H1N1) virus, a new variant of influenza virus. Its viral strains contain gene segments of three types of influenza viruses, namely swine influenza virus, avian influenza virus and human influenza virus. And the virus is mainly transmitted among humans via direct and indirect contact or respiratory tract.

This new virus is originated from pigs. Initially, WHO nominated such influenza as "human-infected swine influenza." However, such a nomination may cause misunderstandings about intake of pork and pork products. And such a nomination may even involve certain issues about religions and beliefs. Therefore, the influenza is known as "North American Influenza" by the World Organisation for Animal Health, "New Influenza Virus" by the European Union, "Mexican Virus" by South Korea and Israel, and "Mexican flu" by New Zealand. In China, it was initially nominated as "human-infected swine influenza," and "New H1N1 influenza" in Taiwan. In order to avoid misleading the public, the WHO declared on 30 April 2009 in Geneva that the nomination of "swine influenza" is terminated and the disease is renamed as "Influenza A (H1N1)."

On 11 June 2009, the WHO raised the pandemic alert level of influenza to Phase 6. By 21 March 2010, according to the WHO official website, the laboratory confirmed cases of influenza A (H1N1) had been reported from more than 213 countries and regions including at least 16,931 deaths. By 7 March 2010, according to data from China, 127,427 confirmed cases had been reported from 31 provinces in mainland, including 8320 severe and critical cases, and 796 deaths. The death rate of the pandemic of influenza A (H1N1) is 0.4–6.77 %, being higher than that from common influenza.

4.1 Etiology

The main pathogen causing influenza is the influenza virus, which can be categorized into the family of Orthomyxoviridae and the genus of influenza virus. Influenza viruses are composed of envelope and segmental single-stranded negative RNA. The virus consists of three parts, namely, from the outside to the inside, the envelope, matrix protein (M protein), and the core. According to matrix protein antigens, genetic characteristics, and virus nucleoprotein particles, the influenza viruses can be classified into type A (A), type B (B), and type C (C). Influenza A can cause seasonal epidemics in certain regions and may even lead to a worldwide pandemic outbreak.

Zeng Hong-Wu (✉)
Department of Radiology, Shenzhen Children's Hospital Guangdong, Shenzhen, China
e-mail: homerzeng@126.com

Yuan Jing
Department of Infection, Shenzhen Third People's Hospital Guangdong, Shenzhen, China
e-mail: 13500054798@139.com

Huang Wen-Xian
Shenzhen Children's Hospital, Futian, Shenzhen, Guangdong, China

Li Hong-Jun
You'an Hospital, Capital Medical University, Beijing, China

Pu-Xuan Lu
Department of Radiology, Shenzhen Third People's Hospital Guangdong, Shenzhen, China
e-mail: lupuxuan@126.com

Le Xiao-Hua • Huang Hua • Wang Hao-Peng • Zhang Qian-Qian
The Shenzhen No.3 People's Hospital, Guangdong College, Shenzhen, China

Mao Xiao-Ming • Zhou Lei
Shenzhen Yantian Hospital, Shenzhen, Guangdong, China

Hu Ya-Nan
Guangzhou University of Chinese Medicine, Baiyun, Guangzhou, Guangdong, China

Sha Ziling
Medical Emergency Center of BaoShan District, Shanghai, China

P.-X. Lu, B.-P. Zhou (eds.), *Diagnostic Imaging of Emerging Infectious Diseases*, DOI 10.1007/978-94-017-7363-8_4

Influenza A (H1N1) virus is a single-stranded RNA virus which is categorized into the family of Orthomyxoviridae and the genus of influenza A virus. According to different antigenic characteristics of hemagglutinin (HA) and neuraminidase (NA) on the surface of virus, influenza A viruses can be classified into several subtypes. HA acts like a key to unlock the door of the host cells for the invading viruses, while NA contributes to destroy the cell receptor, which renders free transmission of the viruses in the body of the host. Both enzymes are highly variant, and the defined influenza A viruses, so far, are nominated based on different combinations of 16 types of HA (H1-16) and 9 types of NA (N1-9), such as H1N1, H1N2, H5N1, etc. Among all the subtypes, HA 1–3 can cause pandemic of human influenza, and H1N1, H1N2, and H3N2 are common and fixed virus phenotypes causing human influenza. In human history, three pandemic outbreaks of influenza occurred in 1918, 1957, and 1968. The prevailing influenza virus in the pandemic of 1918 was influenza A (H1N1) virus. Due to common existence of most influenza A (H1N1) virus strains in pigs, the WHO once nominated the influenza as swine influenza at the beginning of its outbreak.

Typical influenza A (H1N1) virus particle is enveloped and spherical whose diameter is 80–120 nm. Many raised glycoproteins (spikes) are radially arranged on the surface of lipid envelope. These spikes are 10–14 nm of erythrocyte hemagglutinin (HA), neuraminidase (NA), and matrix protein M2. Matrix protein (M1) is located inside the envelope of the virus. The nucleocapsids inside the viral particle are spirally symmetrical whose diameter is 10 nm. Such nucleocapsid contains RNA segments and polymerase proteins (PB1, PB2, PA). Certain enzymes (including glycoproteins hemagglutinin and neuraminidase) play a vital role in the entire life cycle of the virus.

The genome of influenza A (H1N1) virus is approximately 13.6 kb and is composed of eight unequally sized independent RNA segments which separately encode ten kinds of proteins: NA, HA, PA (RNA polymerase subunit PA), PB1 (RNA polymerase subunit PB1), PB2 (RNA polymerase subunit PB2), M (matrix protein, including M1 and M2, encoded by the same RNA segment), NS (nonstructural proteins, including N1 and N2, encoded by the same RNA segment), and NP (nucleoprotein). Influenza A (H1N1) virus is composed of three kinds of gene segments from swine influenza virus, avian influenza virus, and human influenza virus, which is a new mutant strain of swine influenza virus (SIV).

Influenza A (H1N1) virus is sensitive to heat and can be inactivated at 56 °C for 30 min. It is also sensitive to ultraviolet rays. But the UV-inactivated swine influenza virus can induce multiple reactivation of the virus. Swine influenza virus is an enveloped virus and is sensitive to ethanol, iodophor, iodine tincture, chloroform, acetone, and other organic solvents.

4.2 Epidemiology

4.2.1 Introduction

In human history, pandemic outbreak of influenza occurred for several times. It has a high incidence, and populations are generally susceptible to it. Its global infection rate is 5–20 % and its mortality rate is 0.1 %. Within the twentieth century, five pandemic outbreaks of influenza occurred in respective years of 1900, 1918, 1957, 1968, and 1977. The pandemic outbreak of influenza A (H1N1) in 1918 in Spain is the most serious, with about 500 million people being infected worldwide and a mortality rate of 2.5 %.

In the year of 2009, an outbreak of influenza firstly occurred in Mexico City. On 18 March 2009, a significant increase of influenza-like cases was reported by the local health agency. On 30 March 2009, a 10-year-old boy in California, USA, experienced fever, cough, and vomiting. Two days later, his conditions deteriorated and the boy was sent to an emergency clinic for treatment. One week later, the boy was cured. On 15 April 2009, the CDC of the USA received the clinical specimens of this boy and then defined a new swine-origin influenza virus, influenza A (H1N1) virus. The WHO and the CDC indicated that the influenza cases in Mexico and the USA were infected by the same strain of H1N1 subtype of swine influenza virus.

After large-scale prevalence of a new influenza virus in human being, persons with a history of infection or vaccination can acquire certain resistance to such virus. When such influenza virus prevails again, its transmissibility and infectivity can be greatly reduced. The influenza A (H1N1) virus has no exception. Its gradually weakened transmissibility and infectivity have changed influenza A (H1N1) into a seasonal flu, and the virus is currently the dominant strain of influenza. The prevalence of influenza A (H1N1) is currently characterized by decreased epidemic intensity and range as well as low incidence rate of severe cases, which have been shown by data from the prevalence of influenza A (H1N1) in 2013.

Influenza A (H1N1) is mainly transmitted via respiratory tract. Its transmission route is various and its transmission is rapid. The virus can survive and spread in densely populated places with poor ventilation and spread widely along with flow of population to cause prevalence of the disease.

4.2.2 Source of Infection

The main source of infection is patients with influenza A (H1N1) and infected asymptomatic person. Although the influenza A (H1N1) virus has been found in the body of pigs, no evidence has been found to prove that the animal is the source of infection.

The infective stage of the patient with influenza A (H1N1) is the period from 1 day prior to the onset of symptoms to day 7 after the onset or to 24 h after the absence of symptoms (the longer one should be defined as the infective stage). The infective stage may be longer in patients of young children, patients with compromised immunity, and patients critically/seriously ill. In some cases, the virus-carrying persons experience no onset of symptoms but can still infect others.

4.2.3 Route of Transmission

The virus is mainly transmitted via respiratory tract after inhalation of virus-containing droplets or aerosols from sneezing or coughing of infected persons. The virus can also be transmitted via direct or indirect contacts to the mucosa of oral cavity, nose, and eyes. Contacts to respiratory secretions, body fluids, and contaminated utensils of the patients can also cause infection. In addition, the fecal-oral transmission should be taken into account, because many patients experience diarrhea, and fecal detoxification is possible. Humans cannot be infected by influenza A (H1N1) virus via contacts to pork or intake of pork products.

On 12 April 2009, a Canadian farm worker feeding pigs experienced some influenza symptoms after traveling Mexico. He was then diagnosed with influenza A (H1N1). The pigs in this farm began to have influenza symptoms since 24 April 2009. On 2 May 2009, Canadian government officially announced that about 220 pigs in this farm were infected by influenza A (H1N1) virus. The swine infection indicated that human-infected swine influenza can be transmitted to pigs.

4.2.4 Susceptible Population

Populations are generally susceptible to influenza A (H1N1), with no specific immunity. Youngsters aged 9–19 years have a high incidence, with clustering cases in affected school within short period of time.

The following are the high-risk populations of influenza A (H1N1), and these populations are likely to develop into severe cases after onset of influenza symptoms. Therefore, these populations should be highly concerned.

- Pregnancies;
- Obese people (BMI ≥40 means a high risk, BMI between 30 and 39 means a risk factor);
- Children under the age of 5 years (young children patients aged under 2 years are more likely to develop serious complications);
- Elderly people >65 years old;
- The patients with the following underlying diseases or conditions: chronic respiratory disease, cardiovascular disease (except hypertension), kidney disease, liver disease, hematological disease, neurological and neuromuscular disease, metabolic and endocrine system disease, and immune suppression (including those with compromised immunity due to use of immunosuppressor or HIV infection); and the patients aged under 19 years with long-term intake of aspirin.

The abovementioned populations with influenza-like symptoms should receive viral nucleic acid test for influenza A (H1N1) and other necessary examinations as early as possible.

4.3 Pathogenesis and Pathological Changes

4.3.1 Pathogenesis

The influenza A (H1N1) virus responsible for the pandemic of influenza in Mexico and southwestern America is a subtype of influenza A virus that is categorized into the family of Orthomyxoviridae. Influenza A (H1N1) is a zoonotic respiratory disease caused by influenza A (H1N1) virus. As a new mutate of influenza virus, influenza A (H1N1) virus differs from those causing human seasonal H1N1 influenza for years in many aspects, such as genetic and antigenic properties. Evolutionary analysis has revealed that the virus is composed of gene segments from three different influenza viruses: avian influenza virus, swine influenza virus, and human influenza virus. The eight different gene segments are originated from different strains of influenza virus, showing genetic properties of NA and M segments of Asian swine influenza virus, PB2, PB1, PA, HA, NP, and NS segments of North American triple reassortant swine H1 influenza. Humans are generally susceptible to influenza A (H1N1) that can spread from human to human. In vitro experiments have demonstrated that influenza A (H1N1) virus cannot only affect respiratory epithelial cells but also infect dendritic cells (DC) and mononuclear macrophages (MC). The pathogenesis of influenza A (H1N1) may involve of the virus itself, the host immune system, and the interaction between them.

Influenza A (H1N1) can be complicated by multiple organ dysfunction (MODS). Its mechanism is as the following: (1) the influenza A (H1N1) virus can invade the lungs to cause severe pulmonary inflammation. And in some cases, the condition may rapidly progress into acute respiratory distress syndrome (ARDS). (2) The patients with influenza A (H1N1) sustain different degrees of hypoxemia, which enhances anaerobic metabolism of tissue cells and reduces the production of ATP and cAMP. Therefore, the energy metabolism in organs is disturbed. Hypoxia can also lead to decreased cardiac output, insufficient circulating blood volume and reduced organ or tissue perfusion. (3) Secondary infection may occur.

4.3.2 Pathological Changes

The influenza A (H1N1) virus can cause acute respiratory infectious disease, which may progress into interstitial pneumonia in some severe cases, with a mortality rate of about 0.1–0.2 %. The pathological changes of severe influenza A (H1N1) mainly include severe pulmonary disease, multiple organ dysfunction, and secondary infection. The main causes of death include (1) progressive respiratory failure induced by diffuse alveolar lesion; (2) the complication of multiple organ dysfunction including the liver, kidney, and heart; and (3) secondary infection.

4.3.2.1 Respiratory System

Observation by Naked Eyes

The pathological changes noticeable by naked eyes include: increased volume of both lungs with increased weight but decreased air content, consolidation of both lungs, and dark reddish lungs with fibrinous exudates on their surfaces.

Observation by Light Microscopy

Under a light microscope, diffuse alveolar lesion can be observed at both lungs, which is mainly acute diffuse exudates with presence of pulmonary tissue necrosis (Fig. 4.1). The alveolar cavity is demonstrated with edema and/or fibrinous and inflammatory exudates (Fig. 4.2), with formation of pulmonary hyaline membrane. In some alveolar cavities, hemorrhages can be observed, with hyperplasia of type II alveolar epithelial cells. Neither megakaryocytes nor inclusions in nucleus or cytoplasm can be observed. Some alveolar septa are demonstrated to be slightly widened, with vascular dilatation, congestion, and necrosis (Fig. 4.3), as well as thrombus in some cases. Pulmonary interstitial fibrosis is present.

Observation by Electron Microscopy

Virus particles can be observed both within and out of the infected cells in alveolar cavity of pulmonary tissue. The virus is round or oval in shape with a diameter of averagely about 88 nm, and some viruses are surrounded by spikelike structure in a length of about 12 nm.

4.3.2.2 Other Major Systems

Cardiovascular System

The heart is slightly heavier. Under a light microscope, myocardial cells are degenerated, with myocardial breakage, myocardial interstitial edema, infiltration of small quantity or no inflammatory cells, and degeneration of atrial ganglion cells (Figs. 4.4, 4.5, and 4.6).

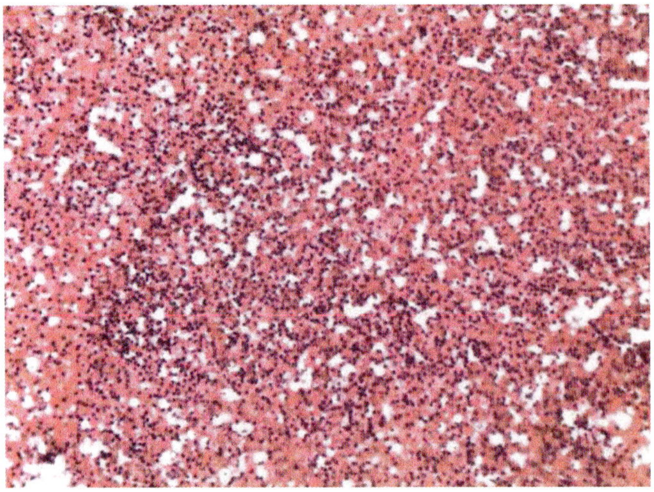

Fig. 4.1 Necrosis of pulmonary tissue and infiltration of inflammatory cells H&E ×100

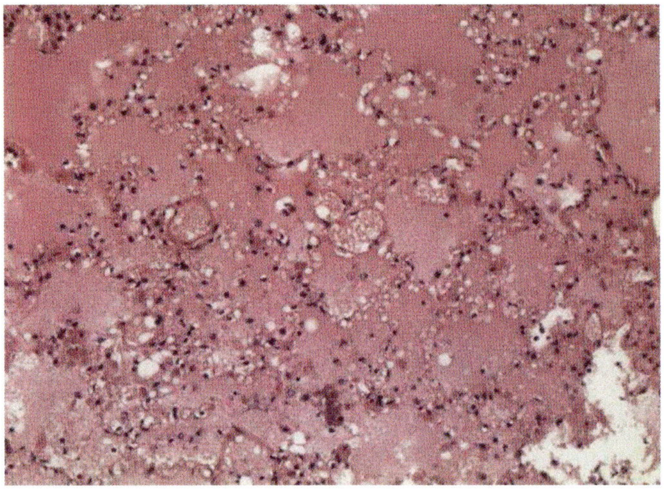

Fig. 4.2 Pulmonary edema, with the alveolar cavity filled by homogeneous acidophilic exudates H&E ×100

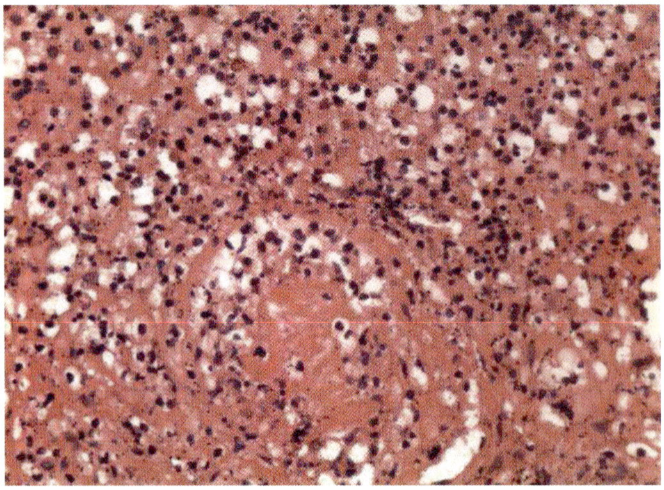

Fig. 4.3 Necrosis of pulmonary vascular wall and infiltration of inflammatory cells H&E ×200

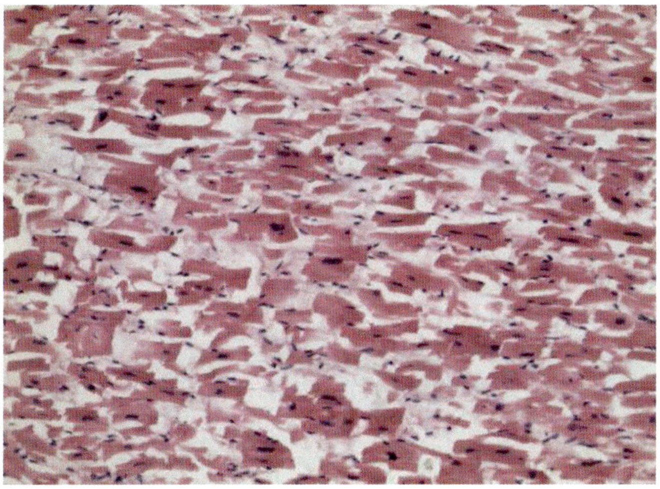

Fig. 4.4 Myocardial breakage, degeneration of myocardial cells, and myocardial interstitial edema H&E ×400

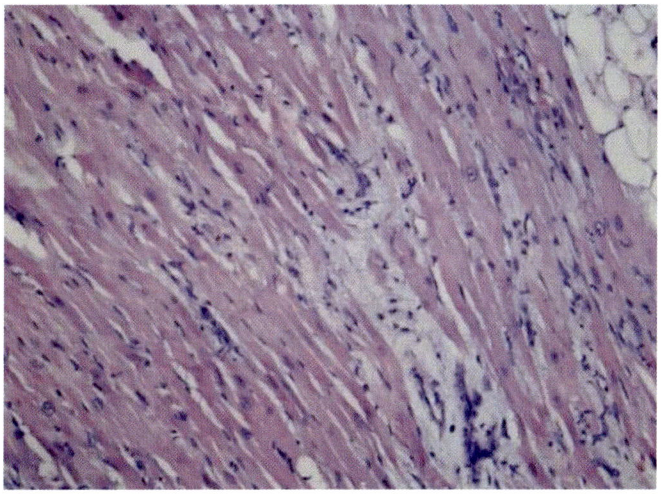

Fig. 4.5 Infiltration of inflammatory cells at the myocardial tissue space H&E ×200

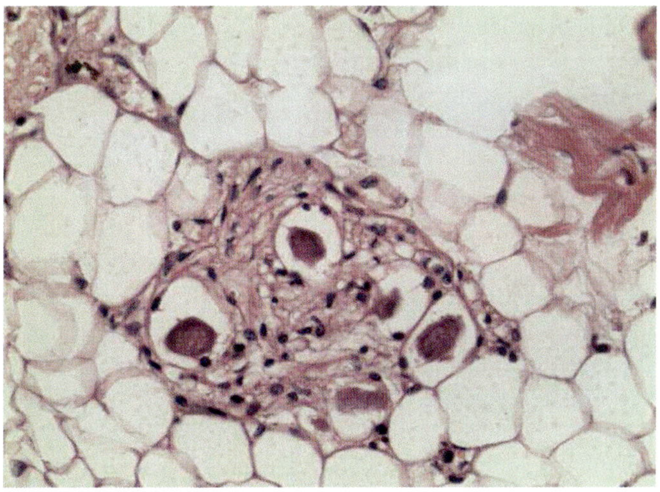

Fig. 4.6 Degeneration of atrial ganglion cell H&E ×200

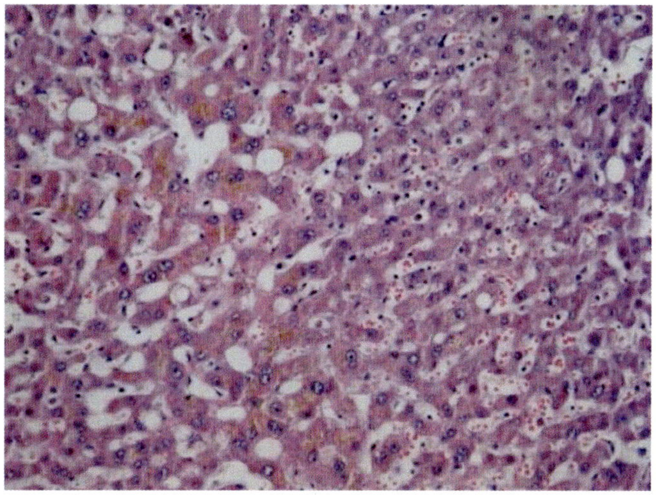

Fig. 4.7 Bullous fatty degeneration of hepatocytes, cholestatic hepatocytes, and dilated hepatic sinus H&E ×200

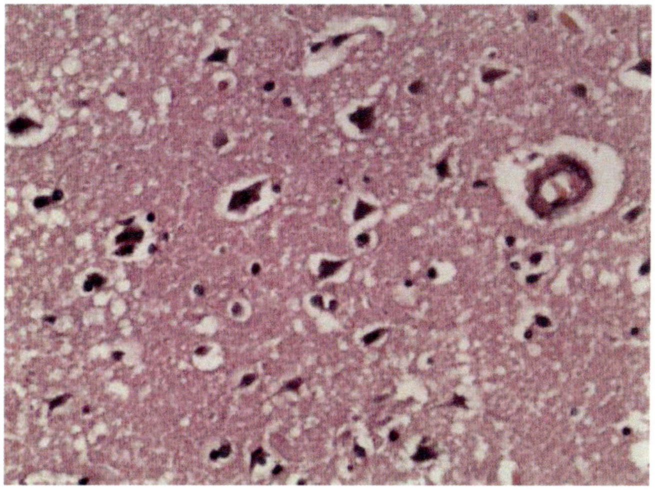

Fig. 4.8 Degeneration of brain nerve cells H&E ×400

Digestive System

The liver can be observed with congestion, focal hepatocytic swelling and fatty degeneration, and infiltration of small quantity mononuclear cells at the portal area. Erythrocytophagy can be observed (Fig. 4.7).

Urinary System

The kidney can be observed with congestion. Under a light microscope examination, glomerular congestion is observed, with edema of renal tubular epithelial cells but no microthrombus and renal tubular necrosis.

Central Nervous System

The pathological changes include cerebral edema and congestion, with visible hemorrhagic focus, focal liquefactive necrosis at the capsule, and neuronal degeneration (Fig. 4.8).

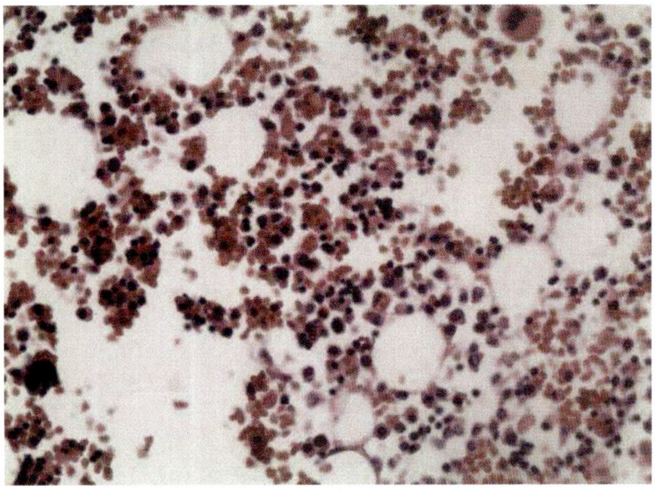

Fig. 4.9 Prominent hemophagocytic phenomenon at bone marrow H&E ×200

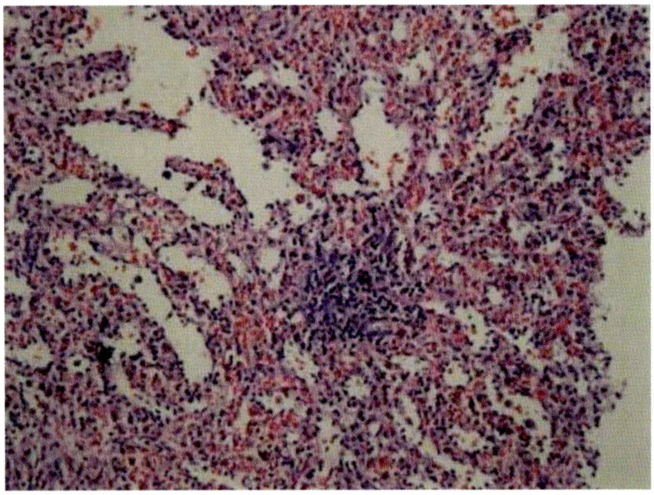

Fig. 4.10 Dilation and congestion of splenic sinus, atrophy of splenic corpuscle, and decreased lymphocytes H&E ×200

Lymphoid Hematopoietic System

Hemophagocytic phenomenon can be observed at some lymph nodes and bone marrow (Fig. 4.9). The spleen can be observed with reduced lymphocytes, histiocytosis, and hemophagocytic phenomenon (Fig. 4.10).

4.3.2.3 Secondary Infection

The patients with influenza A (H1N1) can develop secondary bacterial and fungal infections. The pathogenic bacteria are mainly gram-positive coccus.

4.3.2.4 Molecular Pathology

The nucleoprotein antigen of influenza A (HIN1) virus is located at the nucleus and cytoplasm of infected cells, including epithelial cells at airway, submucosal glands of airway, and detached and lining epithelial cells at alveolus. In addition, the antigen can also be found at the hyaline membrane and rarely vascular endothelial cells. Double labeling has revealed that the target cell of viral infection is pulmonary epithelial cells, predominantly type II alveolar epithelial cells (co-labeled with cytokeratin) and occasionally macrophages.

No viral antigen of influenza A (H1N1) virus is immunohistochemically detected in nonrespiratory tissue. By RT-PCR, the nonrespiratory tissue is also detected negative for influenza A (H1N1) virus.

4.4 Clinical Symptoms, Signs, and Laboratory Tests

Influenza A (H1N1) is a self-limited respiratory disease. Its clinical manifestations resemble to those of seasonal influenza, being mild in most patients. However, the patients from high-risk populations are more likely to develop into severe cases and even death.

4.4.1 Incubation Period

The incubation period of influenza A (H1N1) generally lasts for 1–7 days, mostly 1–3 days, which is longer than that of common influenza and avian influenza.

4.4.2 Clinical Symptoms and Signs

The patient usually experiences influenza-like symptoms, including fever (axillary temperature ≥37.5 °C), sore throat, runny nose, nasal congestion, cough, expectoration, headache, general soreness, and fatigue. In some cases, the patients experience vomiting and/or diarrhea. In rare cases, the patients only experience mild upper respiratory symptoms with no occurrence of fever.

The signs mainly include pharyngeal congestion and swollen tonsils.

4.4.3 Laboratory Tests

4.4.3.1 Peripheral Blood Test

Total WBC count is commonly within or lower than normal range. In some severe pediatric cases, the total WBC count may increase. The common cases commonly show normal or lower WBC count, while the severe cases show normal or increased peripheral WBC count. The increase of WBC count in severe cases may be related to complicated infections. It should be paid close attention that, compared to common cases, the severe cases have obviously decreased percentage and absolute count of peripheral blood lymphocytes. Peripheral blood lymphocyte count <800 cells/ml is a high-risk factor for patient with influenza A (H1N1) to develop respiratory failure. The decrease of both percentage and absolute count of peripheral lymphocytes is an indicator for early prediction.

4.4.3.2 Blood Biochemistry

Blood Biochemistry

The blood biochemistry for liver function is commonly normal in most patients. Only in rare cases, the levels of aspartate aminotransferase (AST), alanine aminotransferase (ALT), and lactate dehydrogenase (LDH) can be tested with increase.

Myocardial enzyme of creatine kinase (CK) exists in the cytoplasm and mitochondria of skeletal muscle, heart, brain, and other tissues, which is an important kinase directly related to intracellular energy transformation, muscle contraction, and ATP regeneration. Its level increases in the cases with myocardial damage.

The blood glucose level in both critical cases and death cases is higher than that in severe cases, which may be related to responses of host to stress.

Electrolyte

In some cases, hypokalemia or hypocalcemia occurs. Relevant studies have demonstrated that hypocalcemia is an important indicator predicting poor prognosis of influenza A (H1N1).

4.4.3.3 Assay for Cellular Immunity

The infection of influenza A (H1N1) virus can cause allergic reaction. In critical cases, the serum cytokine significantly increases, with increased permeability of pulmonary and cerebral vascular vessels, to cause respiratory failure and pulmonary edema. Therefore, the test for serum cytokines plays an important role in assessing conditions of influenza A (H1N1) and guiding clinical prevention and treatment.

4.4.3.4 Etiological Examination

Test for Viral Nucleic Acid

The test for viral nucleic acid is currently the main diagnostic examination for influenza A (H1N1). The respiratory specimens, including throat swabs, nasal swabs, nasopharyngeal or tracheal extracts, and sputum, are tested by using RT-PCR (more favorably real-time RT-PCR). The cases of influenza A (H1N1) show positive results.

Virus Isolation

In the cases of influenza A (H1N1), the pathogenic virus can be isolated from respiratory specimens. In the cases with influenza A (H1N1) complicated by viral pneumonia, the virus can also be isolated from the lung tissue.

Serum Antibody Test

In the cases of influenza A (H1N1), dynamic tests of double sera specimens show at least four times increase of the neutralizing antibody specific to influenza A (H1N1) virus. The result may facilitate to define the diagnosis and the retrospective diagnosis.

4.5 Clinical Diagnosis

The patients with influenza A (H1N1) experience different degrees of fever, cough, expectoration, chest distress, shortness of breath, fatigue, headache, and myalgia, all of which are collectively referred to as the flulike symptoms. Although the influenza A (H1N1) virus is a new mutant of influenza virus, the symptoms of infected patients can be hardly distinguished from infections of respiratory syncytial virus, parainfluenza virus, rhinovirus, adenovirus, *Coronavirus*, and *Legionella pneumophila*. Therefore, the diagnosis cannot be defined based only on the symptoms, but needs to combine findings of specific laboratory tests, such as serological test, viral nucleic acid test, and pathogen isolation.

4.5.1 Suspected Cases

The case with the following ONE condition can be diagnosed as a suspected case:

1. The patient has a history of close contact to patient suspectively or definitively diagnosed with influenza A (H1N1) at its infectious stage within 7 days prior to the onset of influenza-like symptoms. Close contact refers to attending to patients with influenza A (H1N1) in its infectious stage with no effective protection; living together with the patient and exposure to the same environment with the patient; and direct contact to the airway secretions, body fluids, and other contaminated utensils from the patient.
2. The patient has a history of visiting the country or region with epidemic of influenza A (H1N1) (continuous spread of virus from person to person and community-based prevalence and outbreak) within 7 days prior to the onset of influenza-like symptoms.
3. The patient experiences influenza-like symptoms and shows positive to test for influenza A (H1N1) virus, but infection of previous influenza virus subtypes has not been further excluded.

The cases with ONE of the above three conditions should be etiologically tested for influenza A (H1N1), if possible.

4.5.2 Clinically Diagnosed Cases

The clinical diagnosis should be made based only on the following condition. During the same epidemic event of influenza A (H1N1), the patient with influenza-like symptoms has not definitively diagnosed by laboratory test but has been excluded from other diseases with influenza-like clinical manifestations. Such patients can be clinically diagnosed as influenza A (H1N1).

Outbreak of influenza A (H1N1) refers to abnormally increased occurrence of influenza-like disease in one region or unit within a short period of time, and the disease is defined to be influenza A (H1N1) by laboratory tests.

If possible, the clinically diagnosed patients should receive etiological examination.

4.5.3 Definitively Diagnosed Cases

The cases with influenza-like symptoms and at least ONE of the following laboratory findings can be definitively diagnosed as influenza A (H1N1).

1. The viral nucleic acid of influenza A (H1N1) virus is tested positive by real-time RT-PCR or RT-PCR.
2. The serum level of neutralizing antibody specific to influenza A (H1N1) is tested with at least four times increase.
3. The influenza A (H1N1) virus is isolated.

4.5.4 Diagnosis of Severe and Critical Cases

4.5.4.1 Severe Cases

The severe cases can be defined based on ONE of the following conditions.

1. Persistent fever lasting from more than 3 days, accompanied by severe cough, purulent and/or bloody sputum, or chest pain
2. Rapid respiratory rate, dyspnea, cyanotic lips
3. Consciousness changes, including delayed response, drowsiness, restlessness, and convulsions
4. Severe vomiting and diarrhea, dehydration
5. Radiological findings of pneumonia-like signs
6. Rapid increases of myocardial enzyme levels, such as creatine kinase (CK), creatine kinase M isoenzyme (CK-MB), etc.
7. Obviously aggravated previous underlying disease

4.5.4.2 Critical Cases

The critical cases can be defined based on ONE of the following conditions:

1. Respiratory failure
2. Septic and toxic shock
3. Multiple organ dysfunction
4. Other severe clinical conditions in need of monitoring treatment

4.6 Selection of Radiological Modalities

Influenza A (H1N1) is commonly complicated by diseases of respiratory and central nervous system. The selection of radiological modalities is mainly based on the two systems.

4.6.1 Radiology of the Respiratory System

4.6.1.1 Chest X-Ray

The suspected cases should receive upright posterior-anterior chest X-ray. For the severe cases of inability going to the radiology department, a bedside chest X-ray can be performed to assess the condition at a posture of sitting or lying. If possible, a special stand for upright chest X-ray or seated chest X-ray can be used. The children patients capable of standing should receive upright chest X-ray. For patients unable of standing due to severe conditions, seated chest X-ray is preferred.

Indications for Bedside Radiological Examination

The indications for bedside radiological examination are as the following:

1. Persistent fever lasting for at least 3 days
2. Cough with/without expectoration
3. Positive finding in viral nucleic acid test for influenza A (H1N1)
4. Signs of pulmonary inflammation by the first radiological examination

When a patient with suspected diagnosis of influenza A (H1N1) experiences above conditions 1, 2, and 4, a bedside radiological examination should be performed. If a patient with suspected diagnosis of influenza A (H1N1) experienced the above condition 3, the bedside radiological examination is NOT necessary.

Protection Principles During Bedside Radiological Examination

The patients, radiological technicians, and other healthcare workers should be protected against radiohazards. Data revealed that the average radiation dose at the chest surface of the patient by a bedside X-ray machine is 1.45 mGy/time, and its maximum dose is 3.39 mGy/time. The radiation dose by other digital chest X-ray machines is about (0.36 ± 0.05)

mGy/time. The radiation dose of bedside X-ray machine is significantly different from that of other digital chest X-ray machine.

Protective Measures Against Cross-Infection

Before entering into the isolation ward, the radiological technicians should receive training for knowledge and skills about disinfection and isolation. The procedures should be constantly improved.

The patients with influenza A (H1N1) experience rapid changes of lung lesions. Therefore, reexamination of chest X-ray within a short period of time facilitates to assess the condition. During the convalescent stage, chest X-ray should be regularly performed to assess the absorption of lesions and the residual lesions.

4.6.1.2 Chest CT Scan

In recent years, based on the application of new detectors and new algorithm for image reconstruction, the low-dose CT scan can be routinely performed. CT scans are favorable in detecting chest lesions and their characteristics, which can be applied for patients whose diagnosis cannot be defined by chest X-ray. CT scan can display occult lesions posterior to the heart shadow and at the posterior costophrenic angle, which can effectively avoid misdiagnosis and increase the detection rate of the lesions.

4.6.2 Radiology for the Central Nervous System

MRI has the absolute advantage in displaying lesions at the central nervous system due to its capabilities in multiparameter imaging, 3D imaging, and functional imaging. Therefore, MRI is the choice of radiological modalities for the examination of central nervous system. CT scan is applied only when MRI is inapplicable.

Influenza A (H1N1) may be complicated by aseptic meningitis, encephalitis, and acute necrotizing encephalopathy. MRI should be performed with conventional plain imaging and contrast imaging. FLAIR and DWI sequences should be additionally performed during contrast imaging to more favorably display meningeal lesions.

When MRI is performed for young children, some measures should be used to keep him/her warm and limit his/her movement. In addition, due to the loud noise generated during MRI, a pair of soundproof earplugs should be plugged into the ears of pediatric patient so as to avoid awakening the child and to prevent hearing damage. For the pediatric patient with poor compliance, oral/enema use of chloral hydrate can be administered to calm down the child prior to MRI.

4.7 Radiological Demonstration

4.7.1 Radiological Demonstrations of the Respiratory System

Influenza A (H1N1) is a new respiratory infectious disease. And respiratory complications, such as pneumonia and pulmonary edema, are important and common. Death may occur in critical cases due to respiratory failure.

For the patients with influenza A (H1N1), abnormalities displayed by chest radiological examinations are always in inpatients and severely ill patients receiving intensive care. The common complications mainly include pneumonia, pleural effusion, pulmonary edema, pneumothorax, and mediastinal emphysema.

4.7.1.1 Pneumonia

Influenza A (H1N1) is commonly complicated by pneumonia, with multiple lesions. Its radiological demonstrations share some commonalities with common pneumonia, such as exudative lesions, lung consolidation, pulmonary edema, and pleural effusion. Meanwhile, pneumonia complicating influenza A (H1N1) is characterized by commonly bilateral lesions as well as rapid change and exacerbation of the lesions and its range.

Radiological Demonstrations

The most common radiological demonstrations are ground-glass opacities and consolidation opacities at lungs. The two types of opacities may be separately or jointly present, commonly with reticular and nodular opacities. In rare cases, the lesions are demonstrated as consolidation opacities at pulmonary segments or lobes with air bronchogram, accompanied by or no segmental atelectasis. The lesions are commonly found at bilateral lower lung fields, which are focal, multiple, or diffusely distributed. Intrapulmonary nodular opacities, interlobular septal thickening, peribronchial patchy opacities, and pleural effusion are rarely found radiological signs (Fig. 4.11).

CT Scan Demonstrations

1. The common chest CT scan demonstrations are unilateral or bilateral ground-glass opacities, with or without singular consolidation or multiple fused consolidations.
2. The intrapulmonary lesions have lobular, segmental, or lobar distribution and often manifest as light thin small flaky or multiple patchy integrated lesions. By HRCT, the ground-glass opacities are commonly distributed at the peribronchovascular or subpleural region. The lesions are mostly located at both lower lung lobes or multiple lobes and segments of both lungs. In severe cases, the

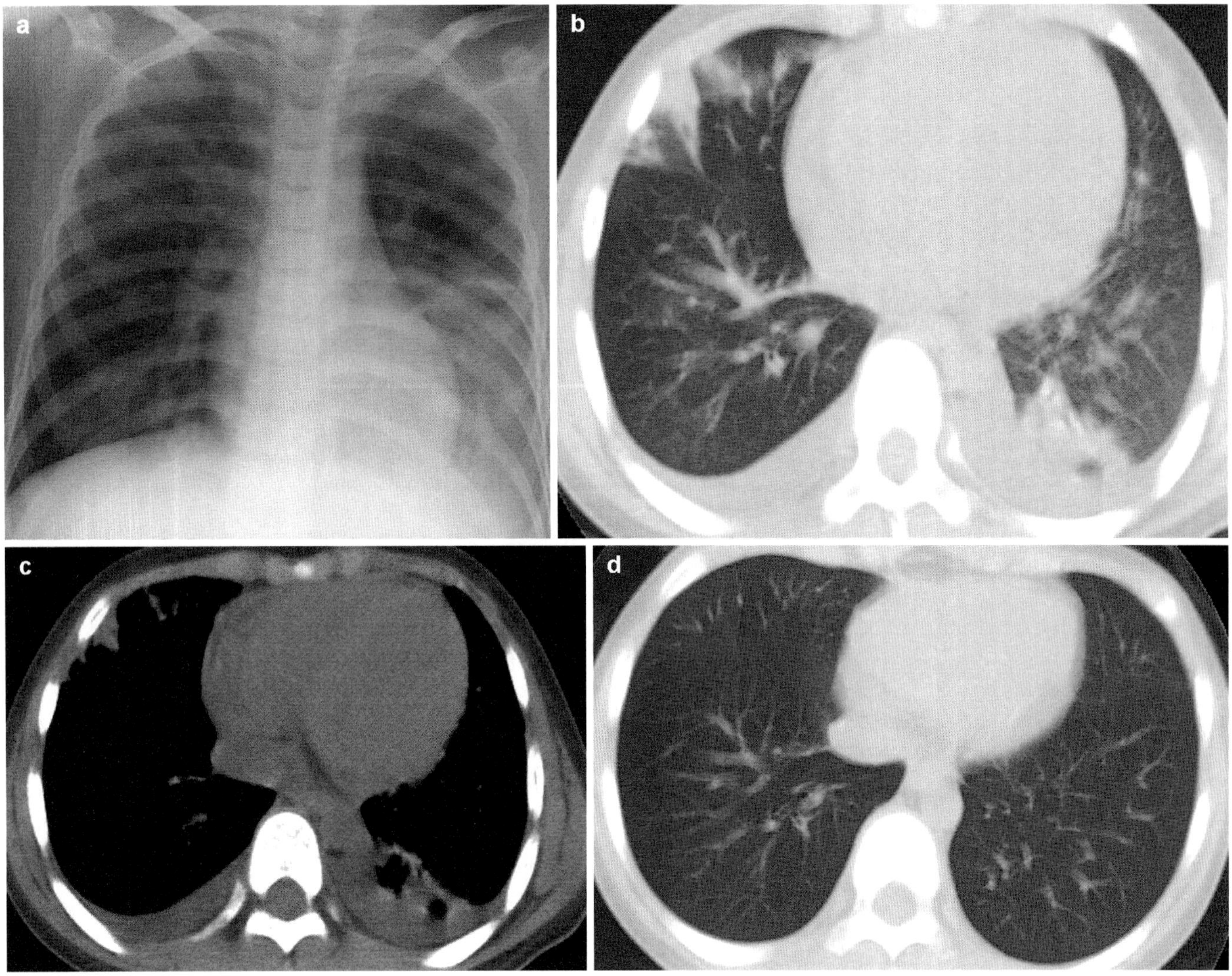

Fig. 4.11 (**a–d**) A boy aged 6 years with a diagnosis of influenza A (H1N1) complicated by pneumonia. (**a**) At d 4 since onset, chest X-ray showed large high-density opacities at the left lower lung field, poorly defined left diaphragmatic surface and absence of left costophrenic angle, and patchy ground-glass opacities at the right lower lung field. (**b**, **c**) At d 5 since onset, plain CT scan (**b** lung window; **c** mediastinal window) displayed flaky consolidation opacities at the basal segment lateroposterior to the left lower lung lobe and subpleural patchy ground-glass opacities at the right middle lung lobe and small quantities of pleural effusion at both lungs. (**d**) At d 16 since onset (1 day before discharge), reexamination by CT scan demonstrated absorption of lesions at both lungs

lesions are always shown as multifocal and integrated consolidation at both lungs with air bronchogram. Otherwise, the severe cases can be demonstrated with atelectasis.

3. The lung lesions can be completely absorbed within a short period of time, generally within 7–15 days. The absorption of lesions commonly lags behind the improvement of clinical conditions. At the early stage of the disease, ground-glass opacities may be integrated as multiple scattering consolidation opacities. Some of the consolidations are not integrated at the onset, but will be integrated within the following several days. The multiple scattering patchy opacities can change into light thin small flaky opacities and gradually disappear.
4. In some cases, the above lesions are accompanied by small quantity of pleural effusion and mediastinal lymphadenectasis (Fig. 4.12).

Typology of Radiological Demonstrations

Pneumonia demonstrated as flaky opacities confined within the lungs is defined as mild. That demonstrated as intrapulmonary flaky opacities with more than two lung lobes involved are defined as moderate. And that demonstrated as intrapulmonary lesions with at least three lung lobes involved are defined as severe. For the patients with mild to moderate pneumonia, pulmonary inflammation can be gradually absorbed after the use of effective therapy. The radiological demonstrations are not necessarily

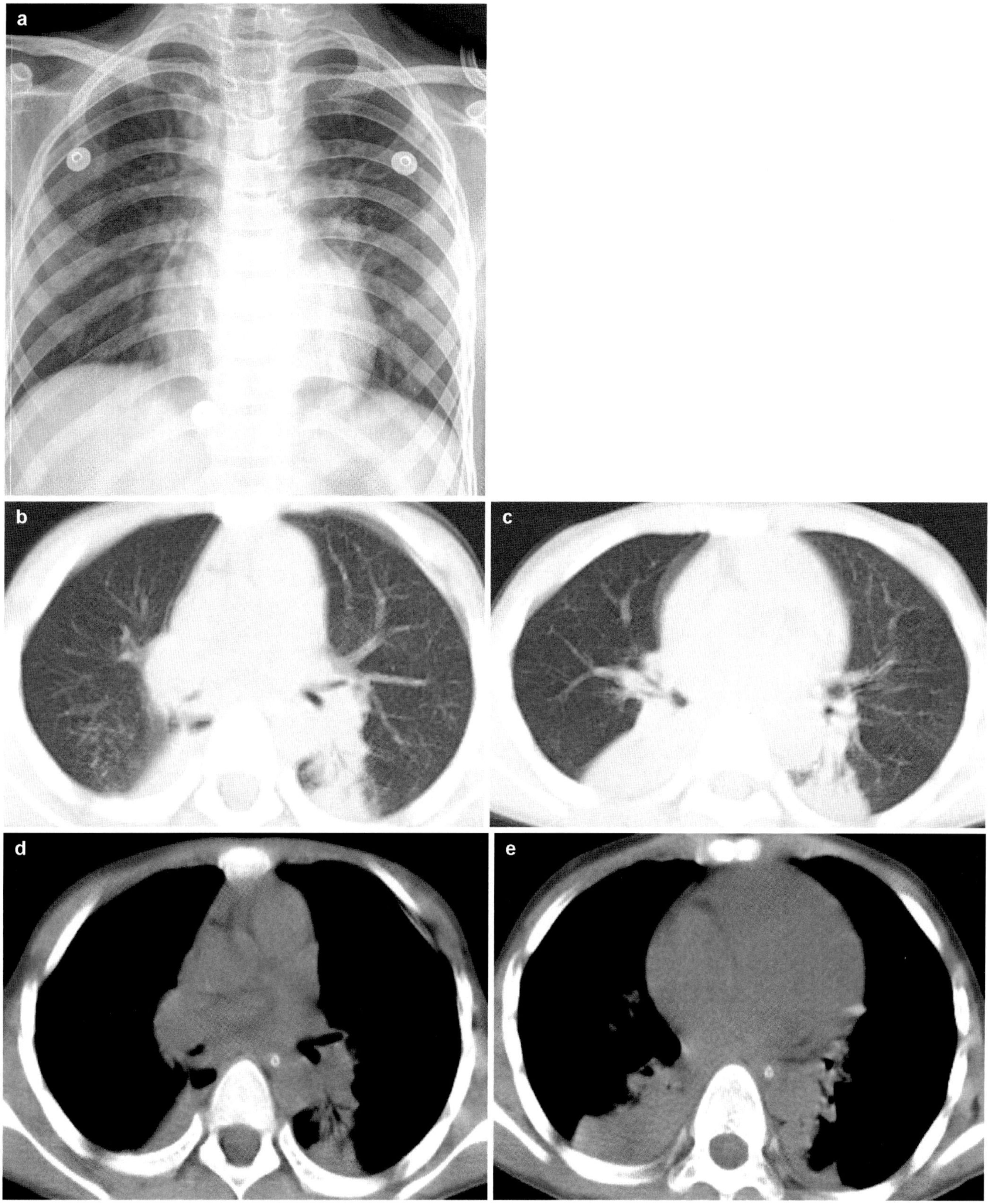

Fig. 4.12 A boy aged 9 years with influenza A (H1N1) complicated by pneumonia. (**a**) At d 3 since onset, chest X-ray showed thickened markings at both lungs and no consolidation opacities at bilateral lung fields. (**b–e**) At d 5 since onset, chest CT scan (**b**, **c**: lung window; **d**, **e**: mediastinal window) showed flaky high-density opacities at the dorsal and lateroposterior basal segments of both lower lung lobes, air bronchogram at the dorsal segment of left lower lung lobe, slightly increased transparency of the right middle lung lobe, and segmental atelectasis at the right lower lung lobe. (**f**) At d 7 since onset, chest X-ray displayed high-density flaky opacities at the middle and inner zone of the right middle and lower lung fields, partial atelectasis at the right lower lung lobe, and basic absorption of inflammation lesions at the left lung

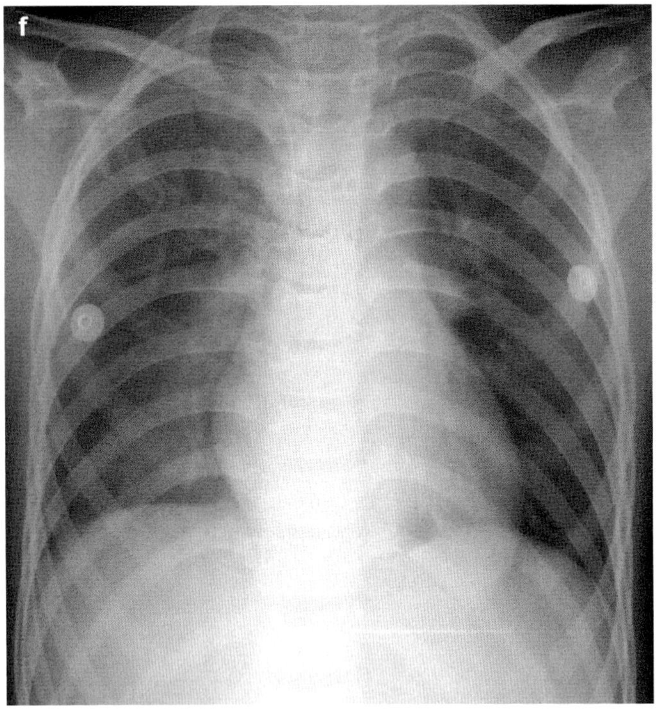

Fig. 4.12 (continued)

correspondent to the clinical symptoms. For severe pediatric cases, radiological examination should be performed to monitor the changes of pneumonia lesions. For the pediatric patients and the patients with severe lung lesions, radiological examination should be performed to assess the short-term absorption of lesions, any delayed absorption, and residual lesions in order to provide the basis for clinical treatment.

The Relationship Between Influenza A (H1N1)/ Complicated by Pneumonia and Viral Load

According to a study of viral load in 20 patients with influenza A (H1N1) whose chest CT scans were normal, the minimum viral load is 2.4 copies/ml, while the maximum viral load is 5.5 copies/ml, with a mean of 4.2 copies/ml. In this study, the dynamic viral load was also measured in 21 patients with influenza A (H1N1) whose chest CT scans demonstrated pneumonia. The average viral load is 7.7 copies/ml. The viral load has statistical difference ($P < 0.05$) between the group without pneumonia and the group with pneumonia. The findings primarily indicated that pneumonia does not occur to complicate influenza A (H1N1) in the cases with a viral load lower than 5.5 copies/ml (Fig. 4.13).

The same study also demonstrated that the severity of pneumonia complicating influenza A (H1N1), with an indicator of CT semiquantitative score, is not significantly related to the viral load. In general, the level of viral load indicates the degree of infection. However, by dynamic chest CT scoring (Radiology, 2003) in 21 cases of influenza A (H1N1) complicated by pneumonia and their viral load measures, it has been found that the severity (chest CT semiquantitative score) of pneumonia complicating influenza A (H1N1) is not related to the viral load, because no statistically significant difference was found ($P > 0.05$). That is to say, a high level of viral load does not necessarily indicate severe lesions of pneumonia.

Influenza A (H1N1) Complicated by Pneumonia in Perinatal Women

1. Location of lesions: commonly at the middle (lingular segment) and lower lobes of both lungs.
2. Morphology of lesions: mostly large or small flaky opacities.
3. Density of lesions: mainly high-density consolidation opacities, light thin opacities, or ground-glass opacities.
4. The lesions are mostly accompanied by unilateral/bilateral pleurisy or pleural effusion or other changes. The pathomechanism underlying pleurisy remains unknown, which may be related to hypoalbuminemia, direct effects of viruses, or endocrine factors.
5. After clinical treatment, the ground-glass opacities at the lungs can be completely absorbed within a short period of time; large high-density consolidation opacities can be obviously absorbed; the residual lesions in the advanced stage can be absorbed slowly (Fig. 4.14).

4.7.1.2 Pleural Effusion

It may develop due to pulmonary edema or pneumonia with the pleura involved. In severe pediatric cases of influenza A (H1N1), the incidence of pneumonia complicated by pleural effusion is relatively higher. By CT scan, the lesions are mostly located at the peripheral lung with the subpleura involved and pleurisy may be demonstrated.

4.7.1.3 Pneumothorax, Mediastinal Emphysema

Pneumothorax and mediastinal emphysema may occur in patients with underlying asthma, and their occurrence is possibly a result of increased intrapulmonary pressure due to shortness of breath caused by influenza A (H1N1) virus. The risk of developing pneumothorax and mediastinal emphysema in severe cases receiving intensive care can be increased due to mechanical ventilation (Figs. 4.15 and 4.16).

4.7.1.4 Mediastinal and Axillary Lymphadenectasis

As a result of inflammatory responses, mediastinal and axillary lymphadenectasis occurs, with no necrosis and integration.

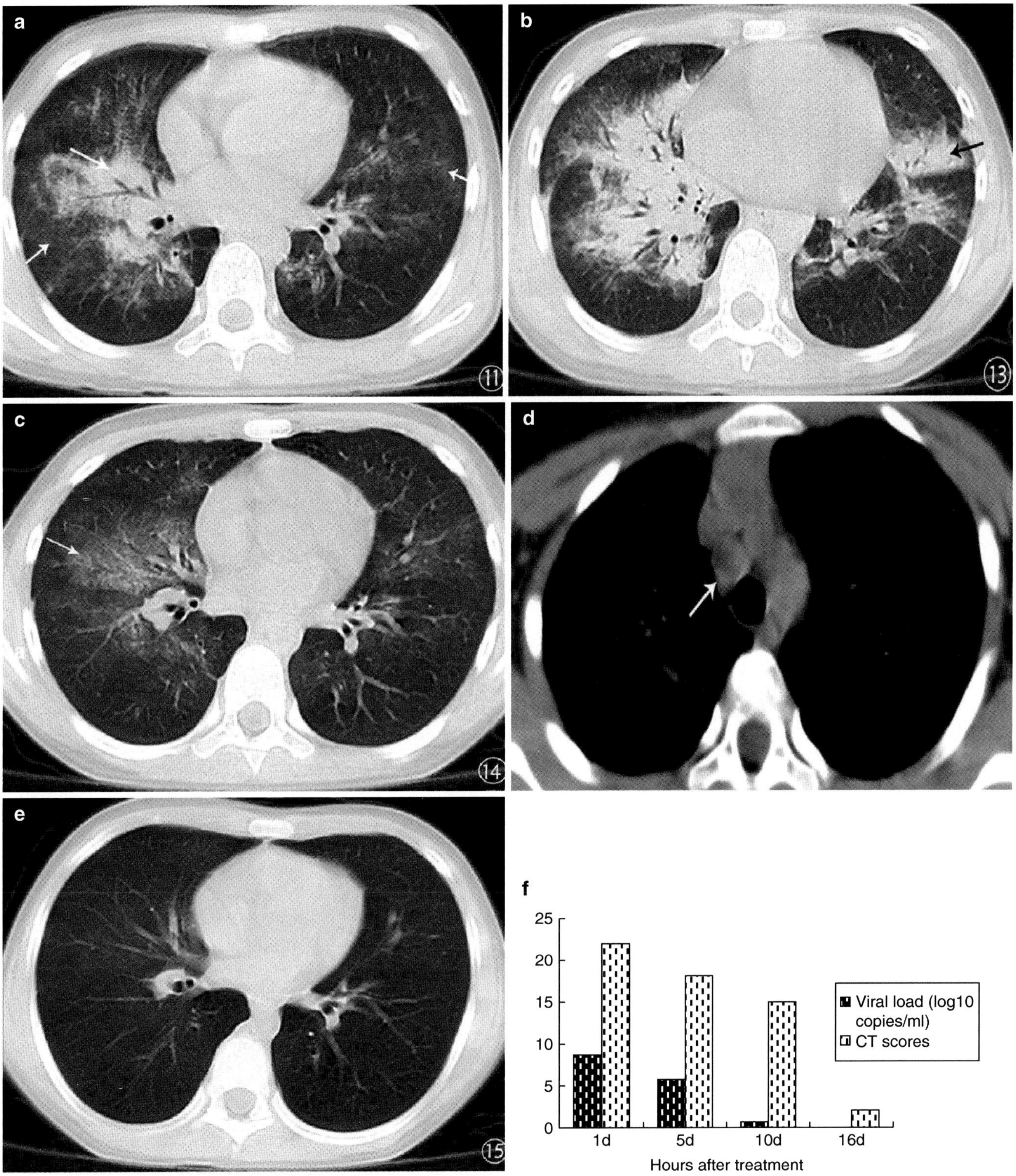

Fig. 4.13 (**a–f**) *A boy aged* 11 years with influenza A (H1N1) complicated by pneumonia. (**a**) At d 4 since onset, chest CT showed scattering ground-glass opacities (*short arrow*) at both lungs, integration of some lesions into flaky consolidation opacities at the right hilum (*long arrow*) with air bronchogram. (**b**) The same CT scan at d 4 also displayed a swollen lymph node (*white arrow*) anterior to the trachea and posterior to the superior vena cava, with uneven density. (**c**) At d 6 since onset, CT scan showed obviously more integrated lesions at both lungs and new patchy integrated lesions at the lingular lobe (*black arrow*) and lower lobe of left lung. (**d**) At d 8 since onset, CT scan demonstrated the obviously smaller range with lesions at both lungs, obviously decreased density of the lesions as ground-glass opacity (*white arrow*). (**e**) At d 14 since onset, CT scan displayed absorption of lesions at both lungs. (**f**) Dynamic changes CT scoring along with changes of the viral load

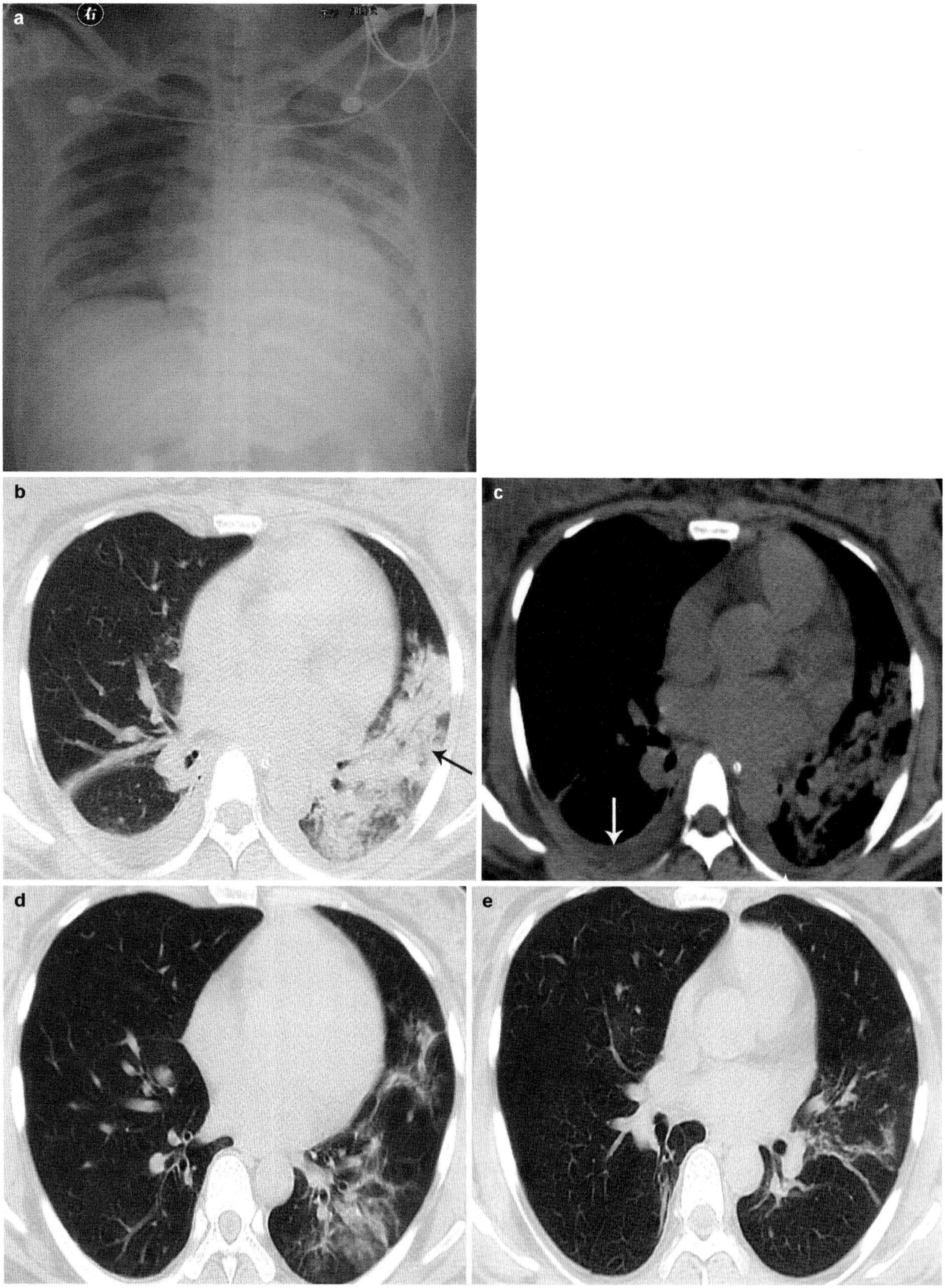

Fig. 4.14 (**a–e**) A pregnant woman aged 26 years with influenza A (H1N1) complicated by pneumonia. (**a**) At d 3 since onset, bedside chest X-ray showed large blurry opacities at left lung, small flaky opacities at the right lower lung near cardiac border, and poorly defined bilateral inferior costophrenic angles. (**b**) At d 5 since onset, the lung window of chest CT displayed large dense consolidation opacities (*black arrow*) at the lingular and lower lobe of left lung, with air bronchogram. (**c**) The same chest CT scan at d 5 demonstrated small quantities of liquid (*white arrow*) in bilateral pleural cavities and right oblique fissure pleura by the mediastinal window. (**d**) At d 7 since onset, chest CT showed decreased density of lesions at the lingular and lower lobes of left lung, and some lesions as ground-glass opacities. (**e**) At d 9 since onset, CT scan displayed obviously smaller range of the lesions and rare ground-glass opacities and cord-like opacities

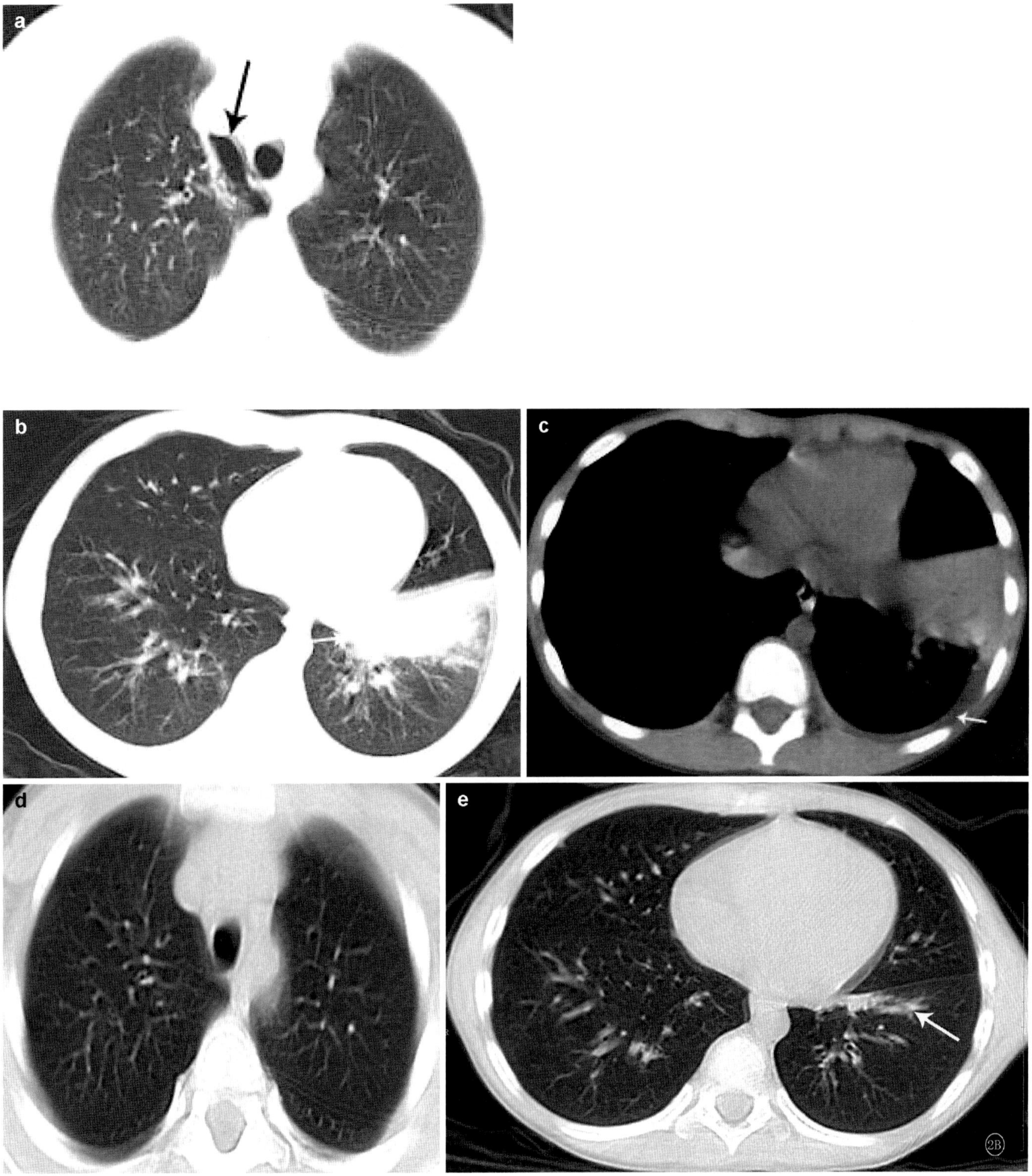

Fig. 4.15 (**a–e**) A boy aged 7 years with influenza A (H1N1) complicated by pneumonia. (**a**) At d 7 since onset, chest CT showed a strip-like area (*black arrow*) next to upper right mediastinum with no lung markings, which was preliminarily diagnosed as right pneumomediastinum; (**b–c**) The same chest CT at d 7 displayed large dense consolidation opacities (*black arrow*) at the left lower lung lobe immediately nearby the oblique fissure pleura, poorly defined border of the dorsal part, a small quantity of liquid (*white arrow*) at the left pleural cavity in the mediastinal window. (**d**) At d 14 since onset, reexamination by CT scan showed absorbed pneumatosis next to upper right mediastinum. (**e**) The same CT scan at d 14 demonstrated rare cord-like opacities (*white arrow*) at the left lower lung lobe

4.7.1.5 Plastic Bronchitis

Plastic bronchitis has an extremely rare occurrence whose diagnosis can be defined by bronchoscopy based on suction of branch-like bronchial casts. Pathologically, it is fibrinous exudation or fibrinous exudation with necrosis and may be accompanied by infiltration of neutrophils, eosinophils, and lymphocytes. Chest X-ray demonstrates some indirect signs, like lung consolidation and atelectasis. Airway reconstruction after CT scan shows higher-density opacities in the cavity (Fig. 4.17).

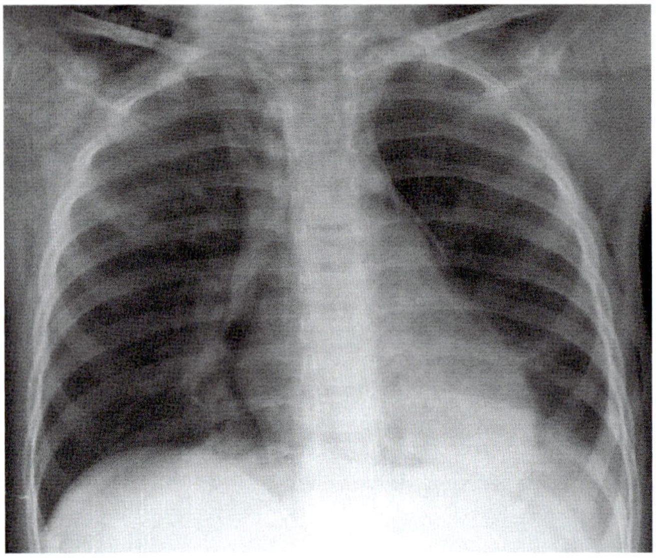

Fig. 4.16 A girl aged 3 years with influenza A (H1N1) complicated by pneumonia. Chest X-ray showed pneumomediastinum, subcutaneous pneumatosis at the neck, and pneumatosis at the left thoracic wall

4.7.1.6 Secondary Fungal Infection

The critical and severe pediatric cases of influenza A (H1N1) with respiratory complications are radiologically characterized by multiple patchy ground-glass opacities and consolidation opacities at both lungs, high incidence of pleural effusion, the more common complications of pneumonia, and pulmonary cryptococcal infection (Fig. 4.18).

4.7.2 Radiological Manifestations of the Central Nervous System

Some critical and severe pediatric patients with influenza A (H1N1) develop diseases of the central nervous system. The common complications of the central nervous system include influenza-related encephalopathy, aseptic meningitis, encephalitis, acute necrotizing encephalopathy, and secondary intracranial fungal infection.

4.7.2.1 Influenza-Related Encephalopathy

Influenza-related encephalopathy has symptoms of the central nervous system and abnormalities on EEG. However, no abnormality can be found by CSF and cranial radiology. The disease is often clinically diagnosed and radiological examination is performed to exclude other possible complications. MRI shows bilaterally symmetrical lesions at the deep white matter and basal ganglia (including the thalamus and brainstem tegmentum) of cerebral hemisphere.

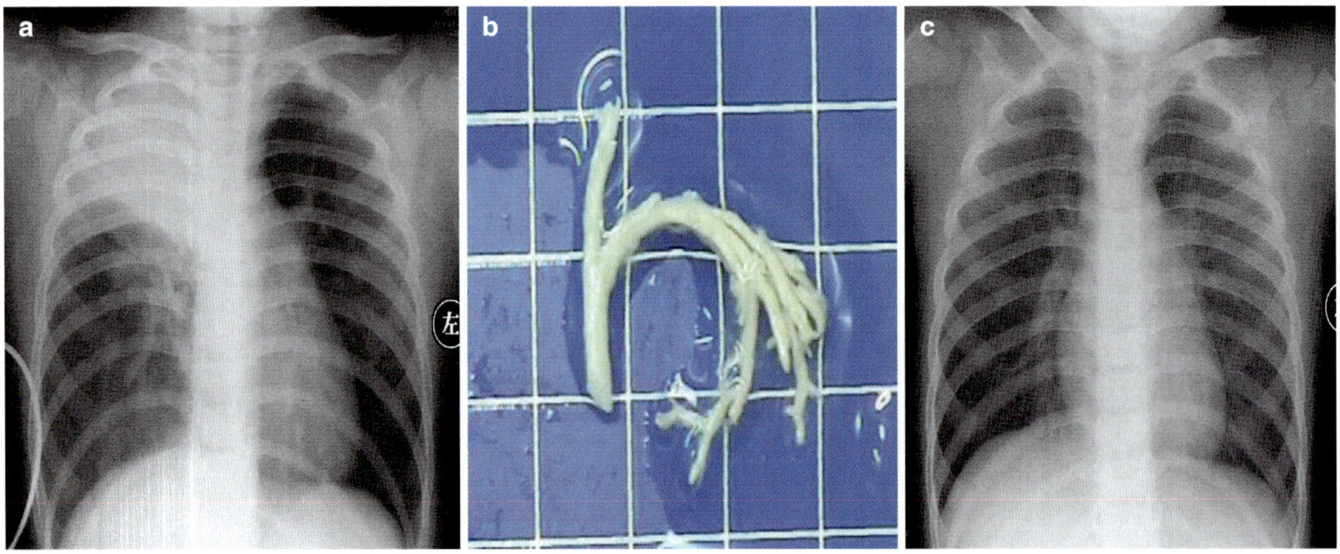

Fig. 4.17 (**a–c**) A boy aged 3 years with influenza A (H1N1) complicated by pneumonia. (**a**) At d 6 since onset, chest X-ray showed inverted triangle-shaped dense opacities at the right upper lung field, indicating lung consolidation and partial atelectasis. (**b**) At d 7 since onset, fibrobronchoscopy showed obstructed bronchi at the right upper lung lobe. Pathological examination of the suctions from bronchi demonstrated fibrinous exudation, large quantities of neutrophils and eosinophils, and no tumor cell, and the pathological diagnosis was plastic bronchitis. (**c**) At d 13 since onset, it was demonstrated that the original inverted triangle-shaped dense opacities at the right upper lung field disappeared

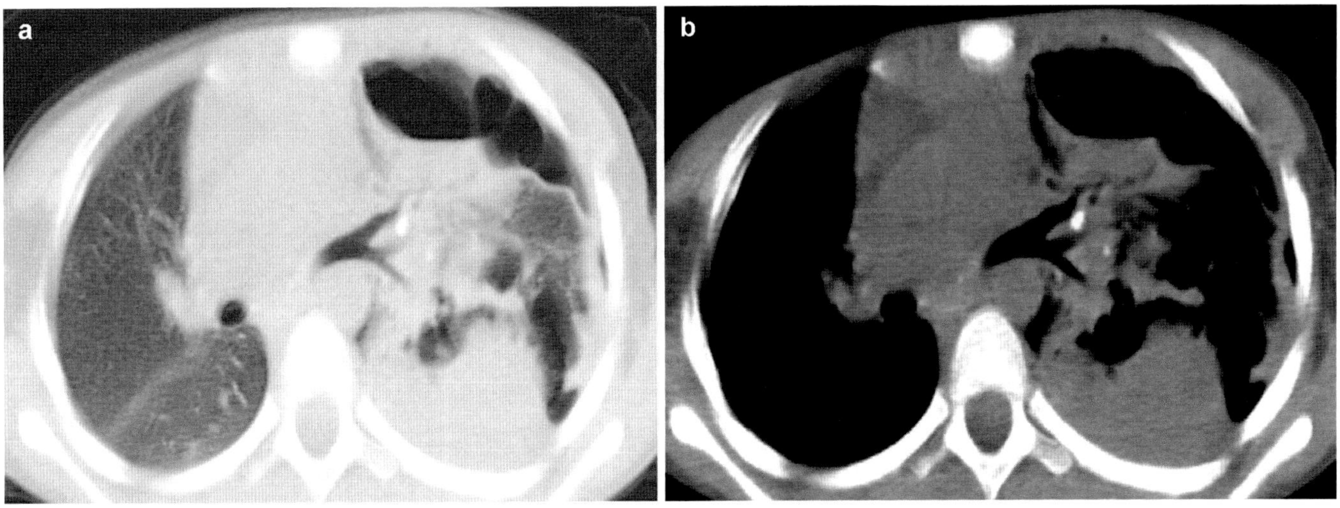

Fig. 4.18 (**a**, **b**) A girl aged 7 years with influenza A (H1N1) complicated by pneumonia and cryptococcal infection. (**a**) At d 7 since onset, plain chest CT scan showed left pneumothorax (*arrow*) in the lung window, shrinkage of the left upper lung lobe, and multiple large flaky high-density opacities at the left upper lung lobe with poorly defined borderline. (**b**) In the mediastinal window, it was demonstrated with flaky consolidation opacities at the dorsal segment of left lower lung lobe, archlike liquid-density opacities (a small quantity of left pleural effusion, *white arrow*) at the left thoracic cavity. Pleural effusion biopsy demonstrated cryptococcal infection

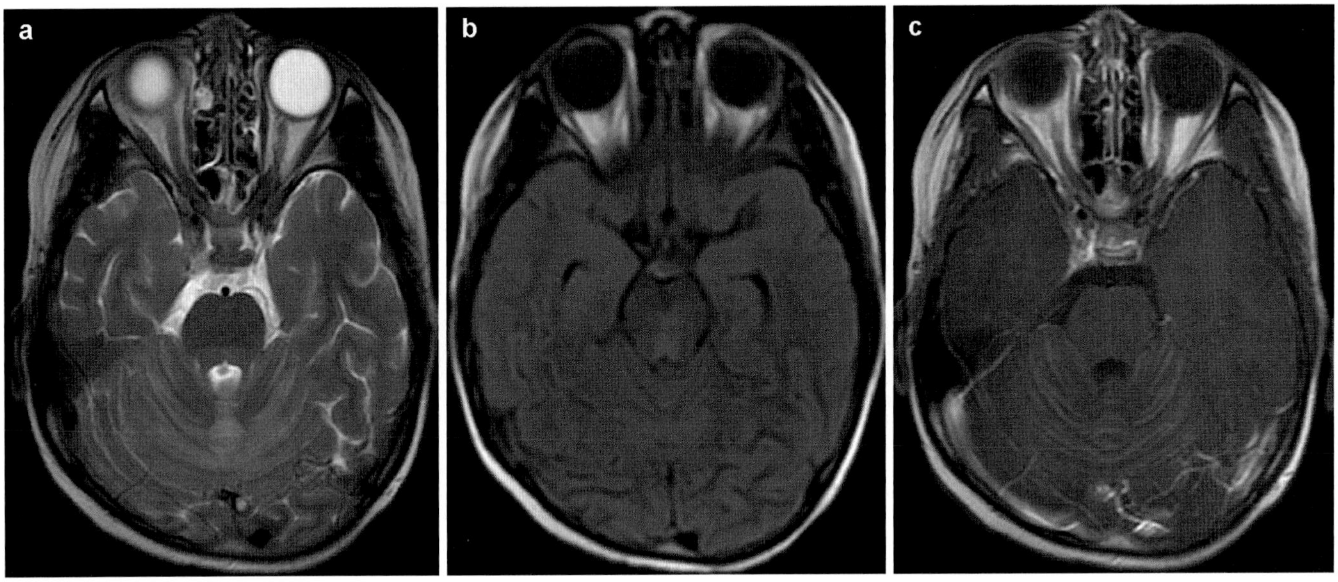

Fig. 4.19 (**a–c**) A boy aged 7 years with influenza A (H1N1) complicated by meningitis. (**a**) T2WI showed widened gyrus of the cerebellum. (**b**) FLAIR displayed increased signals at the sulci of cerebellum. (**c**) Contrast imaging demonstrated obvious enhancement of the cerebellar meninges

4.7.2.2 Aseptic Meningitis

Aseptic meningitis is often clinically diagnosed *Plain* MRI scan is often negative, and contrast MRI occasionally shows meningeal enhancement at both cerebrum and cerebellum that is nonspecific. The pediatric patients with aseptic meningitis commonly have a good prognosis (Fig. 4.19).

4.7.2.3 Encephalitis/Meningoencephalitis

Both have extremely rare occurrence. The lesions may be located at the frontal lobe, parietal lobe, occipital lobe, and other parts, which may involve cortical and subcortical tissues, corpus callosum, and the thalamus. The area with lesions is demonstrated with low density by CT scan, long T1 and long T2 signals by MRI, and slight or no enhancement by contrast imaging.

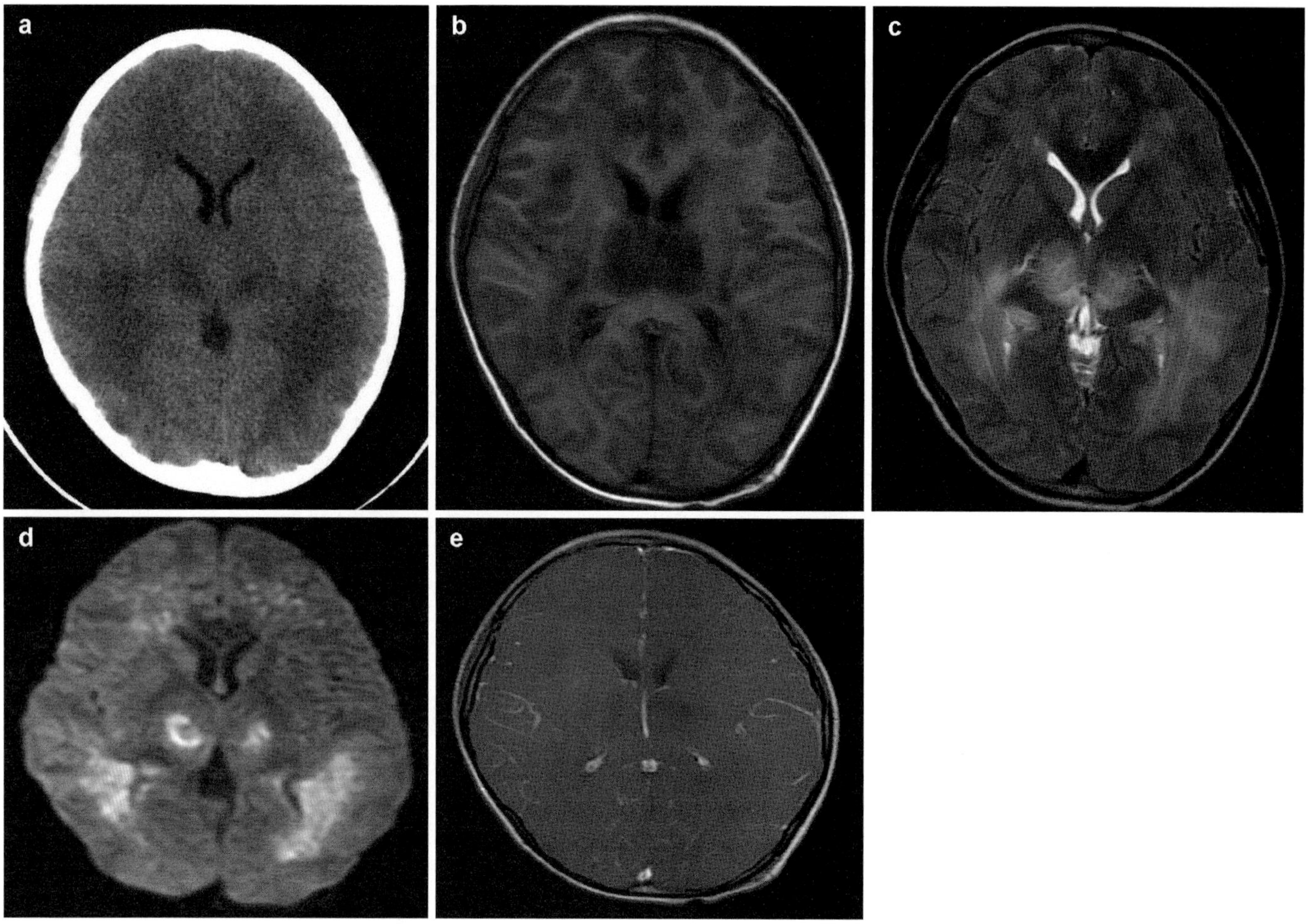

Fig. 4.20 (**a**–**e**) A boy aged 9 years with influenza A (H1N1) complicated by acute necrotizing encephalopathy. At d 4 since onset, the patient received CT and MRI scans. (**a**) Head CT scan showed symmetric low-density opacities at the bilateral thalami, posterior limb of internal capsule, lenticular nucleus, globus pallidus, optic radiation, and frontal white matters. (**b**) Head MRI showed symmetric slightly low T1WI signals at the bilateral thalami, posterior limb of internal capsule, lenticular nucleus, globus pallidus, optic radiation, and frontal white matters. (**c**) T2WI showed high signals of the above lesions;. (**d**) DWI showed centrally low signal and marginal ring-shaped high signal at the bilateral thalami and high signals of other lesions. (**e**) No enhancement of the lesions by contrast scans

4.7.2.4 Acute Necrotizing Encephalopathy

The radiological manifestations are characteristic, showing multifocal and symmetric brain lesions that are characterized by symmetric involvement of bilateral thalami. The internal capsule, lenticular nucleus, brain stem, and cerebral and cerebellar medullary substances can also be involved. The area with lesions is demonstrated with low density by CT scan, long T1 and long T2 signals by MRI, and high signals by FLAIR. By DWI, signals from the area with lesions are special, with centrally low signal and peripherally high signal of the bilateral thalami. ADC shows slightly high signal at the center that is surrounded by ring-shaped low signal (Fig. 4.20).

4.7.2.5 Secondary Intracranial Fungal Infection

Secondary intracranial fungal infection occurs in the pediatric patients mainly due to immunosuppression and long-term use of antibiotics or glucocorticoid. It may be mucor or cryptococcal infection, which is radiologically demonstrated as common fungal infection. MRI demonstrates fungal meningitis as obvious meningeal enhancement and fungal granulomas as round-like slightly long T1 and long T2 signals with marginal enhancement by contrast imaging (Fig. 4.21).

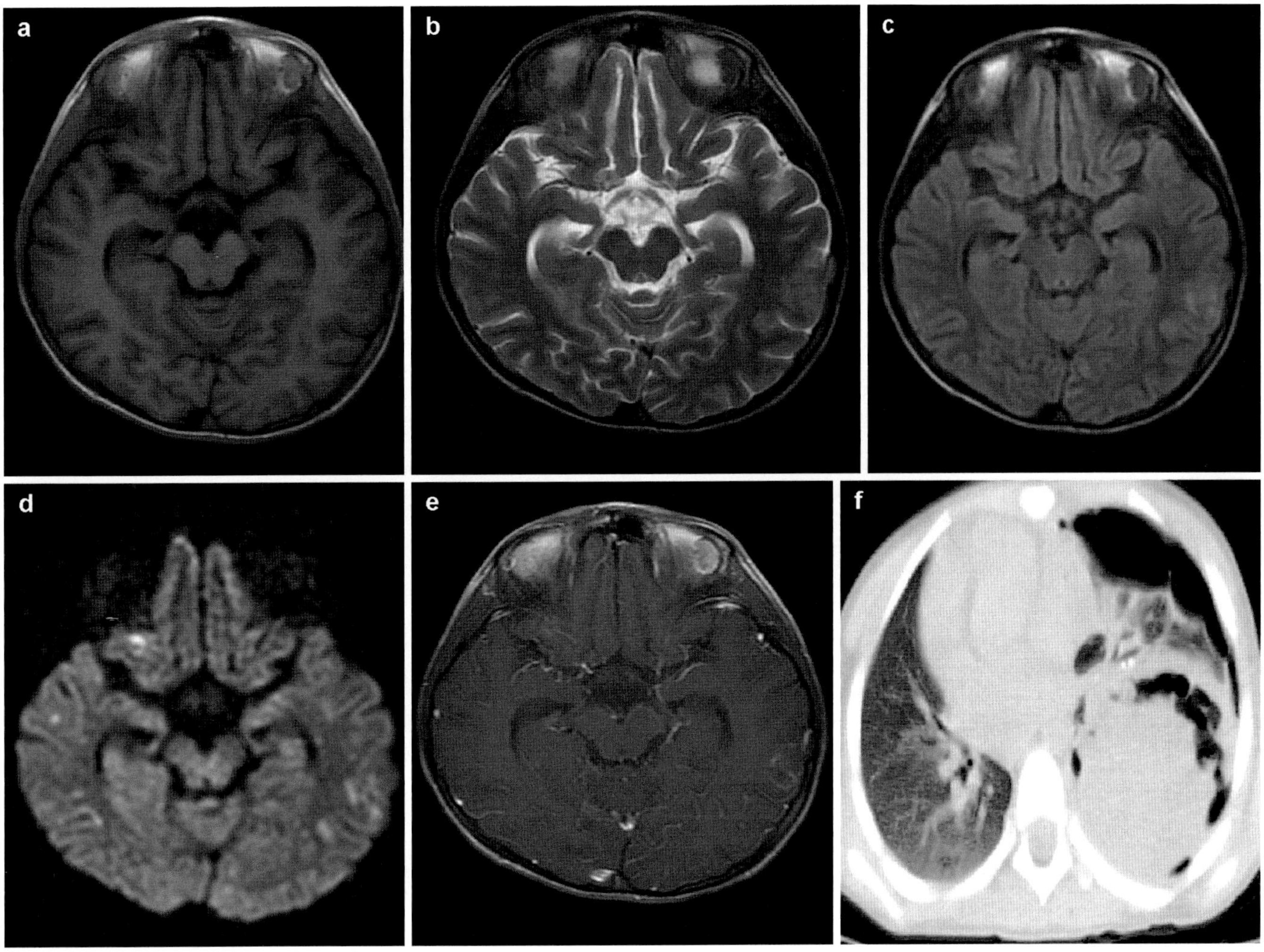

Fig. 4.21 (**a–f**) A boy aged 8 years with influenza A (H1N1) complicated by pneumonia and intracranial mucor infection. At d 21 since onset, the patient received head MRI. (**a**) Round-like low signal opacity at the left temporal lobe; (**b**) slightly high T2WI signals; (**c**) slightly high FLAIR signals; (**d**) high DWI signals and spotlike high signals at the right temporal lobe; (**e**) slight marginal enhancement at the left temporal nodules by contrast imaging. (**f**) The patient was diagnosed with fungal infection, with pneumothorax and large flaky opacities at the chest

Further Reading

1. Perez-Padilla R, de la Rosa-Zamboni D, Ponce de Leon S, et al. Pneumonia and respiratory failure from swine-origin influenza A (H1N1) in Mexico. N Engl J Med. 2009;361(7):680–9.
2. Cai C, Zhong N. Recent studies on outbreak of influenza A (HINI) in 2009. ChinEmerg Med. 2009;29(6):553–5.
3. Lu PX, Deng YY, Yang GL, et al. Relationship between respiratory viral load and lung lesion severity: a study in 24 cases of pandemic H1N1 2009 influenza A pneumonia. J Thorac Dis. 2012;4(4):377–83.
4. Fraser C, Donnelly CA, Cauchemez S, et al. Pandemic potential of a strain of influenza A (H1N1): early findings. Science. 2009; 324(5934):1557–61.
5. Liu YX, Yang DG, Xie JJ, et al. Epidemiology and clinical manifestations of definitively diagnosed cases of influenza A (HINl) in Shenzhen. Chin J Infect Dis. 2009;27(10):582–5.
6. Li CR, Yang J, Jia S, et al. Changes of immune function in pediatric patients with influenza A (HlNl) in 2009. Chin J Pediatr. 2010;48(12):947–53.
7. He YX, Gao ZF, Lu M, Sui GJ. Histopathological study on death cases of critical and severe influenza A (H1N1). J Peking Univ Health Sci. 2010;42(2):137–9.
8. Yuan H, Yang GL, Liu YX, et al. Clinical manifestations, viral load and viral detoxification duration in patients with mild or severe influenza A (HINI). Chin J Infect Dis. 2010;28(12):722–6.
9. Fang MT, Chong YT, Yang GL, et al. The effect of Th17 lymphocytes on clearance of influenza A (H1N1) virus. Chin J Infect Dis. 2010;28(10):593–6.

10. Fang MT, Yang GL, Liu YX, et al. Cellular immunity of patients with influenza A (HlNl) complicated by pneumonia. Chin J Exp Clin Virol. 2010;24(6):412–4.
11. Shieh WJ, Blau DM, Denison AM, et al. 2009 pandemic influenza A (H1N1) pathology and pathogenesis of 100 fatal cases in the United States. Am J Pathol. 2010;177(1):166–75.
12. Chowell G, Bertozzi SM, Colchero MA, et al. Severe respiratory disease concurrent with the circulation of H1N1 influenza. N Engl J Med. 2009;361(7):674–9.
13. Belser JA, Gustin KM, Maines TR, et al. Pathogenesis and transmission of triple-reassortant swine H1N1 influenza viruses isolated before the 2009 H1N1 pandemic. J Virol. 2011;85(4):1563–72.
14. Thomas PG, Brown SA, Morris MY, et al. Physiological numbers of CD4+ T cells generate weak recall responses following influenza virus challenge. J Immunol. 2010;184(4):1721–7.
15. Dawood FS, Jain S, Finelli L, et al. Emergence of a novel swine-origin influenza A (H1N1) virus in humans. N Engl J Med. 2009;360(25):2605–15.
16. Echevarria-Zuno S, Mejia-Arangure JM, Mar-Obeso AJ, et al. Infection and death from influenza A H1N1 virus in Mexico: a retrospective analysis. Lancet. 2009;374(9707):2072–9.
17. Ohman T, Rintahaka J, Kalkkinen N, et al. Actin and RIG-1/MAVS signaling components translocate to mitochondria upon influenza A virus infection of human primary macrophages. J Immunol. 2009;182(9):5682–92.
18. Patel M, Dennis A, Flutter C, et al. Pandemic (H1N1) 2009 influenza. Br J Anaesth. 2010;104(2):128–42.
19. Girard MP, Tam JS, Assossou OM, et al. The 2009 A (H1N1) influenza virus pandemic: a review. Vaccine. 2010;28(31):4895–902.
20. Kang YM, Song BM, Lee JS, et al. Pandemic H1N1 influenza virus causes a stronger inflammatory response than seasonal H1N1 influenza virus in ferrets. Arch Virol. 2011;156(5):759–67.
21. Belser JA, Wadford DA, Pappas C, et al. Pathogenesis of pandemic influenza A (H1N1) and triple-reassortant swine influenza A (H1) viruses in mice. J Virol. 2010;84(9):4194–203.
22. Chien YS, Su CP, Tsai HT, et al. Predictors and outcomes of respiratory failure among hospitalized pneumonia patients with 2009 H1N1 influenza in Taiwan. J Infect. 2010;60(2):168–74.
23. Pizzorno A, Bouhy X, Abed Y, et al. Generation and characterization of recombinant pandemic influenza A (H1N1) viruses resistant to neuraminidase inhibitors. J Infect Dis. 2011;203(1):25–31.
24. Dalvi PS, Singh A, Trivedi HR, et al. Adverse drug reaction profile of oseltamivir in children. J Pharmacol Pharmacother. 2011;2(2):100–3.
25. Liu YX, Yang DQ, Li HJ, et al. Detoxification and antiviral therapy in patients with influenza A (HlNI). Chin J Exp Clin Virol. 2010;24(4):279–81.
26. Yu H, Feng Z, Uteki TM, et al. Risk factors for severe illness with 2009 pandemic influenza A (H1N1) virus infection in China. Clin Infect Dis. 2011;52(4):457–65.
27. Libster R, Bugna J, Coviello S, et al. Pediatric hospitalizations associated with 2009 pandemic influenza A (H1N1) in Argentina. N Engl J Med. 2010;362(1):45–55.
28. Louie JK, Gavali S, Acosta M, et al. Children hospitalized with 2009 novel influenza A (H1N1) in California. Arch Pediatr Adolesc Med. 2010;164(11):1023–31.
29. Belser JA, Kortney M, et al. Pathogenesis and transmission of triple-reassortant swine H1N1 influenza viruses isolated before the 2009 H1N1 pandemic. J Virol. 2011;85:1563–72.
30. Girarda MP, Tamb JS, Assossou OM, et al. The 2009 A (H1N1) influenza virus pandemic: a review. Vaccine. 2010;28:4895–902.
31. Denney L, Aitken C, Li CK, et al. Reduction of natural killer but not effector CD8 T lymphocytes in three consecutive cases of severe/lethal H1N1/09 influenza A virus infection. PLoS One. 2010;5(5):e10675.
32. Zeng H, Gan Y, Huang W, et al. Clinical and radiological manifestations in pediatric patients with acute necrotizing encephalopathy. Chin J Radiol. 2010;44(11):1209–11.
33. Lindstrom S, Garten RJ, Gubareva LV, et al. Emergence of a Novel Swine-origin Influenza A (H1N1) Virus in Humans. N Engl J Med. 2009;360(25):2605–15.
34. Deng YY, Lu PX, Yang GL, et al. Semi-quantitative scoring of chest CT scan and its relationship with viral load in patients with influenza A (H1N1) complicated by pneumonia. Radiol Pract. 2010;25(9):965–8.
35. Deng YY, Lu PX, Liu YX, et al. Chest CT findings and their dynamic changes in patients with influenza A (H1N1) complicated by pneumonia. Chin J Med Radiol Technol. 2010;26(6):1108–11.
36. Sachedina N, Donaldson LJ. Paediatric mortality related to pandemic influenza A H1N1 infection in England: an observational population-based study. Lancet. 2010;376(9755):1846–52.
37. Lee EY, McAdam AJ, Chaudry G, et al. Swine-origin influenza a (H1N1) viral infection in children: initial chest radiographic findings. Radiology. 2010;254(3):934–41.
38. Lu PU, Deng YY, Yang GL, et al. Viral load in patients with influenza A (H1N1) and its relationship with chest CT findings. Chin J Tuberc Respir Dis. 2010;33(10):746–9.

AIDS

5

Pu-Xuan Lu, Feng Tie-Jian, Wang Hui, Lu Xing-Xian, Xiao Yong, Huang Shao-Biao, Liu Yan, Le Xiao-Hua, Zhu Wen-Ke, Zhang Fan, and Wang Qing

5.1 Introduction

Acquired immunodeficiency syndrome (AIDS) is an infectious disease of class B caused by infection of human immunodeficiency virus (HIV). Due to constant duplication and spread of HIV in the body, CD4+T-lymphocytes are destructed to cause its significant decrease, which further leads to loss or compromised immunity of human body. Therefore, patients with AIDS or HIV infection are susceptible to various opportunistic infections and neoplasms. HIV is transmitted primarily via sexual intercourse, blood, and vertical transmission from mother to fetus.

In October 1980, a male patient aged 31 years was admitted to the medical center at the University of California, Los Angles. This male homosexual patient was suffering *Pneumocystis carinii* pneumonia (PCP) due to severely compromised immunity. Since then, another four such patients were consecutively admitted to the center. On June 5, 1981, CDC of the United States published the case report at Morbidity and Mortality Weekly Report (MMWR), and the day was later designated as the discovery day of AIDS.

In 1983, Prof. Montagnier at the French Pasteur Institute isolated a type of antiretrovirus from a homosexual male patient with lymphadenopathy syndrome, which was nominated as lymphadenopathy-associated virus, LAV. In 1984, Dr. Callo at the National Institute of Cancer (NIC) of the United States isolated a virus resembling to a previously found HTLV-I/II from the body fluid of patients, which was then named as human T-cell lymphotropic virus type III, HTLV-III. Also in 1984, Levy reported a virus named AIDS-related virus, ARV. Based on the following studies, LAV, HTLV-III, and ARV were confirmed to be the same *Retroviridae*. In 1986, therefore, the International Committee on Taxonomy of Virus (ICTV) nominated the virus as human immunodeficiency virus, HIV.

In 1986, Montagnier and his colleagues at the French Institute of Pasteur isolated HIV-2. Compared to HIV-1, HIV-2 has a longer incubation period and weaker infectivity. And the two types of HIV virus only have 40 % similarity in gene sequence. Currently, HIV-2 only prevails in some countries in western Africa.

The prevalence of AIDS/HIV has been a major concern of public health and a serious social problem, and AIDS/HIV is one of the most serious threats to human health. AIDS/HIV has spread worldwide, still with increasing occurrence in middle and eastern Europe, middle Asia, Middle East, and northern Africa. And Africa is the most seriously affected area, with the most rapid spreading rate and the largest infected population.

HIV and Simian immunodeficiency virus (SIV) are pathogens that can infect both humans and animals. The animal-borne pathogen is firstly transmitted from animal to human and then from person to person. Thereafter, the spreading pathogen is more likely to undergo variation and recombination to evolve into a stable pathogen that can adapt itself to the new host. Under the comprehensive effects of heredity, society, economy, environment, life habits (such as eating

Pu-Xuan Lu (✉)
Department of Radiology, Shenzhen Third People's Hospital
Guangdong, Shenzhen, China
e-mail: lupuxuan@126.com

Feng Tie-Jian
Department of Infection, Chronic Diseases Hospital, Shenzhen, China
e-mail: fengtiej@126.com

Wang Hui • Liu Yan • Le Xiao-Hua • Zhu Wen-Ke • Wang Qing
The Shenzhen No.3 People's Hospital, Guangdong College, Shenzhen, China

Lu Xing-Xian
Changzhou No.2 People's Hospital, Changzhou, China

Xiao Yong
Shenzhen Armed Police Hospital, Shenzhen, China

Huang Shao-Biao
Guangxi Nanning the Fourth People's Hospital, Nanning, Guangxi, China

Zhang Fan
Women's Hospital of Zhejiang University School of Medicine, Shangcheng, Hangzhou, Zhejiang, China

P.-X. Lu, B.-P. Zhou (eds.), *Diagnostic Imaging of Emerging Infectious Diseases*, DOI 10.1007/978-94-017-7363-8_5

wild animal and keeping pets), and behaviors (such as sex, drug abuse, and migration), its pathogenicity reaches the threshold to cause spread and prevalence.

5.2 Etiology

HIV is the pathogen of AIDS, which is categorized into the family of *Retroviridae* and the genus of *Lentivirus*. Under an electron microscope, the viral particle is spherical whose diameter is 100 nm enveloped by panniculus adiposus consisting of glycoprotein-rich lipid bilayer (mainly gp41 and pg120). The lipid mainly comes from the adventitia of host cells. And its conical core is made up of proteins p24 and p18. In the core, a genomic RNA chain is attached with reverse transcriptase, which speeds up the reverse transcription of viral RNA.

Each HIV genome contains two single positive strand RNA, and each RNA genome is about 9.7 kb. A cap structure (m7G5ppp5' GmpNp) is located at the end of RNA 5', and a poly (A) tail at the end of 3'. Like other retroviruses, the structure and combination of basic HIV genes are composed of a 5' long terminal repeat area (LTR), a structural protein coding area (gag), a protease coding area (pro), a protein coding area with multiple enzymes activity (pol), outer membrane protein (env), and a 3' terminal long repeat area. HIV is more complex than other retroviruses as it has comparatively more regulatory genes. Therefore, it is also known as complex retrovirus to distinguish it from those retroviruses with few or no regulatory genes.

Based on the genetic differences, HIV can be categorized into two subtypes, HIV-1 and HIV-2, with homology of amino acid being 40–60 %. Almost all the patients with AIDS/HIV are infected by HIV-1 and some viral strains originated from western Africa are HIV-2. HIV-1 can be further divided into various genotypes, including group M (major genotype), group O, and group N. Group M is made up of 11 subtypes, namely A, B, C, D, E, F, G, H, I, J, and K. Group O was isolated in Cameroon and in Gabon and France as well. While in other countries, infection by such group of virus has been seldom reported. The homology of group O and group M is 55–70 %. A new genotype of HIV-1 reported in 1998 was nominated as group N. In addition, there are at least 43 circulating recombinant forms (CRF). With only 45 % homology with Simian immunodeficiency virus (SIV), HIV-1 is highly pathogenic, being the major pathogen for the prevalence of AIDS throughout the world. Although HIV-2 resembles to HIV-1 in biological properties, it spreads slowly and is less pathogenic. Its vertical transmission rarely occurs, and its infection causes less serious symptoms that progress slowly. HIV-2 is found mainly in western Africa, with a homology of up to 75 % with SIV. HIV-2 has at least 8 genotypes, namely, A, B, C, D, E, F, G, and H. In addition, based on the biological properties and the receptors used after its access to the host cells, HIV can be also divided into biological HIV and molecular HIV.

HIV mainly infects T-lymphocytes and macrophages, with the virus membrane protein, gp120, binding to the receptor protein CD4 on the surface of host cells. After the binding of HIV to the receptor, the virus core protein and the two RNA chains gain their access into the host cell. With the virus RNA as a template, the reverse transcriptase synthesizes single-stranded DNA, followed by synthesis of double-stranded DNA (pre-virus) by DNA polymerases within the cell. The pre-virus invades the nucleus after cyclization to integrate with the chromosomes under the effects of HIV integrase. Along with the cell division, the virus nucleic acid is transmitted to daughter cells, with long-term latency.

Once away from the host, HIV shows very weak viability in the external environment, as it has very weak resistance to the physical and chemical factors in the natural environment. Its resistance to the physical and chemical factors is even weaker than hepatitis B virus (HBV). Therefore, any effective measures to disinfect and inactivate HBV are applicable to disinfect and inactivate HIV.

5.3 Epidemiology

5.3.1 Worldwide Prevalence of HIV/AIDS

Based on the data released by the Joint United Nations Programme on HIV/AIDS (UNAIDS) and World Health Organization (WHO) in 2012, about 34 million patients (ranging from 31.4 million to 35.9 million) with HIV/AIDS are alive at the end of 2011, including approximately 14 million adult males, 16.7 million adult females, and 2.3 million children aged under 15 years. Sub-Saharan Africa continues to be the most seriously affected area, with an infection rate of 4.9 % among adults, accounting for 69 % of the total infected population worldwide. Concerning the infection rate, the sub-Saharan Africa is followed by Caribbean, Eastern Europe, and Central Asia, with an infection rate of 1 % among adults. And an estimated five million cases of HIV/AIDS are surviving in South Asia, Southeast Asia, and East Asia. The latest epidemiologic data indicated that the incidence of HIV/AIDS reached its peak in 1999; 2011 saw a decrease of 20 % compared with 2001; the mortality rate in 2011 was approximately 24 % lower than that of 2005. In the year of 2011, about 0.33 million cases of new infection were reported in children aged under 15 years, with a decrease of 34 % compared with 0.5 million cases of new infection in 2001.

The transmission route of HIV/AIDS is gradually changing. In Eastern Europe and Central Asia, for instance, HIV previously spread mainly via intravenous drug abuse, but currently via sexual contact. And the infection rate in male homosexuals is rapidly increasing. In some high-income countries, male homosexual contact has been the most common route of transmission.

5.3.2 The Distribution of HIV-1 and Its Variety

Although both HIV-1 and HIV-2 were originated in Africa, different subtypes of HIV are prevailing in different geographical regions. Groups O and N of HIV-1 and HIV-2 only prevail in some regions of Africa, but group M of HIV-1 prevails throughout the world. The most commonly found viral strains are subtypes A and C, followed by subtype B and then recombinant viral strains of A/E and A/G. By molecular epidemiology, all subtypes of HIV are prevailing in Africa, but the most commonly subtypes A and C. In North America, Europe, and Australia, the subtype B is the most commonly found pathogenic virus in reported cases of HIV/AIDS. Although infections of other subtypes of group M and group O have also been reported in the United States and several European countries, most of the infected patients were found to be immigrants from Africa. In South America, subtype B is most predominant prevailing viral strain, and the subtypes C and F are also prevailing. In Argentina and Brazil, infection by recombinant B/F strain has been reported. In Asia, various subtypes of HIV-1 are prevalent in various regions, with subtype C predominantly spreading in India, where subtypes A and B are simultaneously prevailing and infection of recombinant A/C strain has also been reported. With the elongation of prevailing period and the change of transmission route, the transmission route and regional distribution of HIV-1 subtypes are shown to be heterogeneous. In the late 1980s, HIV gained its access into China and the first group of infection was reported to be intravenous drug abusers in Yunnan province by subtype B originated from Europe and/or North America and subtype B' from Thailand. The subtype B was initially the most commonly found pathogenic strain in China, which was then gradually replaced by subtype B'. In the early 1990s, subtype C originated from India prevailed in intravenous drug abusers in Yunnan province, which was then spread rapidly throughout the southern, northern, and central China via behaviors of sharing syringe. Since then, the subtypes C and B' recombined to derive into subtypes CRF07-BC and CRF08-BC, which further spread into southern and northwestern China.

5.4 Pathogenesis and Pathological Changes

5.4.1 Pathogenesis

AIDS is a fatal infectious disease caused by HIV infection and is characterized by severe systemic immunodeficiency. HIV, as a retrovirus, can be categorized into two major types: HIV-1 and HIV-2. HIV-1 is responsible for overwhelmingly majority of HIV infections.

Pathogenesis of HIV infection and its progress into AIDS are as the following:

1. After HIV gains its access into human body, it is assisted by the receptor on the cell surface to selectively adhere to the target cell. So far as we know, the key receptors include CD4+, CXCR4, and CCR5. CD4+ molecule located on the surface of human cells is the primary target of HIV attack.
2. HIV infection can trigger humoral and cellular immune responses in human body.
3. The damage to the immune system caused by HIV infection is indicated by the direct and indirect effects of HIV on CD4+T-cells. As a result of such damages, CD4+T cells are functionally impaired in a large quantity, which further leads to cellular immunodeficiency.
4. Other immune cells containing CD4+receptor, such as B-lymphocytes, monocytes, macrophages, glial cells, bone marrow cells, brain capillary endothelial cells, intestinal pheochromocytes, epidermal Langerhans cells, follicular dendritic cells, and kidney glomerular cells, are also more or less affected by HIV infection.
5. The proapoptotic proteins encoded by HIV genome induce apoptosis of both infected and uninfected cells, resulting in a substantial quantitative decrease of CD4+T cells and development of immunodeficiency.

During the long-term incubation period, the protective immune response and the destructive response of HIV in an infected person maintain a relative balance. As the immunity further compromises and HIV mutates, the balance is damaged, with the latent HIV in the body activated to massively replicate and disseminate. The activated HIV extensively attack immune cells and other target cells to functionally impair cells such as CD4+T cells, monocytes, macrophages, B-lymphocytes, dendritic cells, and NK cells. Immunodeficiency or even loss of immunity, therefore, occurs to cause AIDS. Patients with AIDS are susceptible to fatal opportunistic infections or neoplasms.

5.4.2 Pathological Changes

The histopathological changes in patients with HIV/AIDS are mainly manifested as primary pathological changes of the nervous system and lymphatic and hematopoietic system resulted from directly damages caused by HIV. Along with the conditions' progress, the histopathological changes also include secondary lesions induced by immunodeficiency, such as opportunistic infections and malignancies.

5.4.2.1 Primary Pathological Changes

Lymph Nodes

Lymph node is the earliest and the most commonly involved by HIV/AIDS. Based on its histological changes, HIV infection can be divided into three stages. The first stage is also known as the acute HIV infection stage which is clinically characterized by systemic lymphadenectasis accompanied by fever and skin rash. The swollen lymph nodes are commonly found at the mesentery, retroperitoneum, mediastinum, and lung hilum. Under a light microscope, the structure of swollen lymph node is present, with some follicles dissolved. Discontinuity of lymphocytes at the mantel zone as well as its focal reduction or thinning can also be shown. The second stage is characterized by reduced lymphoid follicles and their hyaline degeneration. Even extinguished lymphoid follicles may be shown. On the cross sections, the lymph nodes are grayish white soft, possibly accompanied by hemorrhage and necrosis. The third stage is the advanced stage of HIV infection, with obviously destructed structure of lymph nodes. The lymph nodes at this stage are hard in deeper color, with no lymphoid follicles and paracortical area but with angiogenesis and marked fibrosis at the lymph sinus. The pathological changes of the above three stages can be observed within a lymph node simultaneously or sequentially.

Spleen

Since pathological examination of the spleen is often performed at autopsy, the description of the splenic pathological changes is mostly about the advanced stage of AIDS. The pathological changes include sparse T cells around the central arteries, lymphocytopenia at splenic corpuscle, absence of B-lymphocyte zone, no germinal centers or complete loss of lymphatic component, and fibrosis of the lymphatic sheath.

Bone Marrow

The bone marrow is demonstrated with granulocytic hyperplasia with left shift of the nucleus at singular or multiple systems as well as hematopoietic disorders with myelodysplastic syndromes (MDS) such as erythroid megaloblastic change or dysplastic changes.

Pathological Changes of the Nervous System

The commonly found pathological changes include HIV-associated encephalitis, aseptic meningitis, vacuolar myelopathy, and leukoencephalopathy. In addition, HIV can directly infect glial cells to cause glial nodules composed of multinucleated giant cells and glial cells, demyelination, vacuolar degeneration, and liquefactive necrosis.

5.4.2.2 Opportunistic Infections and Malignancies

When the immunity is impaired to a certain degree, the patients with HIV/AIDS are vulnerable to opportunistic infections and malignancies.

Opportunistic Infections

The pathogens inducing opportunistic infections in patients with HIV/AIDS are various, which can be categorized into four types: viruses, bacteria, fungi, and parasites. Mixed infection by several types of pathogen is common in patients with HIV/AIDS.

Virus Infection

Cytomegalovirus infection is the most common HIV-associated opportunistic viral infection, followed by herpes simplex virus (HSV) infection and EB virus infection. CMV infection is histologically characterized by the presence of giant cells and intranuclear inclusions (Fig. 5.1). HSV infection commonly involves the skin and mucosa. Microscopic examination reveals vascular dilatation and congestion, inflammatory cells infiltration, edema, and degeneration of the skin, basal mucosa, and peri-epithelium cells. The HSV-infected cells commonly fuse into multinucleated giant cells with eosinophilic intranuclear inclusions. The incidence rate of EB infection is high in patients with HIV/AIDS. In patients with AIDS complicated by malignant lymphoma, the positive rate of EB infection is about 60–70 %.

Bacterial Infections

The incidence rate of bacterial infection in patients with AIDS is 13–40 %. The most common pathogens are mycobacterium tuberculosis (MTB) and mycobacterium avium complex (MAC) that spread via the respiratory tract.

1. AIDS complicated by MTB infection is commonly demonstrated with atypical pathological changes of tuberculosis (Figs. 5.2 and 5.3).
2. AIDS complicated by MAC infection.

MAC, composed of *Mycobacterium avium* and *Mycobacterium intracellulare*, mainly causes pulmonary lesions, with the liver, spleen, gastrointestinal tract, lymph

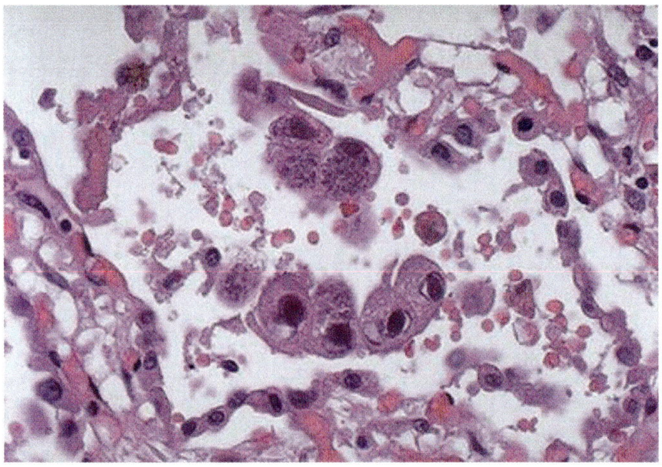

Fig. 5.1 Viral inclusions at the lung induced by CMV infection. H&E×200

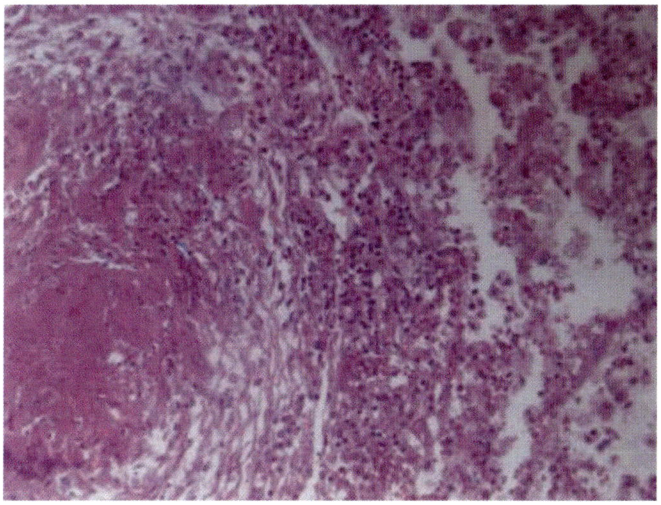

Fig. 5.2 Pulmonary TB, with observable tuberculosis nodules, caseous necrosis, and inflammatory exudates at lung tissue. H&E × 100

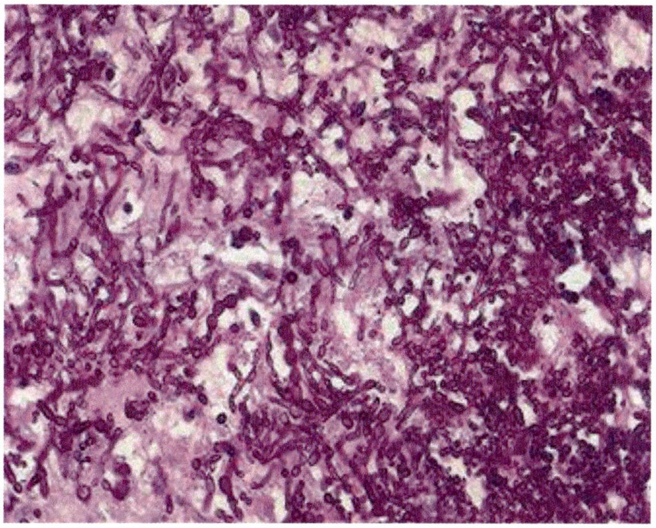

Fig. 5.5 Esophageal *Candida albicans* infection. PAS staining × 200

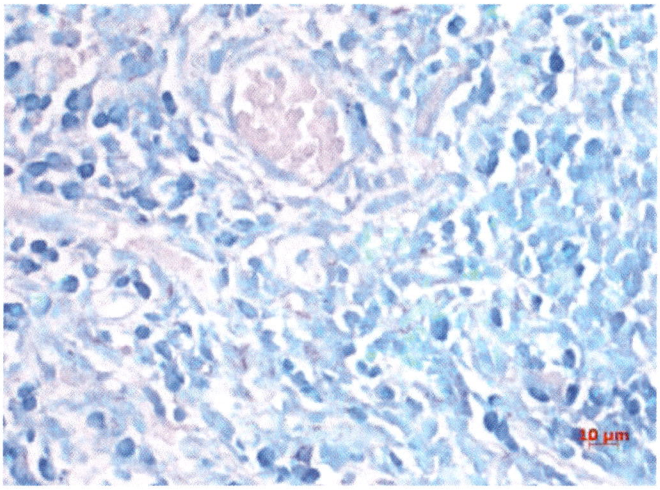

Fig. 5.3 Red short rod-shaped acid-fast bacilli after acid-fast staining

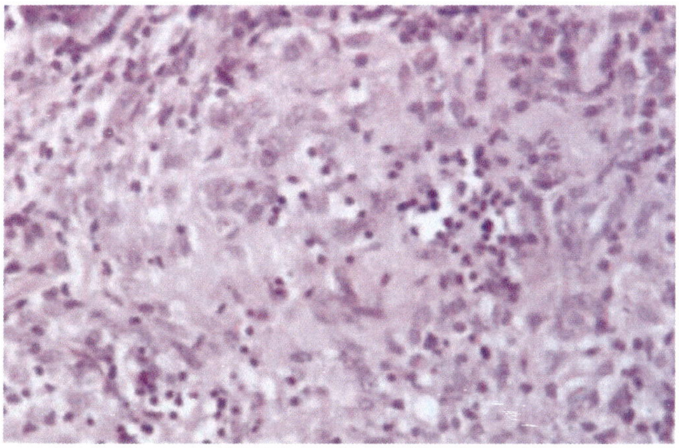

Fig. 5.4 MAC infection in lymph nodes of AIDS patients, with poorly defined nodular lesions due to hyperplasia of epithelioid cells but no non-caseous necrosis. H&E × 400

nodes, and other organs/tissues possibly involved. Nontuberculous mycobacteriosis is pathologically the same as tuberculosis. However, nontuberculous mycobacteriosis shows mild lesions like nodular hyperplasia of epithelioid cells, formation of non-caseous granulomas, hyperplasia and hyaline degeneration of collagen fibers, multifocal histiocytosis, and abundant vacuolated or foamy cytoplasm (Fig. 5.4). Acid-fast staining demonstrated a large quantity of red mycobacteria in the cytoplasm.

AIDS Complicated by Fungal Infections

1. Moniliasis

   Moniliasis is the most common fungal infection in AIDS patients. The lesions are commonly found at the oral cavity, throat, esophagus, and lungs, occasionally involving the central nervous system. Otherwise, disseminated moniliasis may occur. Pseudomycelium and blastospore can be detected in the affected tissue (Fig. 5.5).

2. Cryptococcosis

   The pathological changes caused by cryptococcosis mainly include exudative or granulomatous responses. Infiltration of macrophages, lymphocytes, plasma cells, and multinucleated giant cells can be observed in the lesion. The granulomas and even macrophages can be found to contain *Cryptococcus*, which has a spherical or ovoid shape with thick capsule surrounded by halo. Cryptococcus is stained red by PAS staining (Fig. 5.6) and black by silver staining.

3. Histoplasmosis

   A considerable number of macrophages proliferate in the lesions to phagocytose histoplasma, and epithelioid cells are formed. And even Langerhans-type multinucleated giant cells aggregate into granuloma. Caseous necrosis may be observed at central part of some lesions, with peripheral fibrosis. The small round or oval yeast-like spores of *Histoplasma* have a diameter

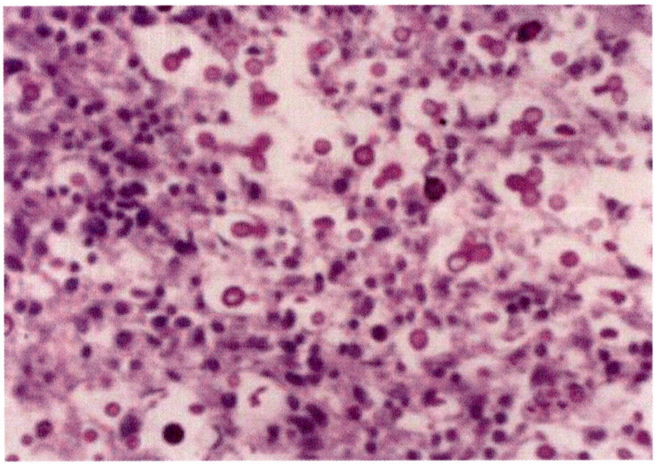

Fig. 5.6 Cryptococcal meningitis, with *Cryptococcus* spores and their budding. PAS staining × 200

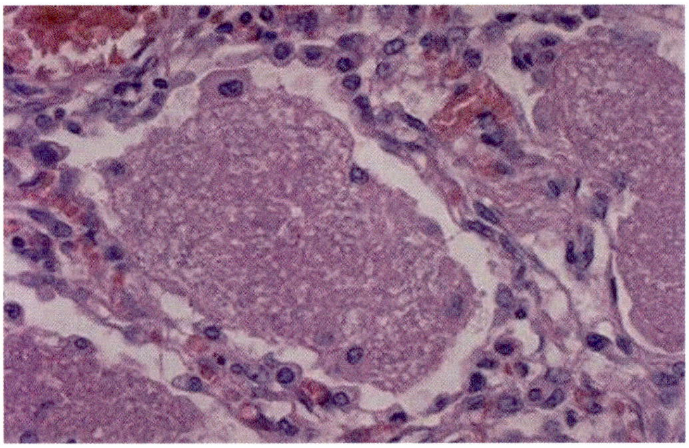

Fig. 5.8 Infection of *Pneumocystis carinii*, with exudates in alveolar space. H&E × 400

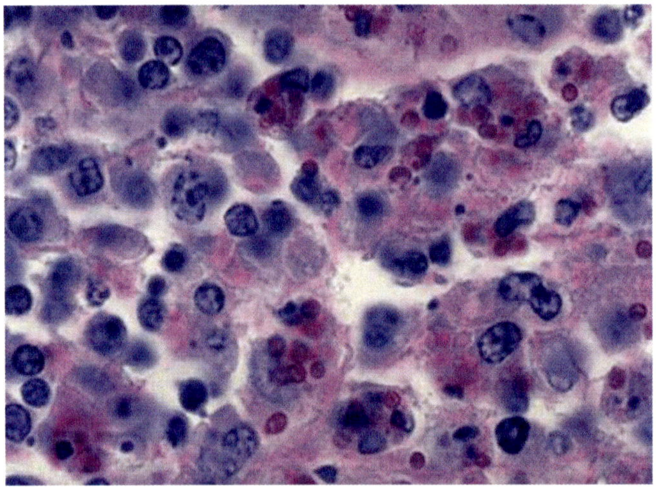

Fig. 5.7 *Histoplasma capsulatum* in Kupffer cells. PAS staining × 400

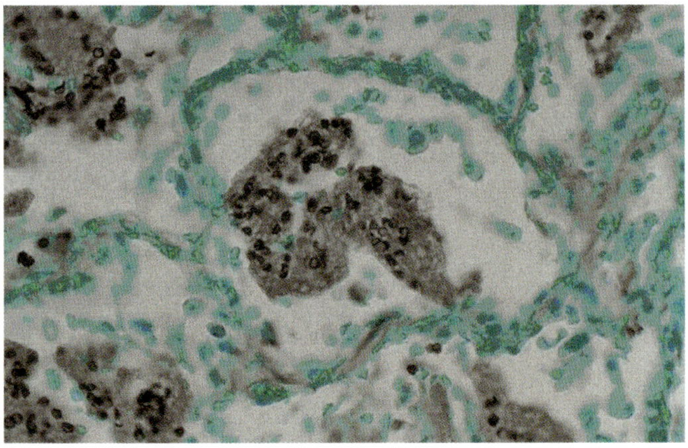

Fig. 5.9 *Pneumocystis carinii* revealed as black cyst in the alveolar exudates. Silver staining × 400

of 1–5 um and are surrounded by non-stainable capsule-like substance. The spores are reproduced by budding (Fig. 5.7).

4. *Pneumocystis carinii* Pneumonia (PCP)
   PCP is clinically characterized by alveolar pneumonia and interstitial pneumonia, with pathological findings of pinkish foamlike or honeycomb-like substances filling in the alveolus (Fig. 5.8). In addition, alveolar epithelial cells, lymphocytes, plasma cells, eosinophils, histiocytes, or alveolar macrophages shed in the alveolus wherein *Pneumocystis* can be identified by methenamine silver staining (Fig. 5.9).

AIDS Complicated by Toxoplasmosis

Toxoplasma gondii is a parasitic protozoa that can cause toxoplasma encephalitis, toxoplasma myocarditis, toxoplasma pneumonia, and other diseases. Toxoplasma encephalitis is more common and is the major cause of death in patients with AIDS. Microscopic examination reveals degeneration and necrosis of nerve cells in the malacia lesion, inflammatory hyperemia surrounding the lesions, infiltration of lymphocytes, as well as hyperplasia of microglia, wherein pseudocapsule and bradyzoite can be found (Fig. 5.10).

5.4.2.3 AIDS Complicated by Malignancies

Kaposi's Sarcoma

Kaposi's sarcoma mainly locates at the skin of limbs. However, in some cases at the advanced stage, the condition may be accompanied by widespread involvement of other organs. The lung, lymph nodes, and gastrointestinal tracts are the commonly involved organs. Microscopic examination reveals the basic histological components of the neoplasm, including tumor blood vessels and sarcoma-type spindle cells (Fig. 5.11).

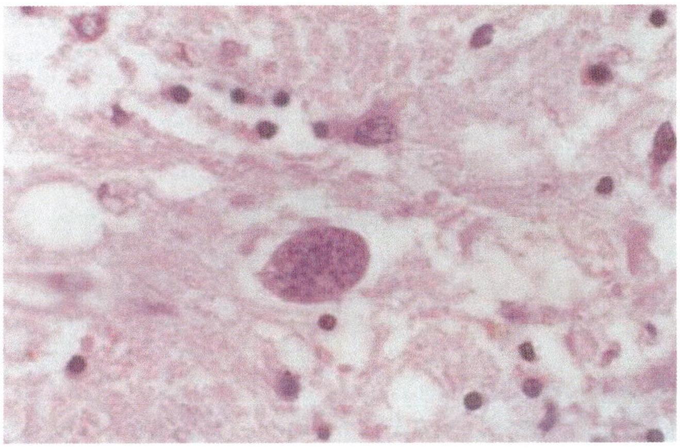

Fig. 5.10 Toxoplasma encephalitis, with a cystic *Toxoplasma* containing a large quantity of *Toxoplasma bradyzoites* that appear like fine particles. H&E×400

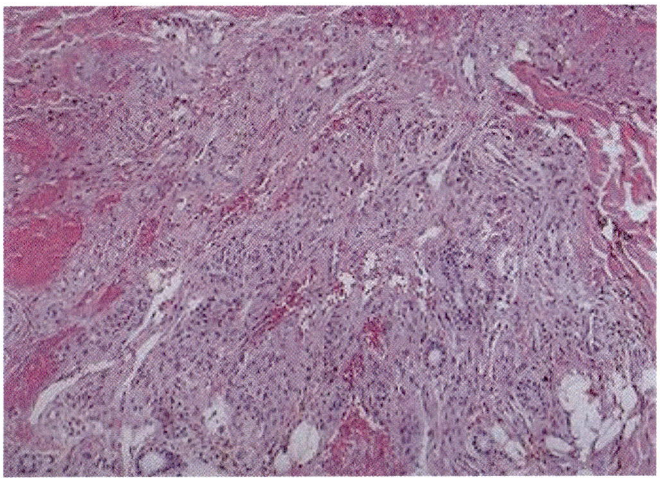

Fig. 5.11 Cutaneous Kaposi's sarcoma that locates in the dermis, with predominant component of spindle cells and with vascular fissure and leakage of red blood cells H&E×200

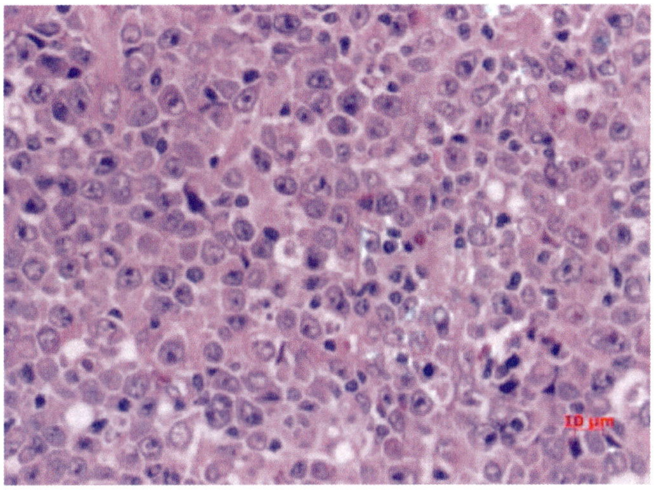

Fig. 5.12 Diffuse large B-cell lymphoma, with a large-sized tumor cells and obvious nuclei. H&E

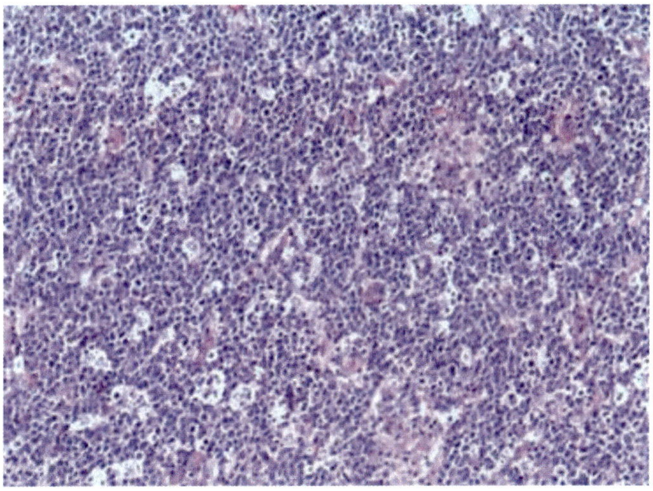

Fig. 5.13 Burkitt's lymphoma of lymph node composed of B cells with uniform morphology and moderate size, with considerable B cells at mitotic phase that appears like stars in the sky. H&E×200

5.4.2.4 AIDS Complicated by Lymphoma

The incidence lymphoma in patients with AIDS is 5–20 %, which is the most commonly non-Hodgkin B-cell lymphoma (NHL) (Fig. 5.12), followed by Burkitt's lymphoma (Fig. 5.13). Other possible lymphomas occurring in patients with AIDS include T-cell lymphoma or non-T-/non-B-cell lymphoma.

5.5 Laboratory Tests

5.5.1 HIV Antibody Test

The commonly used HIV antibody tests include standard HIV screening test and confirmatory test. Standard HIV screening test, with a higher sensitivity and comparatively lower specificity, includes enzyme-linked immunosorbent assay (ELISA), rapid HIV test, and particle agglutination test. The confirmatory test, which is commonly achieved via Western blot (WB) and less commonly by strip immunoblot assay (SIA) or linear immunoblot assay (LIA), has a higher specificity but lower sensitivity. ELISA with a higher sensitivity in combination with WB with a higher specificity shows a diagnostic accuracy of up to 99 % and a false-positive rate of 0.0006 %. By such a combination test, there is almost no chance of misdiagnosis.

5.5.2 HIV P24 Antigen Detection

Various methods can be used to detect P24 antigen, including ELISA, immune complex dissociation (ICD), ultrasensitive enzyme immunoassays (UEI), immunosorbent electron microscopy (ISEM), and lineal immunoenzymatic assay. HIV P24 antigen detection acts primarily as an assistant examination for the diagnosis of HIV infection during its window period. Meanwhile, it plays an important role in early diagnosis of HIV infection, monitoring the disease progression, predicting the prognosis, identifying neonatal infection, assessing the possibility of mother-to-child vertical transmission, evaluating therapeutic efficacy or newly developed vaccines, and basic mechanism of HIV/AIDS.

5.5.3 HIV Nucleic Acid Detection

HIV nucleic acid can be quantitatively or qualitatively detected, and the commonly used methods include RT-PCR, NASBA NucliSENS, bDNA, and real-time PCR. It is performed for the following purposes:

The diagnosis of infant HIV infection
The early diagnosis of HIV infection
The diagnosis of highly suspected cases with primary infection but negative or uncertain results by HIV antibody test
The assistant test for the diagnosis of cases with high-risk behaviors or exposure history, especially the cases with corresponding clinical manifestations
The assessment of disease progress and therapeutic efficacy of antiviral therapies

5.5.4 CD4 T-Cell Count and CD8 T-Cell Count

CD4 and CD8 T-cell count can be examined by flow cytometry assay and non-flow cytometry assay. Automatic detection is commonly performed by using flow cytometer (poly-platform or mono-platform) and specialized cell counter.

CD4 T-cell count and CD8 T-cell count are used for staging HIV infection, grading pediatric immunosuppression, assistantly assessing the therapeutic efficacy and disease progression, as well as evaluating the risk of opportunistic infections.

5.6 Clinical Diagnosis of HIV/AIDS

5.6.1 Principles of Diagnosis

The diagnosis of HIV/AIDS can be defined in combination with the epidemiologic history, including history of unsafe sexual behavior, history of intravenous drug abuse, history of infusing blood or blood products that are not tested for HIV, children of anti-HIV-positive parents, and history of occupational exposure. The clinical symptoms and laboratory test results should be comprehensively and diligently analyzed for the diagnosis. The cases that are tested HIV/AIDS positive should receive confirmative test. Nucleic acid test and HIV p24 antigen test facilitate the diagnosis of HIV/AIDS, which can help to effectively shorten the "window period." Meanwhile, both tests can also facilitate the early diagnosis of neonatal HIV infection.

5.6.2 Diagnostic Criteria

5.6.2.1 Acute Stage

A patient who has a recent epidemiological history and symptoms, in combination to positive finding of anti-HIV antibody, can be diagnosed with HIV infection. Otherwise, based only on positive laboratory finding of anti-HIV antibody, the diagnosis can be made.

5.6.2.2 Asymptomatic Stage

A patient with an epidemiological history, in combination to positive finding of anti-HIV antibody, can be diagnosed with HIV infection. Otherwise, based only on laboratory finding of positive anti-HIV antibody, the diagnosis can be made.

5.6.2.3 AIDS Stage

A patient with an epidemiological history, in combination to anti-HIV antibody positive and the following one condition, can be diagnosed with HIV/AIDS. Otherwise, based on the laboratory findings of HIV antibody positive and CD4 T-cell count <200 cells/μl, the diagnosis can be made.

1. Persistent and irregular fever with no known cause and a body temperature > 38 °C for above 1 month
2. Chronic diarrhea, with a frequency of > 3 times per day, for above 1 month
3. A weight loss by at least 10 % within 6 months
4. Repeated occurrence of oral candida infection
5. Repeated occurrence of herpes simplex virus or herpes zoster virus infection
6. *Pneumocystis carinii* pneumonia (PCP)
7. Occurrence of bacterial pneumonia
8. Development of active TB or non-mycobacterium tuberculosis
9. Deep fungal infection
10. Experiencing symptoms of central nervous system lesions
11. Developing dementia in young and middle-aged adults patients
12. Developing active cytomegalovirus infection
13. Toxoplasma encephalopathy
14. Occurrence of penicillium (such as *Penicillium marneffei*) infection
15. Repeated occurrence of sepsis
16. Kaposi's sarcoma at skin mucosa or organ, lymphoma

5.7 Radiological Demonstrations

5.7.1 Chest

The lesions at chest of patients with HIV/AIDS diversify and the lungs are the most affected organ. The related pathogens include parasite, fungus, mycobacterium, virus, bacteria, and *Toxoplasma gondii*.

5.7.1.1 Opportunistic Infection

Pneumocystis carinii **Pneumonia (PCP)**

Pneumocystis carinii pneumonia is the most common pulmonary condition complicating HIV/AIDS, which often causes disabilities or even death. Pathologically, it is characterized by diffuse lesions at both lungs, filled pulmonary alveoli and bronchiole by foamy substances that are composed of dead bacteria and immunoglobulin and alveolar exudates with plasma cells, leukocytes, and histiocytes. The disease develops rapidly, with formation of typical alveolar effusive lesion within several days.

Typical CT Demonstrations of *Pneumocystis carinii* Pneumonia

The diagnostic sensitivity, specificity, positive predictive value, and negative predictive value of high-resolution CT for *Pneumocystis carinii* pneumonia are 100 %, 83.3 %, 90.5 %, and 100 %, respectively. And the most characteristic demonstration is intrapulmonary ground glass opacity, which represents the early stage of alveolar infiltration (Fig. 5.14).

It was once believed that lung air sac is uncommon in patients with HIV/AIDS complicated by *Pneumocystis carinii* pneumonia. However, with the development of detection techniques, the occurrence of lung air sac in patients with HIV/AIDS complicated by PCP is increasing, with an incidence rate of 10–34 %. It is, therefore, another common CT demonstration in addition to ground glass opacity characteristically of *Pneumocystis carinii* pneumonia. The demonstration of lung air sac in such patients is diverse, with thin sac wall, intact and smooth lining and outer wall, no liquid, and other substances in the sac cavity. The lung air sac may be demonstrated as singular, multiple, or honeycomb-like lesion that is commonly located at the subpleura or

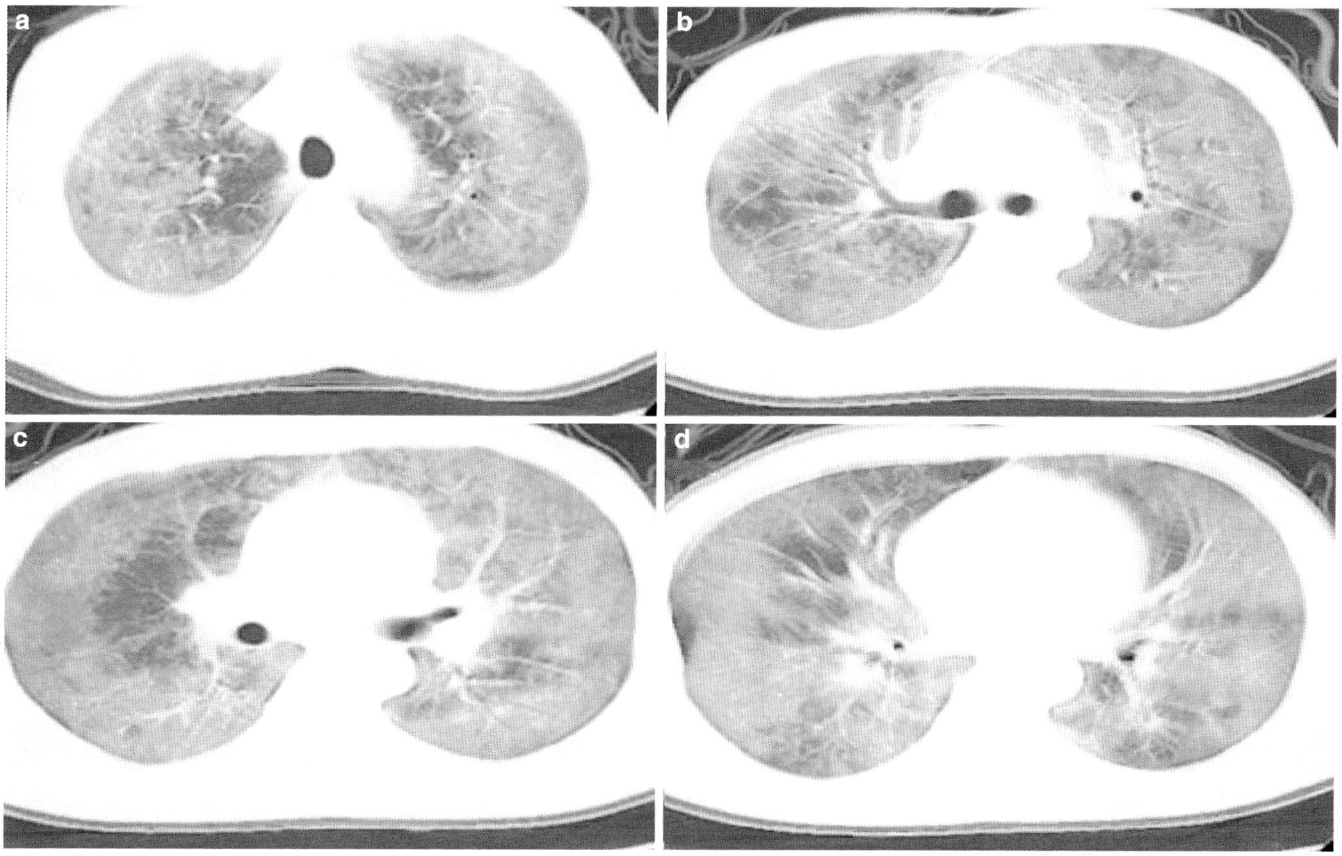

Fig. 5.14 (**a–d**) A male patient aged 31 years with AIDS complicated by *Pneumocystis carinii* pneumonia. Chest CT showed extensive ground glass opacity in both lungs

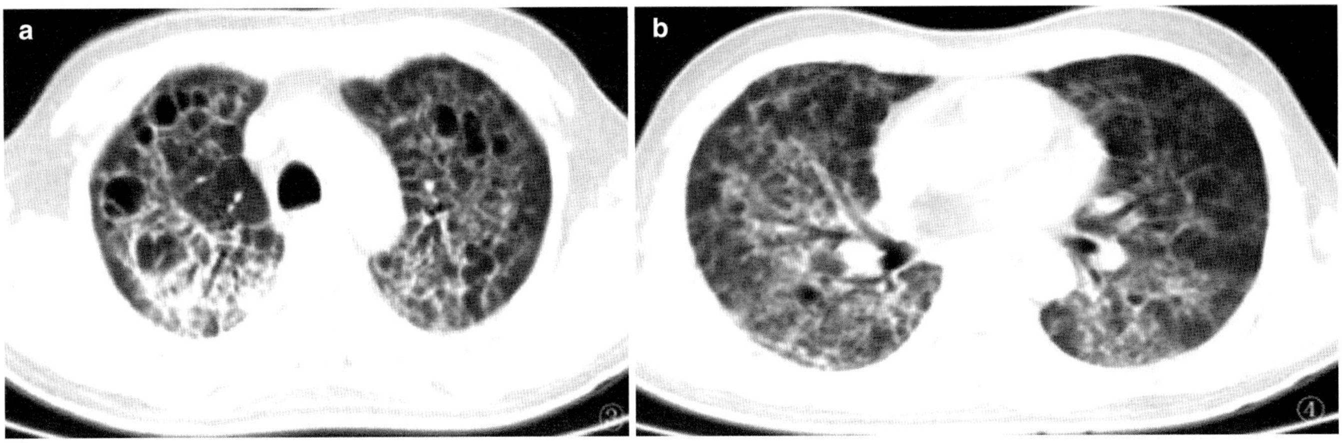

Fig. 5.15 (**a**, **b**) A female patient aged 23 years with AIDS complicated by *Pneumocystis carinii* pneumonia. Chest CT demonstrated extensive lung air sac and ground glass opacity in both lungs

pulmonary parenchyma. The lung air sac is commonly distributed at the upper lung lobes, possibly with any lung lobes involved (Fig. 5.15). The mechanism underlying its occurrence remains unknown, which is speculated to be a pulmonary parenchymal response to *Pneumocystis carinii*. The response exhibits pulmonary alveolar or interstitial inflammation and different degrees of fibrosis that leads to remodeling of lung structures to develop cystic or honeycomb-like lesion. Lung air sac may occur at any stage of infection, commonly surrounded by different degrees of ground glass opacity. After effective treatment, lung air sac can repair itself and be cured.

Rupture of some subpleural lung air sacs may cause pneumothorax. Therefore, the finding of lung air sac or pneumothorax at the area of ground glass opacity in patients with AIDS strongly indicates *Pneumocystis carinii* pneumonia.

Atypical Demonstrations of *Pneumocystis carinii* Pneumonia

The atypical demonstrations of *Pneumocystis carinii* pneumonia are various and non-characteristic, which present challenge for its radiological diagnosis. The abnormalities at pulmonary parenchyma include:

1. Pulmonary nodule or mass.

   The diameter ranges from 2 to 3 mm miliary nodule to over 1 cm nodule with solitary or focal distribution. Histologically, the nodule manifests as granulomatous inflammation and its incidence rate is about 5 % in patients with *Pneumocystis carinii* pneumonia. At the chronic stage, the nodule is calcified. In the cases with disseminated infection, it may occur at the liver, spleen, or kidney.
2. Segmental inflammation.

   It commonly occurs at upper lobes of both lungs with one lobe or segment as a unit.
3. Interstitial fibrosis.

   It occurs in patients with chronic *Pneumocystis carinii* pneumonia that lasts for several months or even several years. And it could also be sequelae of fibrosis or pulmonary cystic lesion after treatment for acute *Pneumocystis carinii* pneumonia. Interstitial fibrosis manifests as thickened interlobular septum, blurry reticular opacity, tractional bronchiectasis, and honeycomb-like lesion.
4. Bronchial abnormalities.

   The bronchial abnormalities include bronchiolitis, bronchiolitis obstruction, and endobronchial lesion.
5. Mediastinal and hilar lymphadenectasis. The lesions are commonly mild.

Types of *Pneumocystis carinii* Pneumonia

Lu PX et al. categorized *Pneumocystis carinii* pneumonia into 5 types based on its CT demonstrations, including ground glass opacity type, lung air sac type, consolidation type, interstitial type, and mixed type. The ground glass opacity type is the most common characteristic, with symmetrically distributed opacities with increased density in the lungs and bronchovascular bundles inside. The lung air sac type shows thin-wall air sac, with intact and smooth lining and outer wall but no liquid level in the sac. The sac is commonly surrounded by different degrees of ground glass opacity and flaky infiltrative opacity. Lung air sac type has multiple lesions at both lungs that are more commonly found at upper lung lobes (Fig. 5.16). The consolidation type displays uneven patches of opacities at both lungs and segmental pneumonia with one lobe or segment as a unit. The interstitial type displays thickened interlobular septum and bilaterally asymmetric diffuse reticular or network-like nodular opacities, which may be complicated by consolidation (Fig. 5.17). The mixed type shows concurrence of above lesions, which is commonly found in patients at the advanced stage.

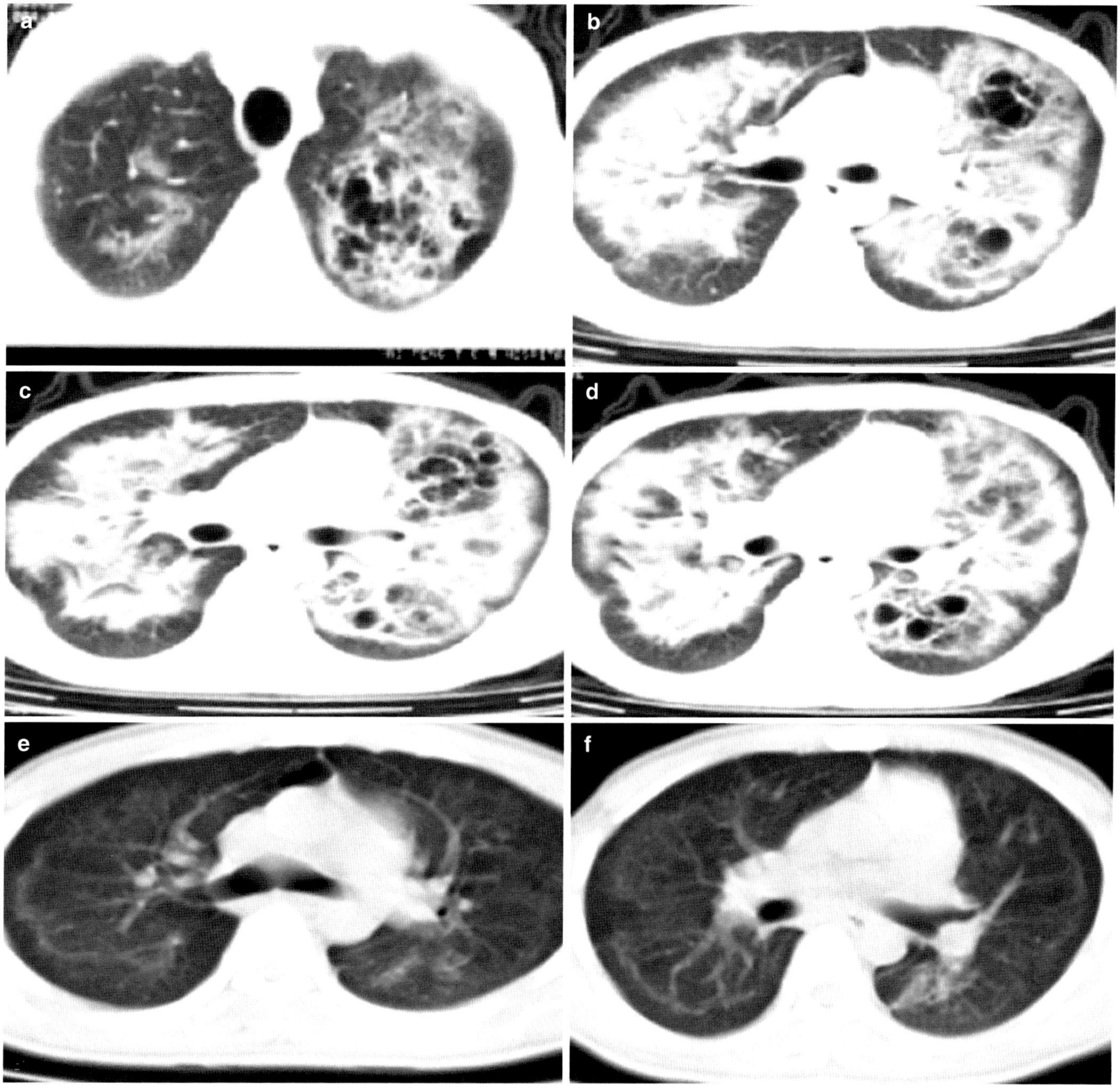

Fig. 5.16 (**a–f**) A male patient aged 39 years with AIDS complicated by *Pneumocystis carinii* pneumonia (lung air sac type). (**a–d**) Both lungs were demonstrated with multiple thin-wall air sacs, with septum in some sacs, surrounded by lung consolidation and ground glass opacity. Thickened interlobular septum and reticular nodular opacities were also shown. (**e**, **f**) Reexamination at d 30 after treatment, the lung air sacs were displayed to be obviously absorbed and improved

The categorization entails the pathological changes and the dynamic CT findings of *Pneumocystis carinii* pneumonia, which is significant for the diagnosis and differential diagnosis of *Pneumocystis carinii* pneumonia.

Tuberculosis

Mycobacterium tuberculosis is still an important respiratory pathogen in patients with HIV/AIDS. HIV infection has been known to be one of the most dangerous factors inducing development of latent tuberculosis into active tuberculosis. The radiological demonstration of HIV/AIDS complicated by tuberculosis is related to the immunity of patient. At the early stage of AIDS, the radiological demonstration resembles to tuberculosis in patients with normal immunity. At the middle and advanced stages of AIDS, the patient's immunity is moderately or seriously suppressed.

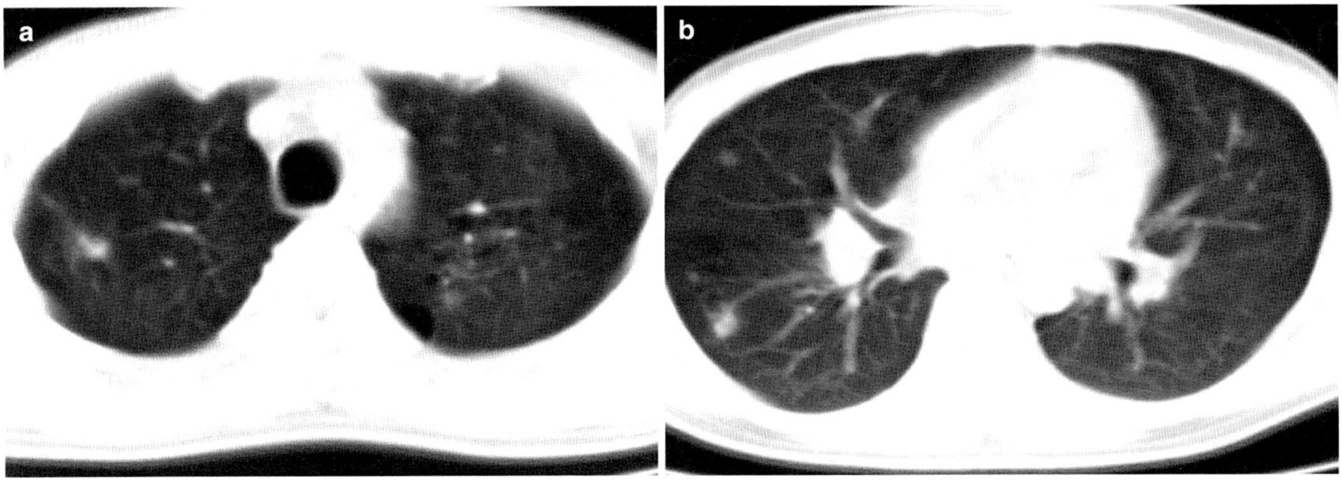

Fig. 5.17 (**a**, **b**) A male patient aged 45 years with AIDS complicated by *Pneumocystis carinii* pneumonia. Both lungs were displayed with small nodular opacity and ground glass opacity

Therefore, tuberculosis is radiologically displayed as intrapulmonary infiltration as well as hilar and mediastinal lymphadenectasis with no definite location.

Primary Tuberculosis

Hilar and mediastinal lymphadenectasis may be singular or multiple. In the cases with multiple hilar and mediastinal lymphadenectasis, the lesions are extensive and may integrate into mass. By CT scan, 70–90 % of patients with primary tuberculosis have hilar and mediastinal lymphadenectasis, and the calcification rate of enlarged lymph nodes is much lower than that of simplex tuberculosis. CT plain scan demonstrated the enlarged lymph nodes with low density. By contrast scan, marginal ring-shaped enhancement is commonly shown, with central low-density caseous necrosis (Fig. 5.18). Intrapulmonary infiltration commonly occurs at vulnerable sites of non-simplex tuberculosis, such as the lower lung lobes or right middle lung lobe. Multiple lung segments and lobes may be concurrently involved. The lesions progress rapidly that are commonly exudative consolidation. In some cases, signs of bronchial dissemination may be demonstrated, such as acinar nodular opacity and tree-bud sign. However, the signs of fibrosis and calcification are rarely shown.

Secondary Tuberculosis

At acute and asymptomatic stages of HIV infection, the radiological demonstration of secondary tuberculosis resembles to tuberculosis in patients with no HIV infection due to slightly suppressed immunity of the patients. The lesions are often located at the apicoposterior segment of the upper lung lobe or dorsal segment of the lower lung lobe, displayed as flaky focal consolidation and nodule opacities. Cavity has an incidence rate of 20–25 %, while lymphadenopathy and extrapulmonary lesions have an incidence rate of 10–15 %. Along with continual decrease of peripheral CD4+T-cell count, patients with AIDS experience increasingly serious cellular immunodeficiency. Therefore, the complication of tuberculosis may be radiologically demonstrated as more extensively severe and atypical lesions. The lesions are radiologically characterized by no definite location, diversified morphology, common progression into thin-wall or irregular no-wall cavity, and common occurrence of hilar and mediastinal lymphadenectasis. CT scans show involvement of multiple lung lobes or segments. Lesions with various morphologies can be simultaneously demonstrated, including infiltrations and military and acinar nodule dissemination. In addition, caseous pneumonia is common (Fig. 5.19). Radiologically, the lesions are generalized into "three multis and three rares": concurrence of multiple lesions (including exudation, proliferation, and cavity), multiple morphology, and multi-segmental distribution but rare occurrence of fibrosis, calcification, and mass-like opacity. The cavity may be singular or multiple and multiple cavities are more common. The cavities commonly scatter within the lungs, especially the upper and middle lung lobes (Fig. 5.20). Lymphadenectasis at lung hilus and mediastinum has a high incidence rate (Fig. 5.21), which is 17–69 % in patients with AIDS complicated by tuberculosis, but only 3–23%in patients with simplex tuberculosis. CT plain scan showed enlarged lymph nodes with homogeneous and slightly low density. By contrast CT scan, irregular ring-shaped enhancement can be displayed but no enhancement of the central caseous necrosis.

Fungal Infection

The fungi invading the lung of patients with AIDS commonly include cryptococcus, histoplasma, candida, aspergillus, yeast, and coccidioides.

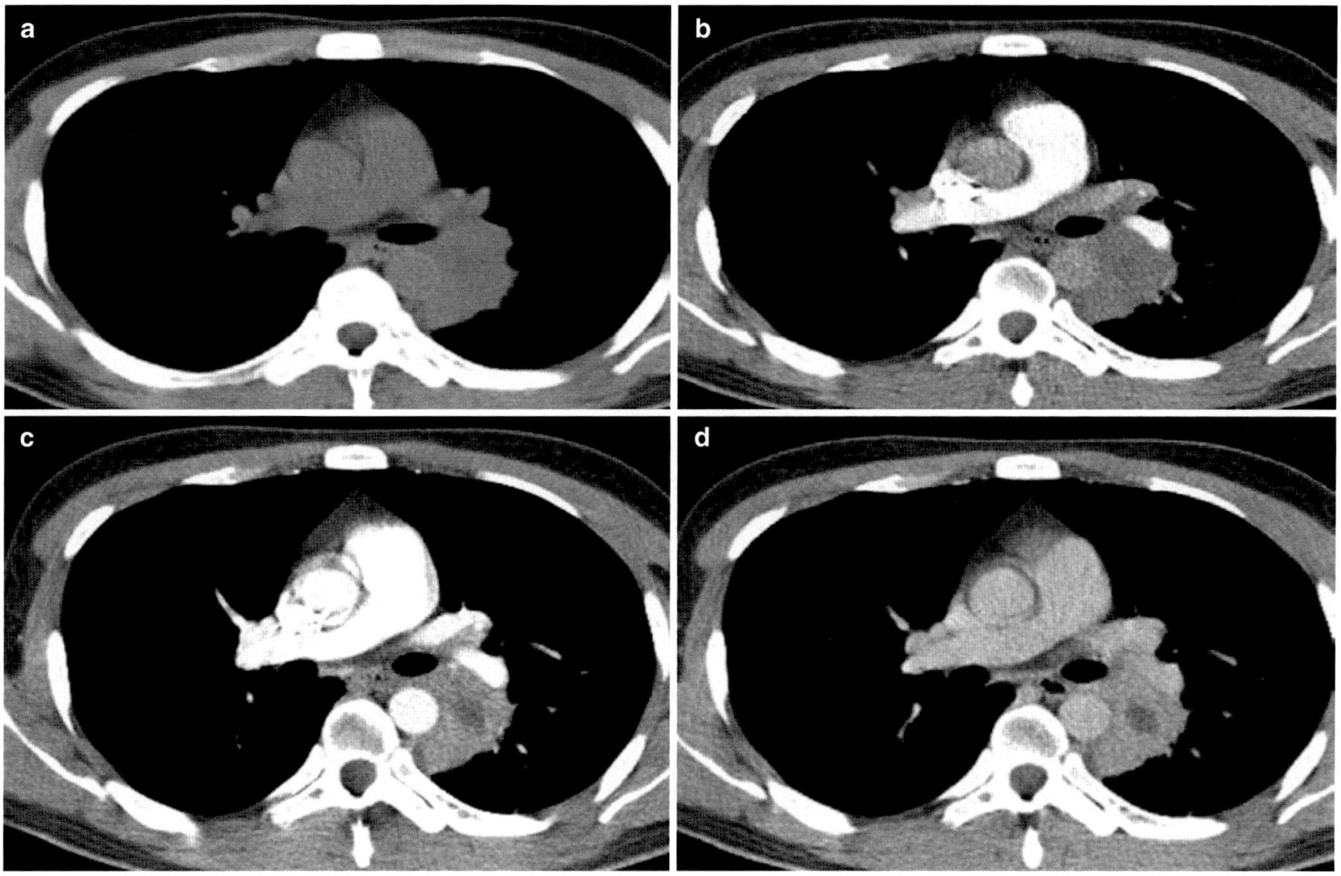

Fig. 5.18 (**a–d**) A male patient aged 34 years with AIDS complicated by lymphoid tuberculosis. Chest CT plain and contrast scan showed integration of multiple enlarged lymph nodes in the mediastinum, posterior to major bronchus and adjacent to thoracic aorta, with obvious enhancement

Pulmonary Cryptococcosis

It is a common deep fungal infection and commonly concurs with meningitis. Radiologically, the lesions are characterized by various shapes, various kinds, and multiple different-sized foci.

By CT scan, pulmonary cryptococcosis manifests solitary mass-like opacity, singular or multiple nodular opacities, singular or multiple patches of infiltration opacity, diffusive miliary nodule opacity, interstitial pneumonia, and diffusive mixed lesions. The nodular opacities are commonly well defined but morphologically irregular with different sizes and a diameter of about 5–60 mm or larger. Some of the nodular opacities are lobulated and have spikes. The patches of infiltration opacity may be demonstrated as small strips or flakes with the singular or multiple lung lobes involved. The opacity is poorly defined with inhomogeneous density, possibly with observable bronchus sign or vacuole sign. By HRCT, the diffuse miliary nodules are displayed as poorly defined acinar nodules with homogeneous density and a size of 3–5 mm, which resemble to lesions of pneumonia or miliary tuberculosis. Diffuse mixed lesions refer to coexistence of nodules, patches, mass, and lobar consolidation, in which solitary or multiple lung nodules are the most common sign by CT scan. The second common signs include mass and consolidation. The rare CT signs include cavity, calcification, hydrothorax, and hilar/mediastinal lymphadenectasis (Fig. 5.22).

Simplex involvement of the lungs is rare, accounting for about 5–10 %. About 40 % of the patients also experience pleuritis.

Histoplasmosis

In patients with AIDS, histoplasmosis may be hematogenously disseminated to involve multiple organs and induce pneumonia. The condition is commonly accompanied by systemic lymphadenectasis, hepatosplenomegaly, meningitis, pericarditis, or endocarditis.

Lung histoplasmosis is more common, with complex and diverse radiological demonstrations. The commonly found radiological signs include flaky or patchy inflammatory infiltration, diffuse miliary lesions, and nodular or mass-like lesion, cavity, and lymphadenectasis (Fig. 5.23).

Lung Aspergillosis

Due to the use of hormones and secondary neutrophilic granulocytopenia, the risk of infecting aspergillosis in patients

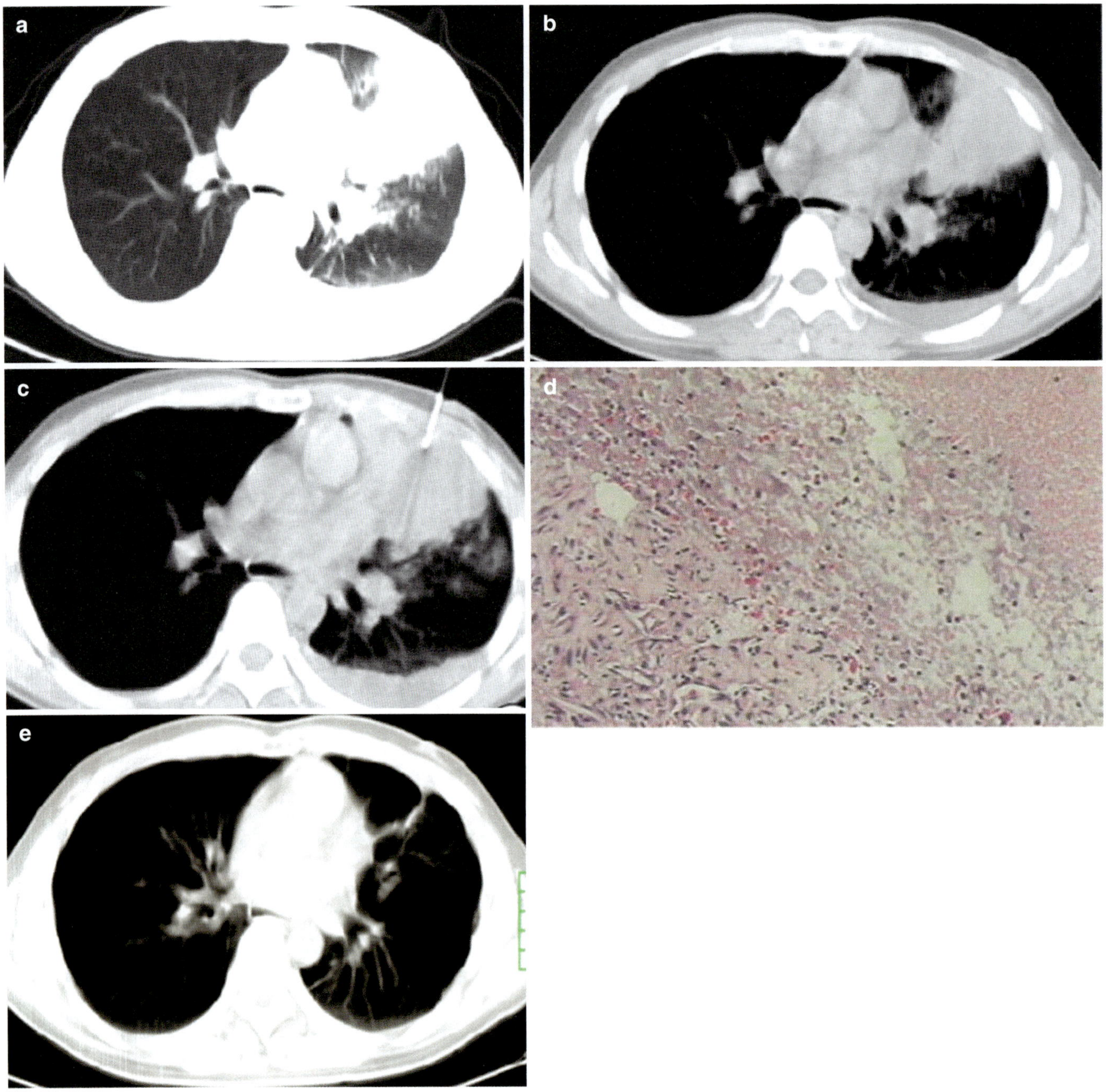

Fig. 5.19 (**a–e**) A female patient aged 24 years with AIDS complicated by consolidation type of tuberculosis and left pleuritis. By sputum culture, the acid-fast bacillus was positive (+); (**a**) consolidation opacity was displayed at the lingual lobe of the left lung that was surrounded by pulmonary acinar nodules; (**b**) a small quantity of pleural effusion was shown in the left pleural cavity; (**c**) biopsy after CT-guided puncture was performed; (**d**) pathology showed granulation tissue and caseous necrosis that are in line with tuberculosis (H&E × 100); (**e**) reexamination after antituberculosis and antiviral therapies for more than 1 year showed cord-like opacity at the lingual lobe of the left lung but no pleural effusion

with AIDS increases, especially invasive aspergillosis. In patients with AIDS, invasive aspergillosis, aspergilloma, bronchial obstructive aspergillosis, and tracheobronchial necrotic aspergillosis occur to complicate the condition.

Chest CT scan showed infiltration and cavity at the lungs, and lung aspergilloma is the most characteristic. The lesion of lung aspergilloma is radiologically displayed as well-defined round shadow in hollow cavity that is mobile along with posture change. *Aspergillus* may invade vascular vessels to cause formation of thrombus and further hemorrhagic infarct. In addition, the lesions of lung aspergilloma include flaky, nodular, or spherical density and opacity, segmental lung

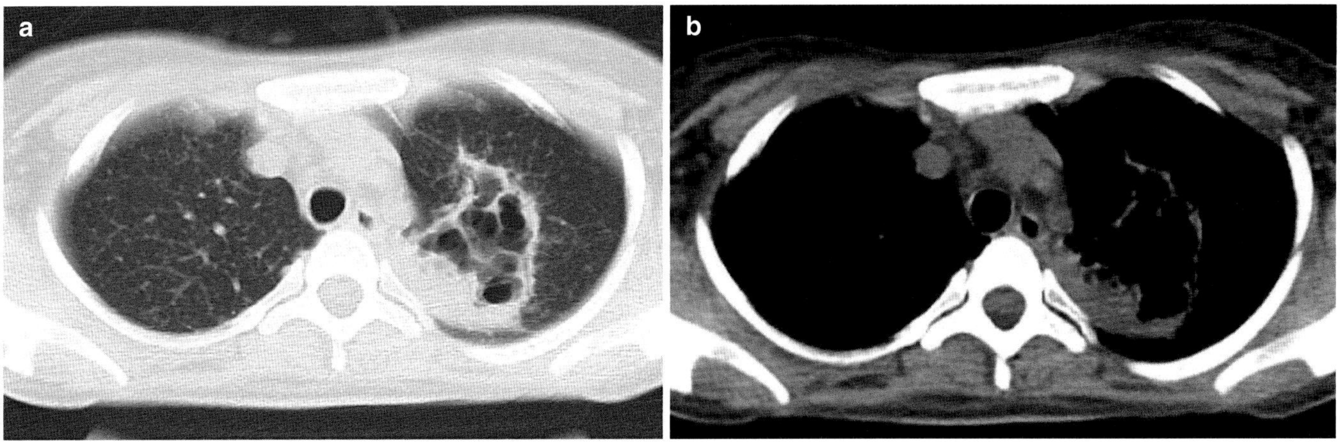

Fig. 5.20 (**a**, **b**) A female patient aged 27 years with AIDS complicated by cavity type of tuberculosis in the left lung. Chest CT scan showed large irregular flaky opacity at the left upper lung lobe with multiple cavities inside

consolidation, and observable cavity or aspergilloma. Other radiological signs of lung aspergillosis include subpleural nodule, consolidation, and pleural effusion (Fig. 5.24).

Pulmonary Candidiasis

In population with fungal infection, candida infection is common, which could induce inflammatory response in the bronchus and lung. Therefore, pulmonary candidiasis is categorized into bronchitis type and pneumonia type. In patients with AIDS complicated by pulmonary candidiasis, candida simultaneously invades the skin, superficial oral cavity, and esophagus.

Based on the location of lesion, pulmonary candidiasis is categorized into bronchitis type and pneumonia type. For bronchitis type, the lesion mainly involves bronchus and its surrounding tissues but with the lung parenchyma unaffected. The radiological signs include increased, thickened, and blurry lung markings and possibly accompanying hilar lymphadenectasis. The pneumonia type is more common. Candida invades the pulmonary alveoli to induce acute, subacute, and chronic inflammatory lesion in the lung parenchyma that is radiologically displayed as bronchopneumonia or lobular/segmental pneumonia. The radiological signs include extensive integrated spots and irregular flakes of consolidation opacity at middle and lower lung fields of both lungs (Fig. 5.25).

Pulmonary *Penicillium marneffei* (PM)

Pulmonary PM commonly occurs in immunity compromised persons, such as patients with HIV infection. In recent years, its incidence is increasing. The pathogen, *Penicillium marneffei*, is inhaled via respiratory tract to cause primary infection at the lungs. The lesions, resembling to those of tuberculosis or bacterial pneumonia, mainly affect the reticular endothelial system and commonly disseminate along with blood and lymph flow.

Radiologically, the cases with predominantly parenchymal change are demonstrated with flaky consolidation opacity at the lungs that commonly progresses into the lung parenchyma along the pleura on the back. In some cases, the condition is also displayed as diffuse oval nodules in different sizes at both lungs. The cases with predominantly interstitial change are demonstrated with grid-like miliary shadows at both lungs. Pulmonary PM is commonly accompanied by hilar/mediastinal lymphadenectasis. The lesions of pulmonary PM are commonly located at the middle and lower lung fields, especially basilar part of the dorsal lower lung lobe. The intrapulmonary lesions change slowly and can be absorbed after effective antifungal therapy for about 30 days (Figs. 5.26 and 5.27).

Mucormycosis

With the increasing incidence rate of AIDS, the occurrence of mucormycosis is increasing but remains a low rate. Therefore, mucormycosis is still a rare opportunistic infection. The diagnosis of lung mucormycosis can be defined based on microscopic fungi examination of the tissue specimen from lesion and pathogen culture to ensure the characteristic mycelium and pathological change.

By CT scan, lung mucormycosis is demonstrated with mediastinal lymphadenectasis, intrapulmonary grid-like opacity or thickened interlobular septum, intrapulmonary infiltrative lesion, miliary nodular lesions at both lungs, pleural effusion, and nodular mass-like opacity (Fig. 5.28).

Viral Infection

AIDS can be complicated by viral pneumonia caused by cytomegalovirus, herpes simplex virus, and varicella zoster virus. *Cytomegalovirus* pneumonia is the most common, with common radiological manifestation of bilateral

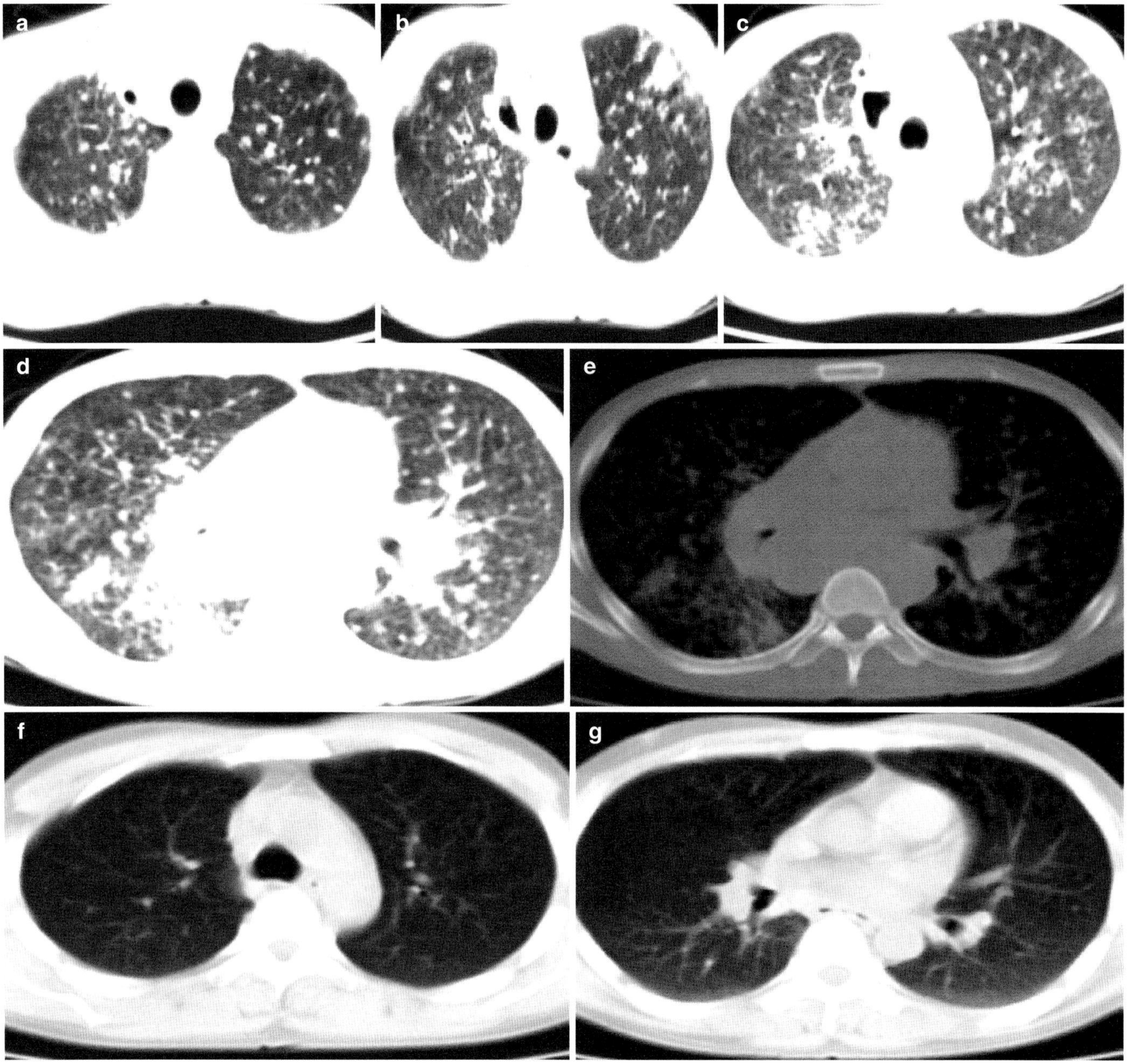

Fig. 5.21 A male patient aged 33 years with AIDS complicated by tuberculosis. (**a**–**e**) Chest CT scan showed multiple patches of and nodular opacities at the upper and middle lobes of both lungs and mass-like high density and opacity at right lung hilum. (**f**, **g**) Reexamination after antituberculosis therapy for 6 months displayed almost complete absorption of lesions

interstitial lesions that can be hardly distinguished from typical PCP. Pathologically, *Cytomegalovirus* pneumonia is characterized by diffuse alveolar lesion, pulmonary interstitial edema, and hematogenous random distribution of nodules. Radiologically, the disease is characterized by reticular or network-like nodules, ground glass opacity, and air cavity consolidation. By antiviral therapy, the lesions are absorbed slowly. CT scan displayed extensive fibrosis in both lungs, with pleural arc-like opacity, thickened interlobular septum, and grid-like opacity (Fig. 5.29).

Bacterial Infection

Rhodococcus equi Infection

By CT scan, pulmonary *Rhodococcus equi* infection is characterized by segmental consolidation with singular or multiple cavities, commonly with the upper lung lobes involved (Fig. 5.30). HRCT demonstrated centrilobular nodules and tree-bud sign, with manifestations of air cavity consolidation, ground glass opacity, centrilobular nodules and tree-bud sign. Recent studies have demonstrated that about 60 %

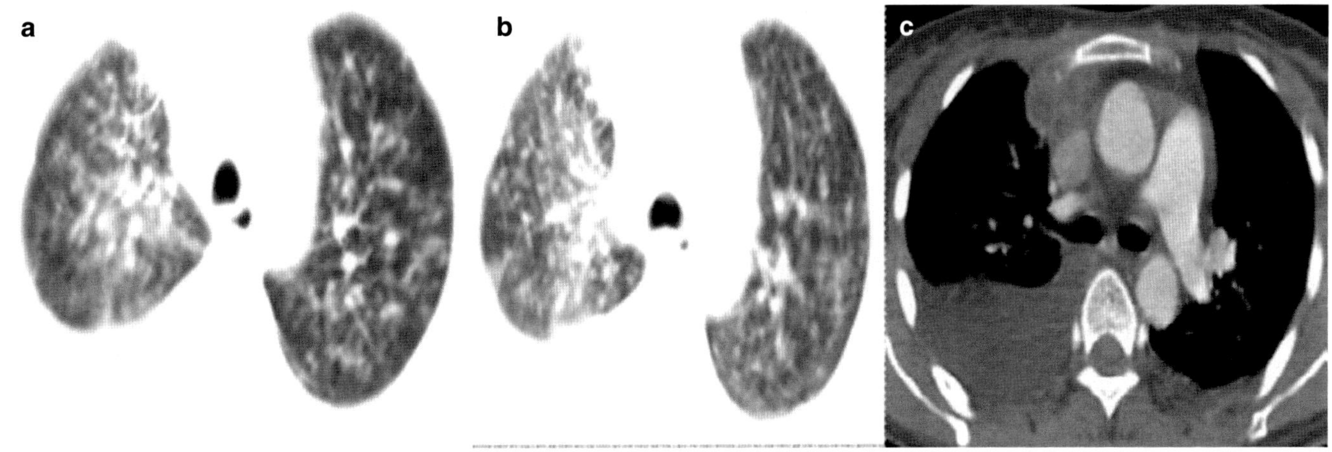

Fig. 5.22 (**a**–**c**) A male patient aged 33 years with AIDS complicated by pulmonary cryptococcosis. Chest CT showed patches and nodular blurry opacities at both lungs, mediastinal lymphadenectasis, and pleural effusion

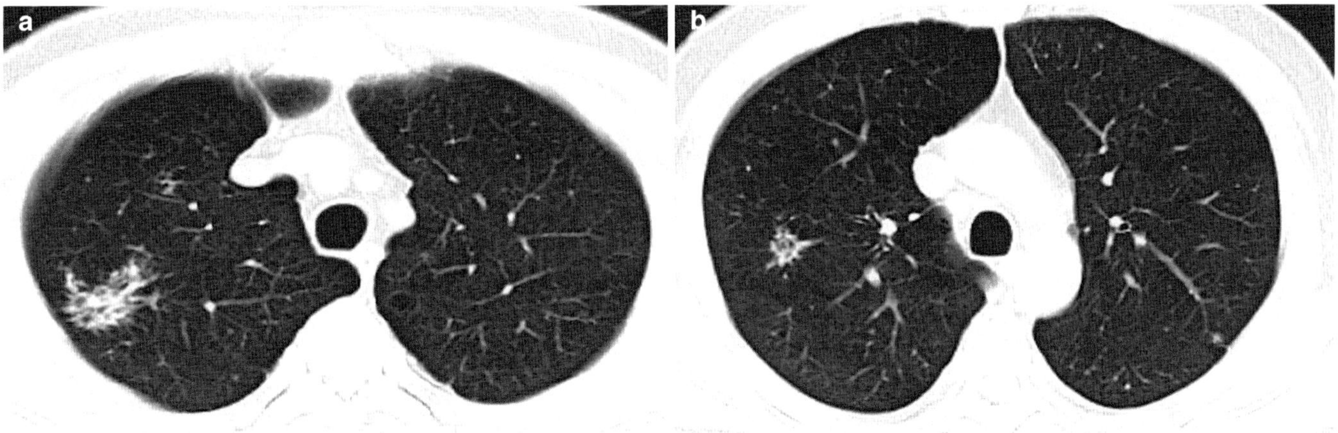

Fig. 5.23 (**a**, **b**) A patient with AIDS complicated by lung histoplasmosis. Chest CT scan displayed spots and grid-like opacity as well as small nodular lesions at the left upper lung

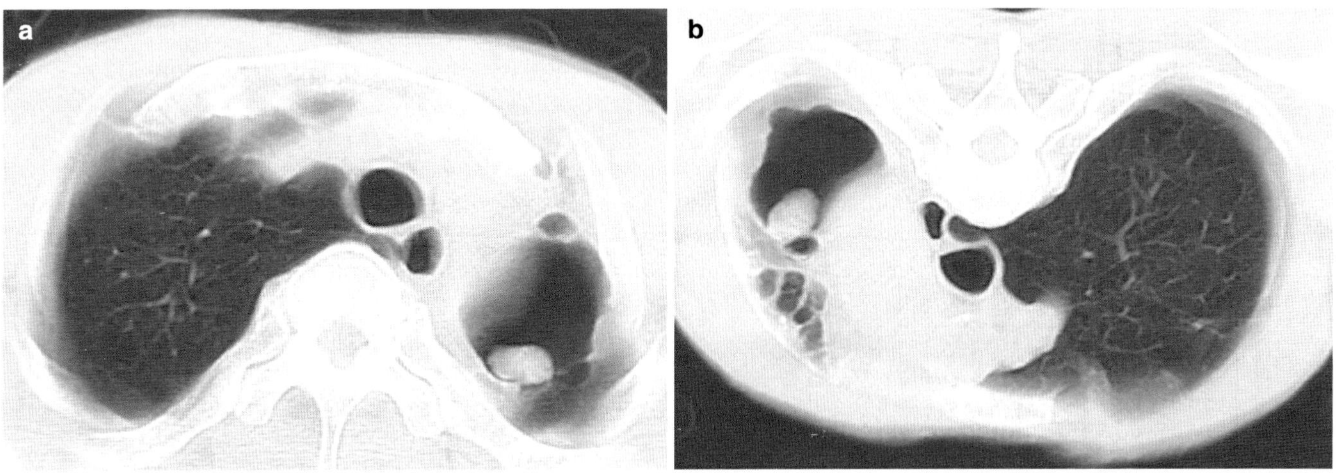

Fig. 5.24 (**a**, **b**) A male patient aged 63 years with AIDS complicated by *Aspergillus* infection. Aspergilloma in the cavity was demonstrated to be mobile along with posture change

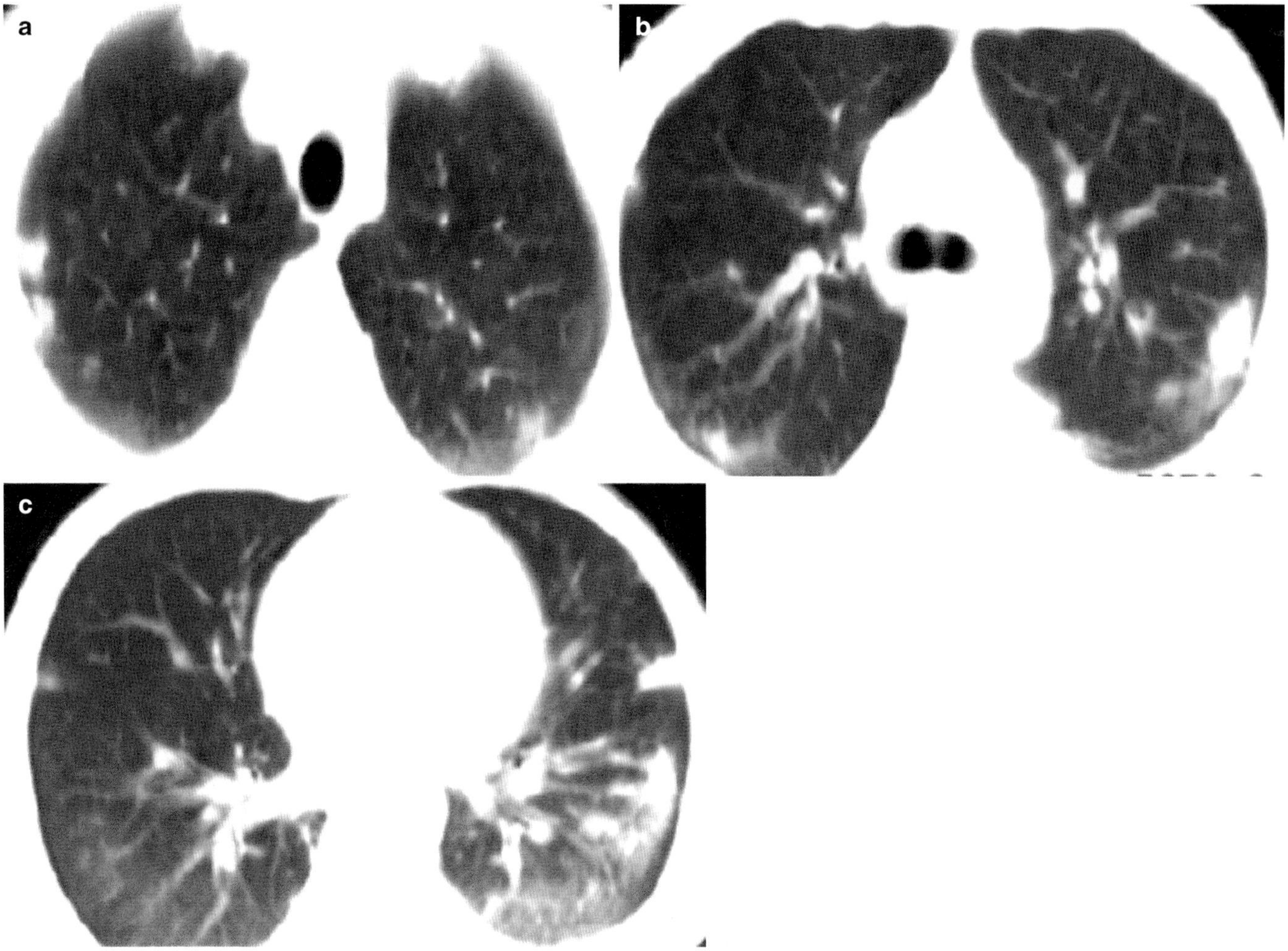

Fig. 5.25 (**a–c**) A male patient aged 31 years with AIDS complicated by *Candida albicans* infection. The pathogen was detected by bronchofiberscope sputum culture. Chest CT scan showed small flaky consolidation and ground glass opacity in both lungs, which was more commonly found at peripheral lungs and under the pleura

of cases with pulmonary *Rhodococcus equi* infection can be displayed with centrilobular nodules and tree-bud sign that are mainly distributed around the consolidation area. It was speculated that the two signs may be caused by dissemination of endobronchial infection. Wicky et al. reported that the multiple nodules have a diameter of 5–20 mm, commonly accompanied by cavity. The condition develops into pulmonary abscess in 5–30 % of the patients, which is commonly singular. By chest CT scan, pulmonary abscess was displayed as round-like thick-wall abscess cavity, possibly with fluid-fluid level inside and irregular lining.

Other Bacterial Infection

AIDS-associated bacterial pneumonia radiologically resembles to bacterial pneumonia in patients with normal immunity. Most cases of streptococcal and *Haemophilus influenza* pneumonia are demonstrated with unilateral focalized segmental or lobar consolidation, occasionally accompanied by pleural effusion. In the cases of pneumonia caused by streptococcus infection, the most common radiological demonstrations include ground glass opacity, grid-like opacity, and lung consolidation at the singular or multiple lung lobes, regardless of the patients' immunity. AIDS complicated by *Staphylococcus aureus* infection is radiologically displayed as multiple pulmonary cavities and nodules. By chest CT, the lesions were demonstrated as segmental/lobar consolidation or lobular infiltration, with singular or multiple lung air sacs or cavities. *Staphylococcus aureus* pneumonia is radiologically characterized by pulmonary infiltration, lung abscess, lung air sac, and empyema/pyopneumothorax. *Pseudomonas aeruginosa* infection is commonly displayed as hollow nodule opacity and mass-like opacity (Fig. 5.31, 5.32, and 5.33)

Klebsiellar pneumonia is radiologically displayed as scattering patches and flakes of high density and opacity at both lungs, some of which are poorly defined. There may be also

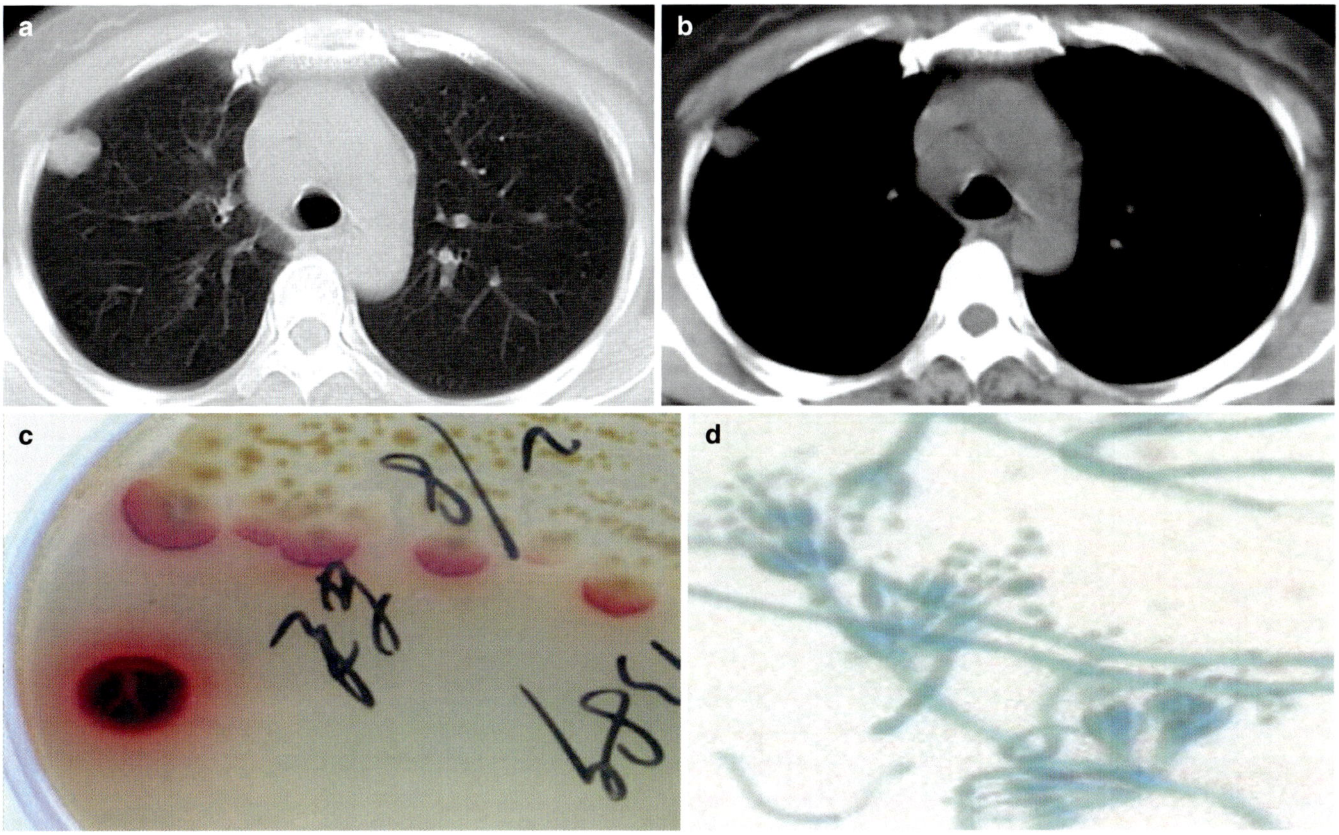

Fig. 5.26 A female patient aged 46 years with AIDS complicated by *Penicillium marneffei* infection. (**a**, **b**) CT scan showed a small nodule under the pleura in the right lung. By tissue culture following puncture, *Penicillium marneffei* was detected. (**c**, **d**) In Sabouraud agar medium at 25 °C, specific rose-colored colony was found to diffuse in the medium. By bacteria culture, characteristic broom-shaped branches were observable

lung air sac shadows and calcified mediastinal lymph nodes. By chest CT scan, Baumannii pneumonia resembles to common bronchopneumonia, predominantly with ground glass opacity. Baumannii pneumonia may also be demonstrated with lobar or flaky infiltration as well as radiological signs of lung abscess and pleuritis (Figs. 5.34 and 5.35).

5.7.1.2 Neoplasm

Kaposi's Sarcoma

Clinically, about 25 % of patients with Kaposi's sarcoma have their lungs involved, whose occurrence is commonly followed by occurrence of skin or mucosa Kaposi's sarcoma. Kaposi's sarcoma is commonly disseminated via lymphatic vessels to invade the interlobular septum, peribronchovascular tissue, and subpleural interstitium. CT scan showed both pulmonary hili with multiple irregular small nodular infiltrations, which is typically lung Kaposi's sarcoma. Nodular thickening at peribronchial and subpleural tissues as well as in lung fissures is a common sign of lung Kaposi's sarcoma. In addition, lymphadenectasis and pleural fluid can also be radiologically demonstrated (Fig. 5.36).

Malignant Lymphoma

In AIDS patients at the advanced stage, the incidence rate AIDS-associated lymphoma is 5–20 %, and non-Hodgkin's B-cell lymphoma (NHL) is the most common. The second common AIDS-associated lymphoma is Burkitt's lymphoma. Other AIDS-associated lymphomas include T-cell lymphoma and non-B-/non-T-cell lymphoma.

Chest CT showed the morphology of the lesions to be nodular or mass-like. By HRCT, ground glass opacity around the nodular or mass-like opacity can be demonstrated, namely, the halo sign. In addition, HRCT also showed air bronchogram sign and/or cavity in the lesions. It has been found that most cases have unilateral or bilateral hilar and mediastinal lymphadenectasis and pleural effusion. In some cases, AIDS-associated lymphoma occurs at the axillary fossa (Figs. 5.37 and 5.38).

Generally, the complications in the chest of AIDS patients may be infective or noninfective, whose radiological demonstrations may be typical, atypical, or even negative. For the cases with atypical radiological and clinical manifestations or with suspected multiple complications, biopsy following puncture or bronchofibroscopy should be performed as early as possible to define the diagnosis.

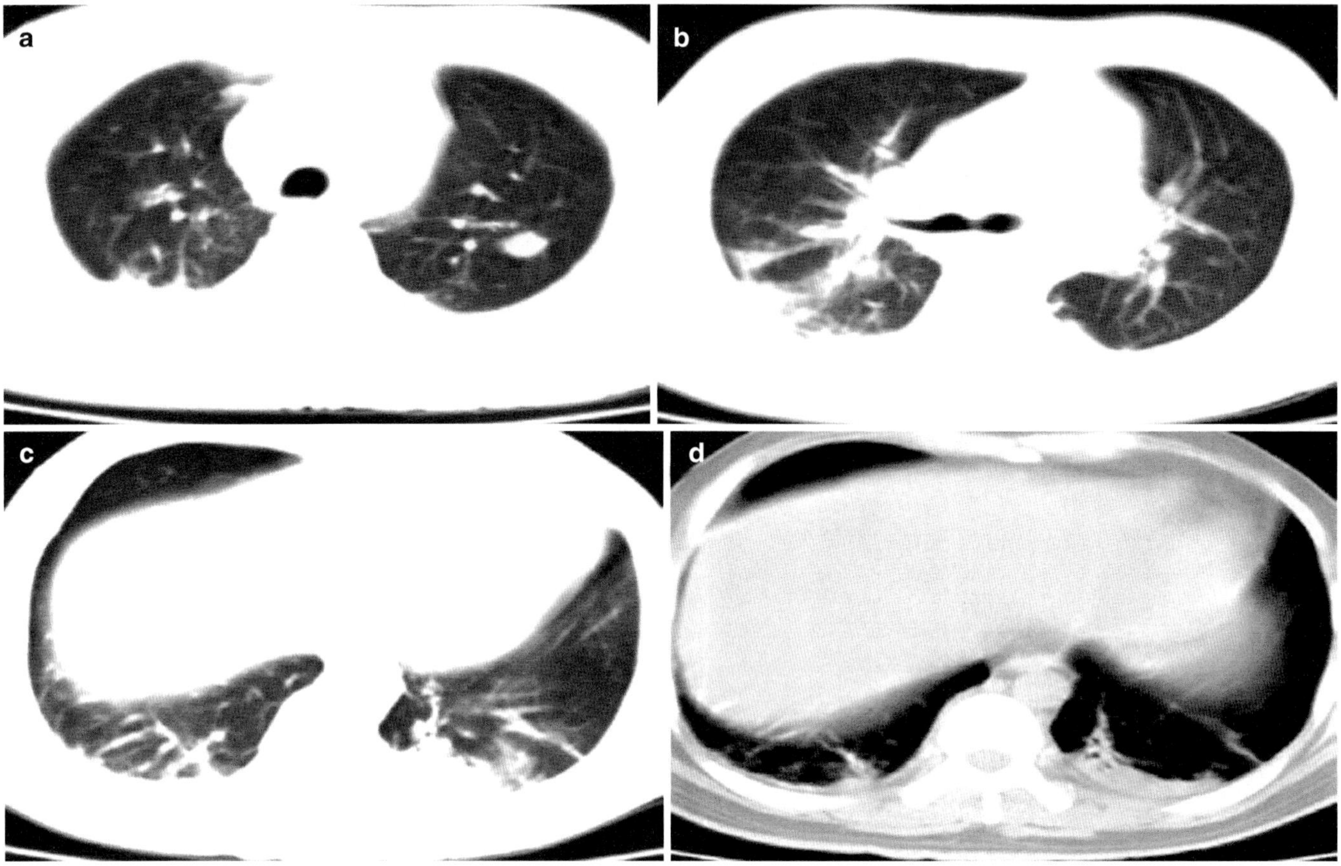

Fig. 5.27 (**a–d**) A female patient aged 40 years with AIDS complicated by *Penicillium marneffei* infection. The lesions were displayed as nodular and strips of shadows, predominantly flaky consolidation opacity at the posterior segment of both lower lungs

5.7.2 Abdomen

5.7.2.1 Gastrointestinal and Retroperitoneal Complications

Gastrointestinal Complications

In patients with AIDS, *Candida albicans*, *Mycobacterium tuberculosis*, *Penicillium marneffei*, and cytomegalovirus can induce gastrointestinal inflammation to complicate AIDS. The inflammation can be caused by one kind of pathogen or simultaneously by different pathogens.

Candida albicans is a type of conditional pathogenic fungus, which is pathogenic to induce infection in people with compromised immunity or imbalanced bacterial colonies. The lesions are commonly found at the oral cavity, throat, and esophagus, with the lungs sometimes involved. Gastrointestinal X-ray showed brush sign, lace sign, and cobblestone sign, which are characteristic X-ray demonstrations of the infection. Gas barium double-contrast radiology showed deranged mucosal structure, with different-sized and diverse-shaped filling defects and niche signs (Fig. 5.39).

Penicillium marneffei in the lungs mainly causes damages to the reticular endothelial system, which is disseminated along with blood flow or lymph flow. In addition to radiological abnormalities at the lungs, the abdominal lymph nodes and intestinal mesentery may also be demonstrated with lesions, specifically lymphadenectasis and intestinal wall edema and adhesion (Fig. 5.40).

Peritoneal and Retroperitoneal Infection

Esophageal tuberculosis rarely occurs, arising from adjacent mediastinal lymph nodes or intrapulmonary lesions. Tuberculosis with small intestinal involvement can be demonstrated with segmental ulceration, thickened intestinal wall, intestinal stenosis, and mass-like lesions, which may be complicated by fistula, obstruction, perforation, and bleeding. In addition to lung infection, tuberculosis often invades retroperitoneal lymph nodes and mesentery. CT scan showed mild intestinal dilatation, regular or irregular thickening of the small intestinal folds, and enlarged lymph nodes with fusion. Abdominal contrast CT scan showed ring-shaped enhancement of the enlarged lymph nodes that is located at the mesentery or retroperitoneum to induce separation of intestinal loop (Fig. 5.41, 5.42, and 5.43).

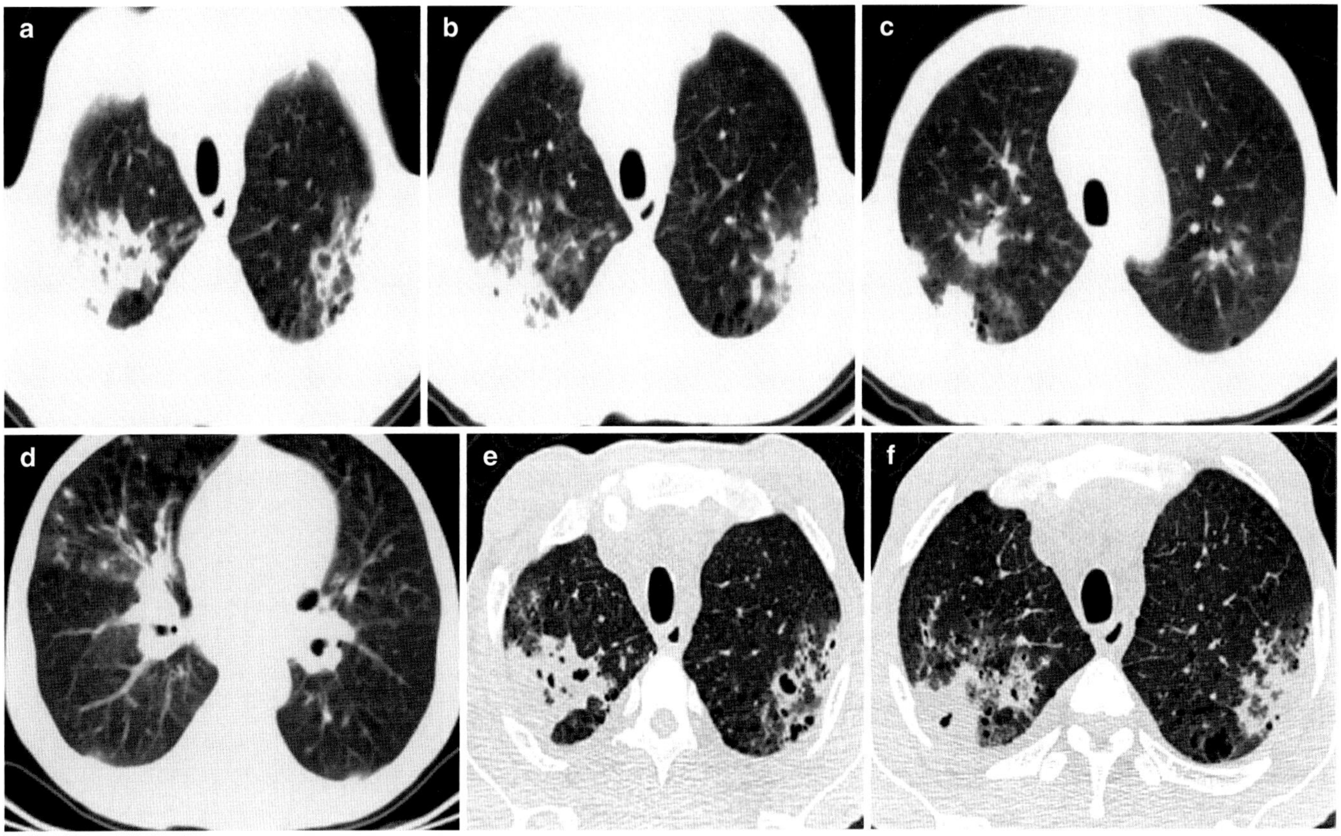

Fig. 5.28 A male patient aged 34 years with AIDS (C3) complicated by mucormycosis. His CD4+cell count was 22/uL, and CD4+/CD8+ was 0.35. By culture of alveolar lavage liquid, mucor infection was defined. (**a–d**) Pulmonary window of CT scan showed multiple poorly defined patchy and nodular increased density shadows at the apicoposterior segment of both upper lung lobes and the right middle lung lobe. (**e**, **f**) HRCT showed multiple small cavities in the lesions and minor bronchial dilation, multiple small air sacs at the peripheral lung tissues, and slight ground glass opacity around the lesions

She complained of intermittent diarrhea for 6 months, weight loss for 46 days, and fever for 2 days. Abdominal CT scan showed extensive enlarged lymph nodes with fusion and intestinal adhesion.

5.7.2.2 Complications in the Liver, Gallbladder, Pancreas, and Spleen

Infection

Tuberculosis

In the cases of AIDS complicated by tuberculosis, most have extrapulmonary infiltration in the liver, spleen, lymph nodes, central nervous system, skeleton, gastrointestinal tract, and kidney. In some cases, no lesions of tuberculosis can be found in the lungs. In most cases, tuberculosis is displayed as focal infection, occurring before the immunity is seriously suppressed. CT scan showed multiple low-density lesions at the liver, spleen, pancreas, and kidney, with mesentery and peritoneal lymphadenectasis. Central necrosis can be found at the enlarged lymph nodes, and segmental thickening of the ileum wall can be also observed. Typical CT demonstrations include central low density and surrounding ring-shaped enhancement (Fig. 5.44).

Bacterial Abscess

The patients with AIDS, especially intravenous drug abusers, are susceptible to sepsis and abscess. And the most common pathogenic bacteria are *Staphylococcus aureus* and *Streptococcus*. The liver, spleen, lung, and kidney can be infected due to the hematogenous dissemination of the pathogen. The radiological findings are nonspecific (Fig. 5.45).

Fungal Infection

Fungal infection is common in patients with AIDS, but it rarely involves the liver and spleen. *Aspergillus* infection could induce multiple abscesses in the liver, spleen, pancreas, and kidney, with low-density lesions and bull's-eye sign by CT scan. Compared to lesions of liver abscess in patients with normal immunity, liver abscess complicating AIDS is characterized by large abscess cavity, more obvious local inflammatory response, and radiological inconsistency with clinical symptoms (Fig. 5.46).

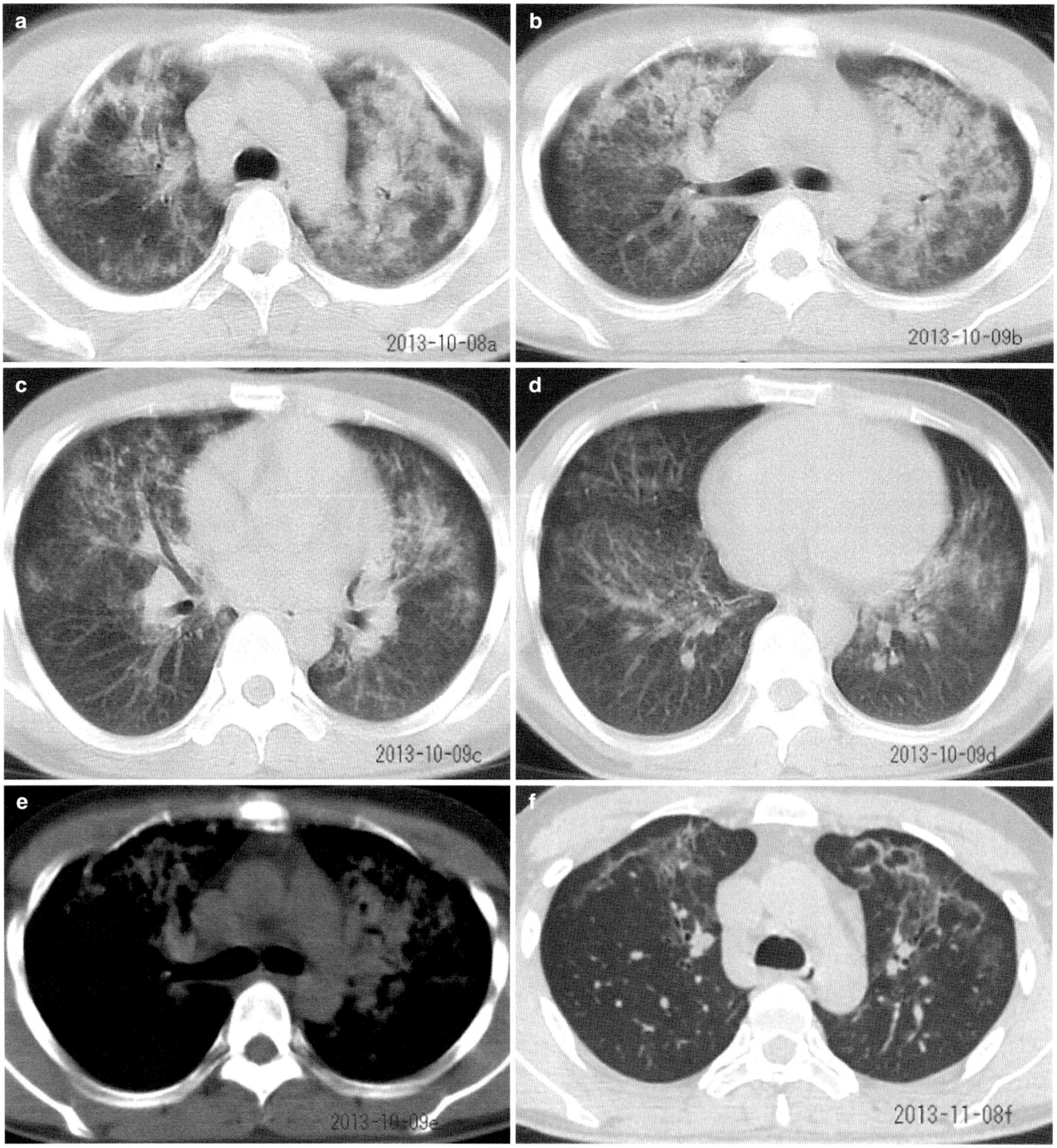

Fig. 5.29 A male patient aged 56 years with AIDS complicated by cytomegalovirus pneumonia. (**a–d**) Pulmonary window by CT scan displayed extensive ground glass opacity and consolidation at both lungs, predominantly at the upper lungs. (**e**) Mediastinal window by CT scan showed irregular patches of consolidation in the upper lungs. (**f–h**) Reexamination after antiviral therapy for 1 month, the consolidation and ground glass opacity in both lungs were shown to be obviously absorbed. Bilateral upper and middle lung lobes were displayed with thickened interlobular septum, subpleural arc-shaped opacity, and grid-like fiber strip opacity that were predominantly under the anterior pleura

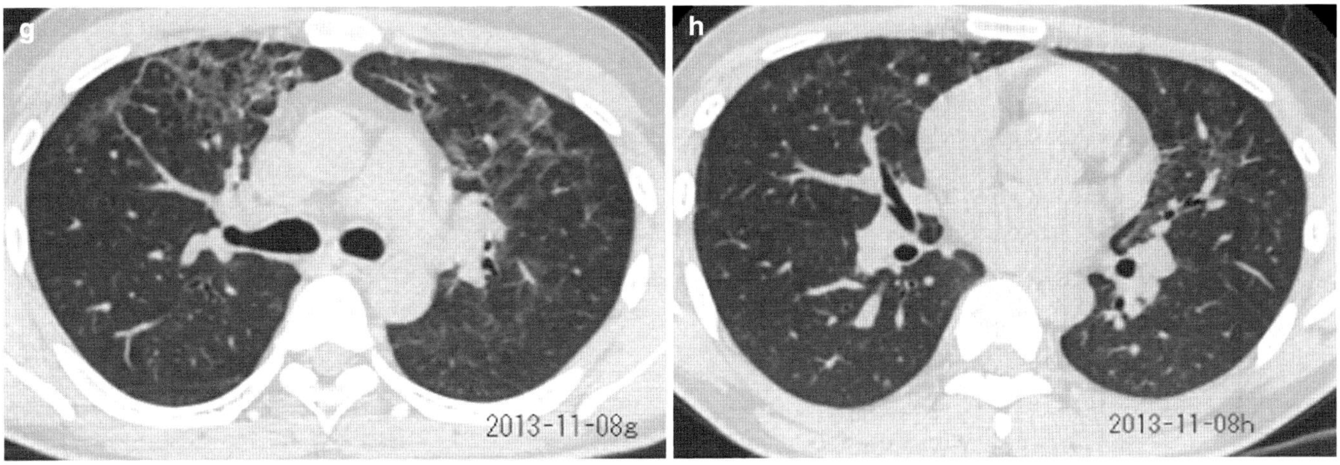

Fig. 5.29 (continued)

5.7.2.3 Neoplasm

Kaposi's sarcoma and lymphoma are common, which may involve the liver and spleen. However, they are commonly a part of multiple systems involvement, rarely occurring alone.

Kaposi's Sarcoma

Kaposi's sarcoma involves the liver, commonly resulting in slight increase of blood alkaline phosphatase but no clinical symptoms. Kaposi's sarcoma is distributed along the vascular vessels of the infiltrated organs, and the invaded lymph nodes are shown with high density. CT scans showed multiple low-density small nodular lesions that tend to distribute around the liver hilus, liver capsule, and perihepatic portal vein, and irregular enlargement of the vascular branches shadows in the liver parenchyma. Contrast scanning in the early stage demonstrated multiple low-density small nodular lesions around the liver hilus, liver capsule, and perihepatic portal vein. In addition to lesions in the liver, Kaposi's sarcoma could also invade the muscles and corresponding soft tissues, with high-density nodule opacity in the soft tissues (Fig. 5.47).

Lymphoma

Compared to non-AIDS-associated lymphoma, lymphoma in patients with AIDS has higher malignancy and poorer prognosis and is more aggressive to abdominal organs. Radiologically, swollen liver, spleen, and kidney are demonstrated. CT scan showed the lesions as multiple nodules or mass opacity with low density but mostly well defined. The lesions may be displayed with lobulation and in some cases multiple round or round-like opacity. In some large lesions, central necrosis can be observed. By contrast scan, the lesions were demonstrated with no or slight enhancement at the arterial phase and better defined lesions at the venous phase with no or slight homogeneous enhancement. The density of lesions is lower than that of liver parenchyma (Fig. 5.48).

5.7.3 Central Nervous System

AIDS-associated central nervous system diseases can be categorized into the following 4 types: HIV infection, opportunistic infection, neoplasm, and other diseases.

5.7.3.1 HIV Infection

HIV is neurotropic and can invade the central nervous system at the early stage of HIV infection to induce acute aseptic meningitis or cerebropathy. Clinically, the patients experience progressive dementia, disturbance in thinking, delayed response, language and motor impairment, concentration inability, and memory loss. HIV infection of the central nervous system can be divided into 2 stages: the asymptomatic early stage and the stage of progressive subacute encephalitis and cerebral atrophy. The first stage is radiologically characterized by multiple white matter lesions in size of lower than 1 cm and demyelination. Cerebral atrophy at the second stage can be sufficiently displayed by MRI and CT, which is commonly central cerebral atrophy and rarely peripheral cerebral cortical atrophy. By radiology, the typical demonstration is diffuse white matter lesion. Demyelination caused by HIV infection has more diffusive and symmetric lesions, which are mostly located adjacent to cerebral ventricles and progress into extensively fused lesion. By plain CT scan, the lesions were demonstrated with low density, while by MRI, with hypointense T1WI signal and hyperintense T2WI signal. The lesions are commonly shown with no space-occupying effect and enhancement (Fig. 5.49).

5.7.3.2 Opportunistic Infection

Toxoplasmosis

MRI displayed multiple lesions, with the deep gray nucleus and interface of gray and white matters involved. Other common sites with lesion include the posterior cranial fossa,

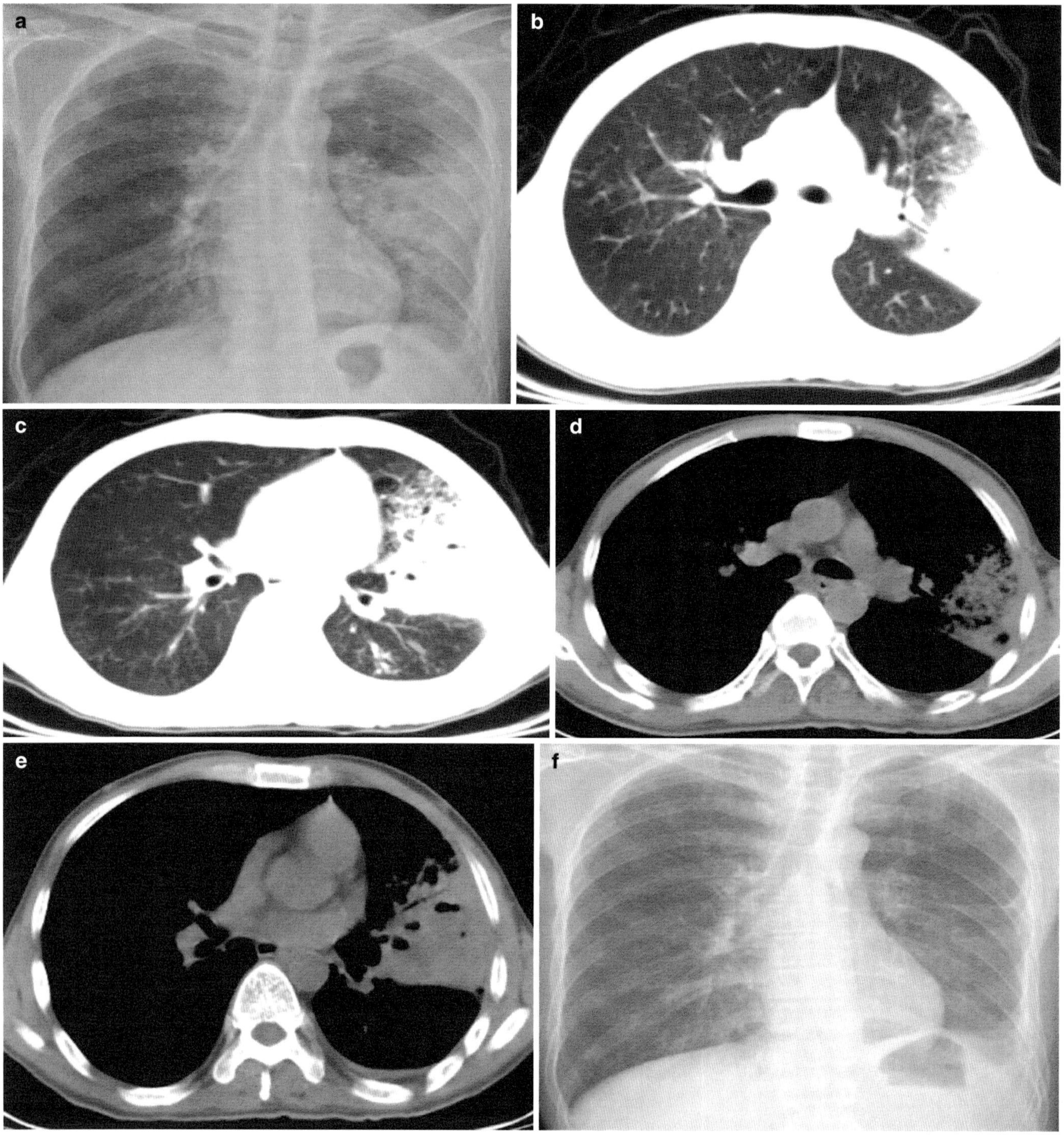

Fig. 5.30 A male patient aged 41 years with AIDS (C3) complicated by *Rhodococcus equi*. infection. CD4+cell count was 77/uL. By cultures of blood and alveolar lavage fluid, the pathogen was defined to be *Rhodococcus equi*. (**a**) Chest X-ray showed a poorly defined large flake of increased density and opacity at the lingual segment of the left upper lung lobe, with small patches of low-density area inside that unevenly distributed and thickened left pleura. (**b–e**) Chest CT scan showed a large area of consolidation at the lingual segment of the left upper lung lobe that was segmentally distributed, with patches of low-density area and small cavities and spots of increased density and opacity at the left lower lung lobe. (**f**) Reexamination after treatment for 10 months, the lesions at the left lung were demonstrated to be almost absorbed. However, rare cords like high density and opacity were locally displayed, with well-defined boundary

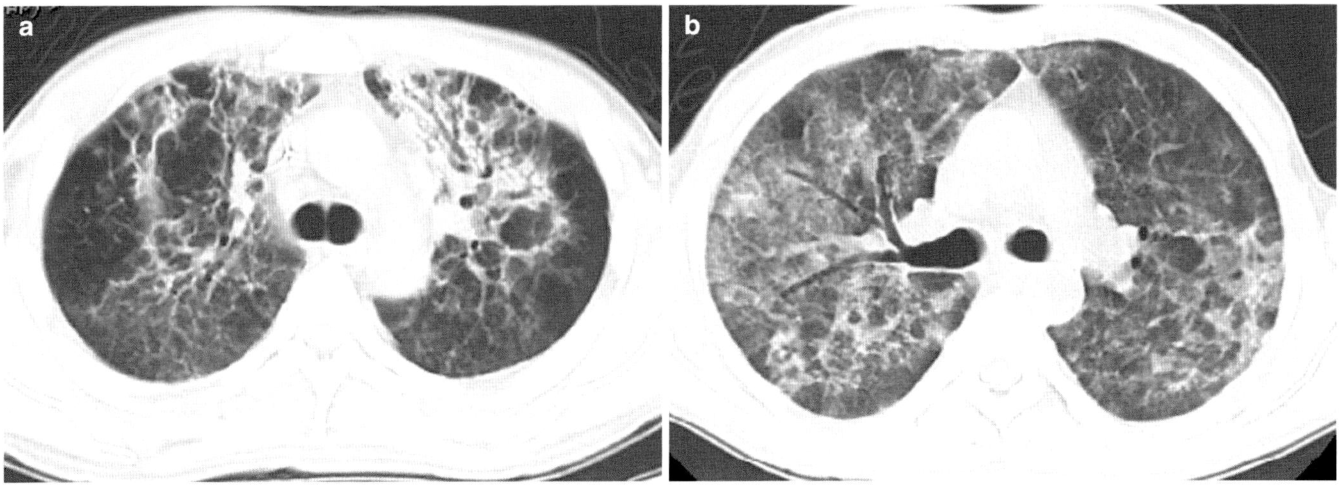

Fig. 5.31 (**a**, **b**) A male patient aged 39 years with AIDS complicated by group A streptococcal infection. Both lungs were demonstrated with ground glass opacity and large grid-like high density and opacity

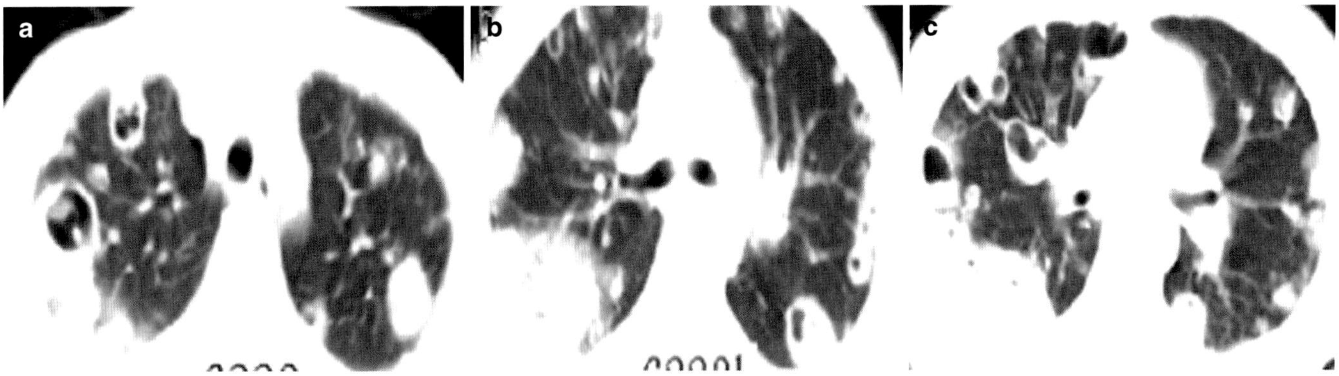

Fig. 5.32 (**a–c**) A female patient aged 35 years with AIDS complicated by *Staphylococcus aureus* pneumonia. By culture of pleural fluid, *Staphylococcus aureus* was detected. Both lungs were demonstrated with multiple cavities and nodules

cerebral cortex, and paraventricular white matter. The lesions are shown with isointense or hypointense T1WI signal and hypointense signal or hyperintense T2WI signal. Around the lesion, typical edema may occur, whose range is in proportional to the size of lesion, with prominent space-occupying effect. By T2WI, the lesions are sometimes hardly distinguished from surrounding edema. Contrast MR imaging demonstrates characteristic enhancement of the lesions, specifically full enhancement of nodules with a size of less than 1 cm and thin ring-shaped enhancement of nodules with a size of over 1 cm. In the cases with seriously compromised cellular immunity, the enhanced ring is shown to be extremely thin that can hardly be observable or even absent. Sometimes spots of hemorrhage can be shown within lesion. MRI also plays important role in assessing therapeutic efficacy during follow-ups after anti-*Toxoplasma gondii* therapy. The lesions are commonly shown with obvious improvement within 2-week treatment, but their complete disappearance may need 3–6-month treatment. However, calcification, brain atrophy, and glial scar commonly remain. MRS is valuable in differential diagnosis of AIDS complicated by lump and infection. MRS demonstrates toxoplasma encephalitis with low choline peak value and N-acetylaspartic acid level, but high levels of Lip and Cr. However, both toxoplasma encephalitis and tuberculous encephalitis are inflammatory granuloma. The value of MRS in defining the pathogen and their differential diagnosis still needs to be assessed (Figs. 5.50 and 5.51)

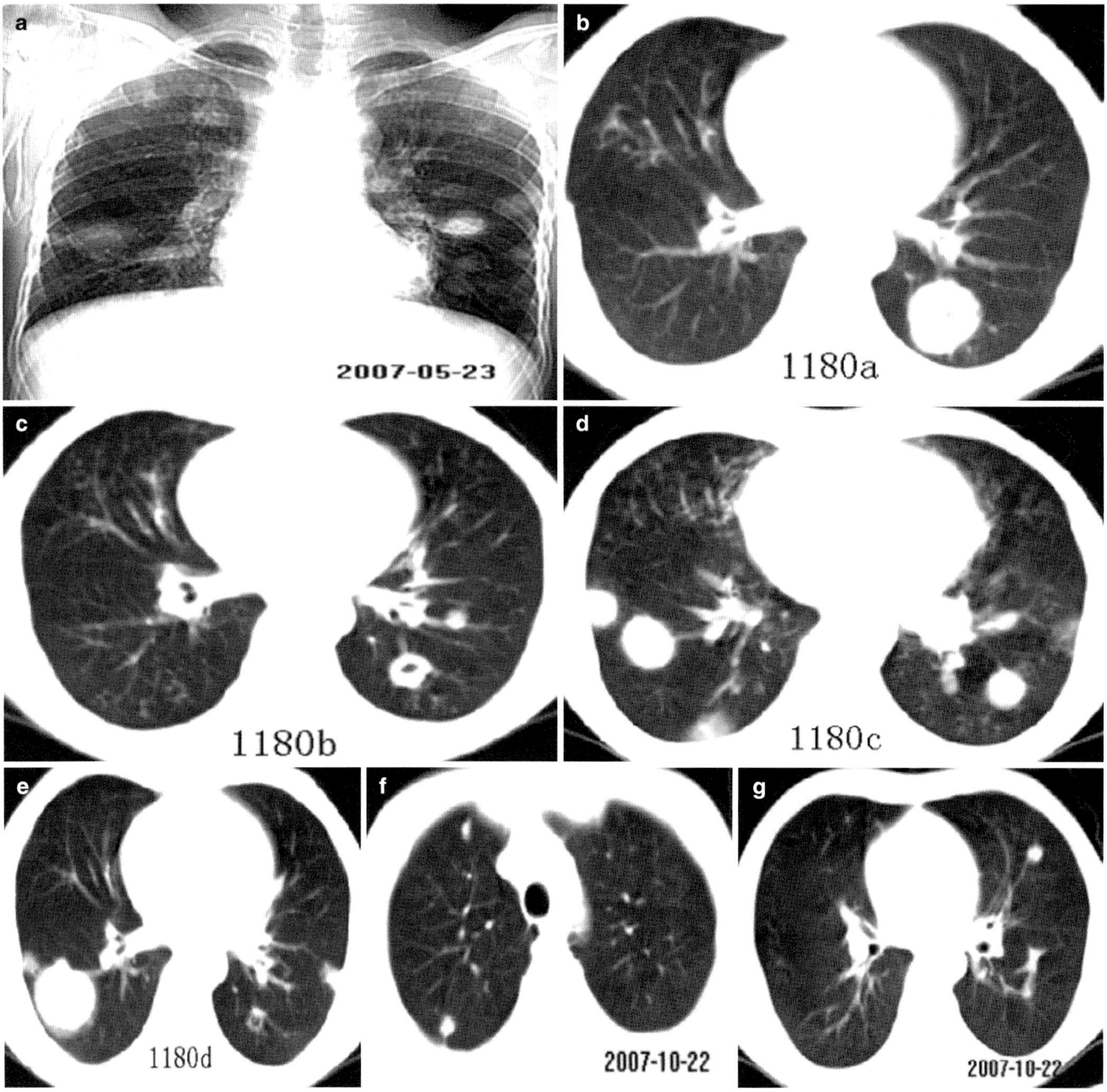

Fig. 5.33 (**a–g**) A male patient aged 38 years with AIDS complicated by *Pseudomonas aeruginosa* infection. (**a**) Chest X-ray showed multiple-nodule opacity. (**b–e**) Chest CT scan showed both lungs with multiple nodules and hollow nodules in different sizes. (**f, g**) Reexamination after treatment for 4 months demonstrated obvious shrinkage and absorption of the lesions

Fungal Infection

In patients with AIDS, cryptococcosis and histoplasmosis are common fungal infection of the central nervous system. Clinically, both are manifested as meningitis with or without brain parenchyma involved. Fungal meningitis is commonly demonstrated with extensive nodular enhancement in basal cistern and accompanying communicating hydrocephalus. The infection disseminates via perivascular space to cause lesions at the basal ganglia or choroid plexus, such as ischemia, encephalitis, and gelatinous pseudocyst. Fungal

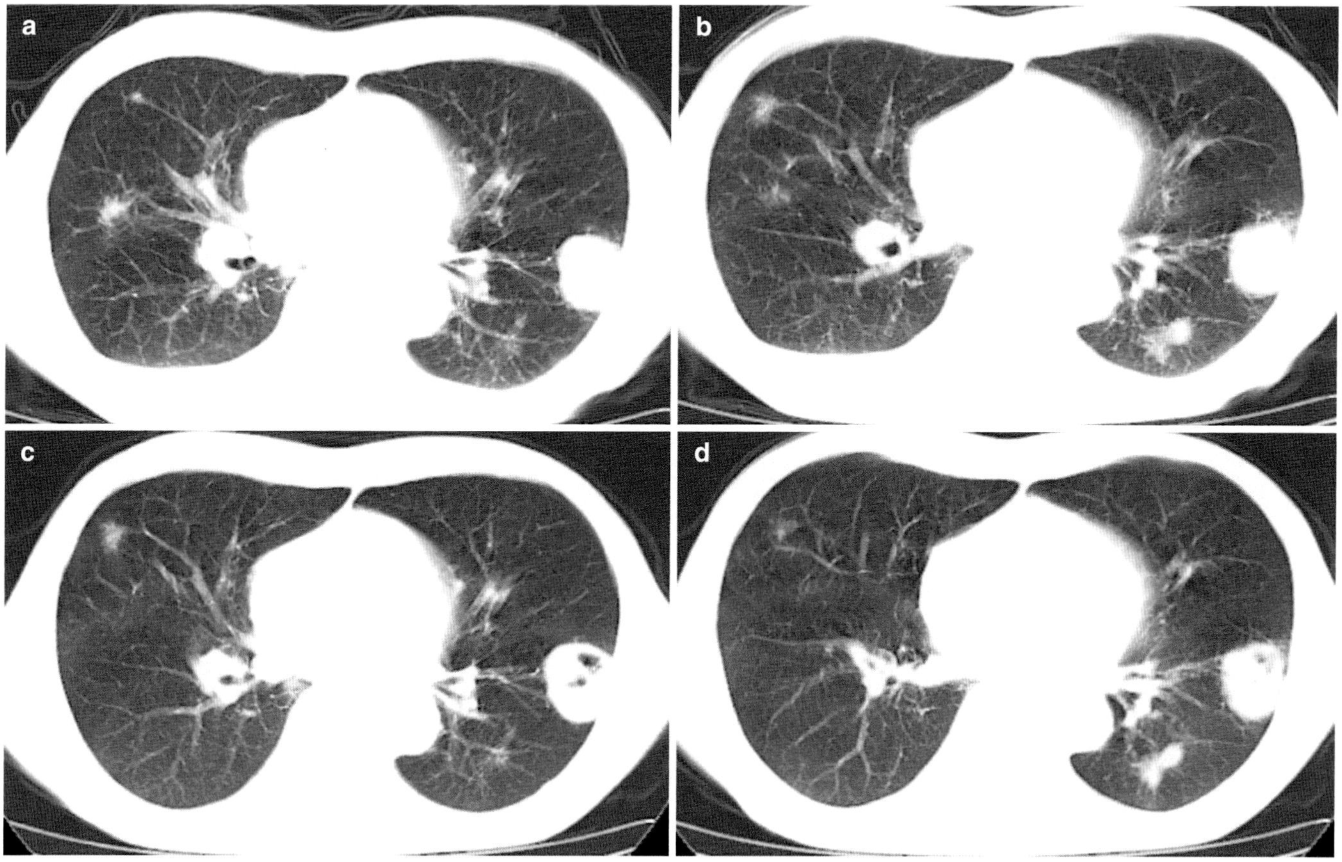

Fig. 5.34 (**a–d**) A male patient aged 70 years with AIDS complicated by *Klebsiella* infection. The patient was HIV positive (+) and his CD4 cell count was 59/ul. By culture of sputum, *Klebsiella* was detected. (**a, b**) Chest CT scan showed both lungs with multiple spots, flakes, and patches of heterogeneously high density and opacity. (**c, d**) Reexamination by chest CT scan after treatment for 18 days showed that the lesions at both lungs were improved and absorbed and small air sac in the lesions of the left lung

infection could also involve the spinal cord, with hypointense T1WI signal and hyperintense T2WI signal by MRI as well as surrounding edema. Ring-shaped enhancement of the lesion by contrast imaging indicates possible cryptococcosis of the central nervous system. However, the value of DWI, ADC, FLAIR, and MRS in distinguishing cryptococcosis from other diseases needs to be assessed (Figs. 5.52 and 5.53).

Tuberculosis Infection

In patients with HIV infection or AIDS, the incidence rates of pulmonary tuberculosis and extrapulmonary tuberculosis are increasing. CT and MRI demonstrations of intracranial tuberculosis are diverse, including meningitis, encephalitis, tuberculous granuloma, encephalitis, and brain abscess. Tuberculous meningitis is commonly manifested as extensive nodular enhancement in the basal cistern and accompanying communicating hydrocephalus. MRI showed intracranial lesion with isointense T1WI signal and mixed hypointense and hyperintense T2WI signal. By contrast MR imaging, the lesion is demonstrated with ring-shaped or homogeneous enhancement (Figs. 5.54 and 5.55).

AIDS Complicated by Progressive Multifocal Leukoencephalopathy (PML)

In patients with AIDS, due to their compromised immunity, human papovavirus (abbreviated as JC virus) can be activated to cause progressive multifocal leukoencephalopathy (PML). Its incidence rate in patients with AIDS is about 4 %.

By CT scan, the white matter is shown with multiple patches of low density and opacity that may be fused and is commonly bilaterally asymmetric. The lesion shows no space-occupying effect and no enhancement, which may involve bilateral lateral paraventricular and subcortical white matter. Occasionally, spotlike or ring-shaped enhancement of the lesion can be observed. Along with progress of the condition, the low-density area continues to expand, with manifestation of cerebral atrophy at the advanced stage.

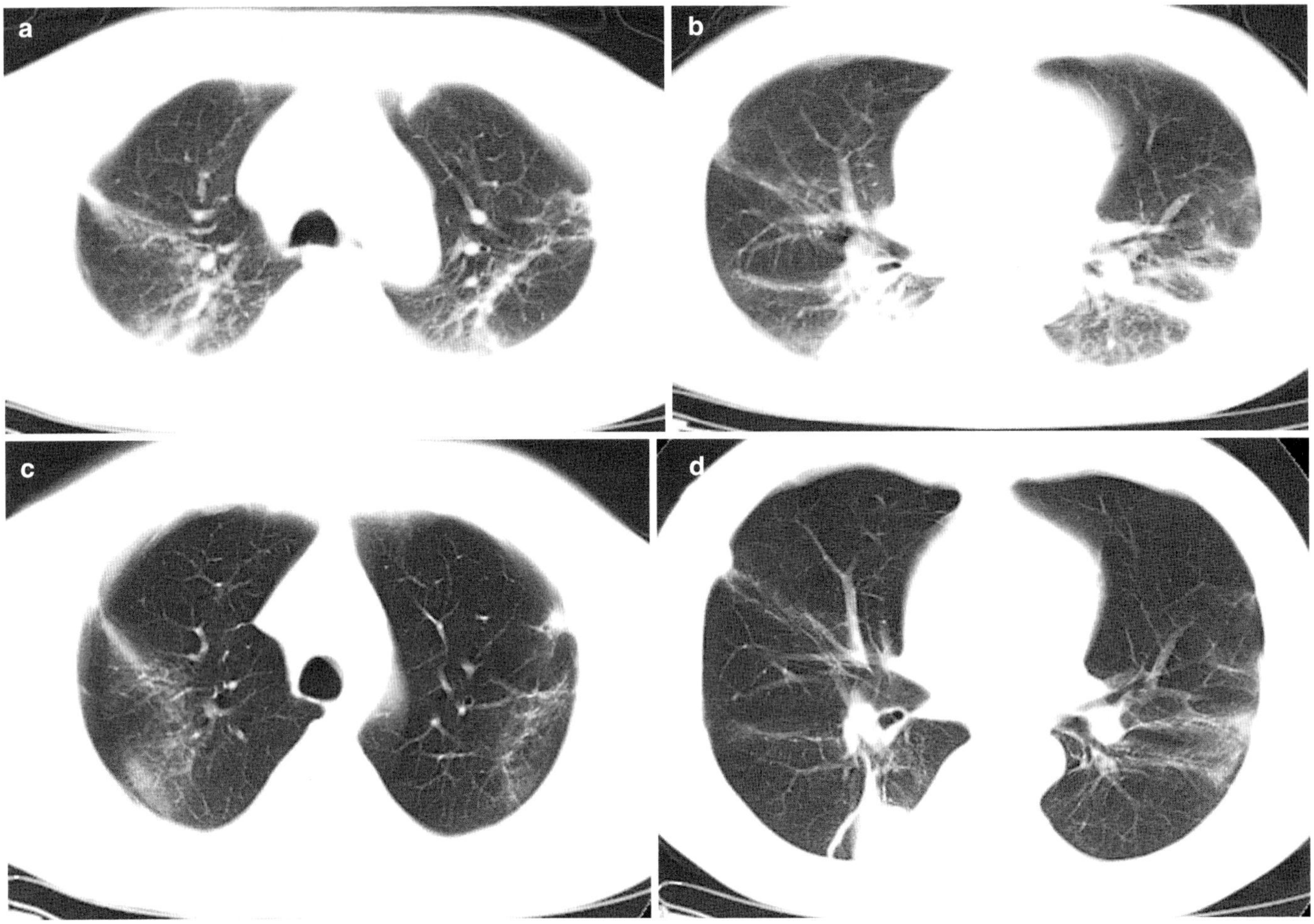

Fig. 5.35 (**a–d**) A male patient aged 49 years with AIDS complicated by baumannii infection. The patient was detected to be HIV positive (+) and his CD4 T-cell count was 772/ul. By culture of sputum, baumannii was detected. (**a**, **b**) Chest CT showed both lungs with flakes of high density and opacity, some of which were ground glass opacity. (**c**, **d**) Reexamination by chest CT scan after treatment for 11 days demonstrated that some of the high-density lesions were absorbed and ground glass opacity at both lungs

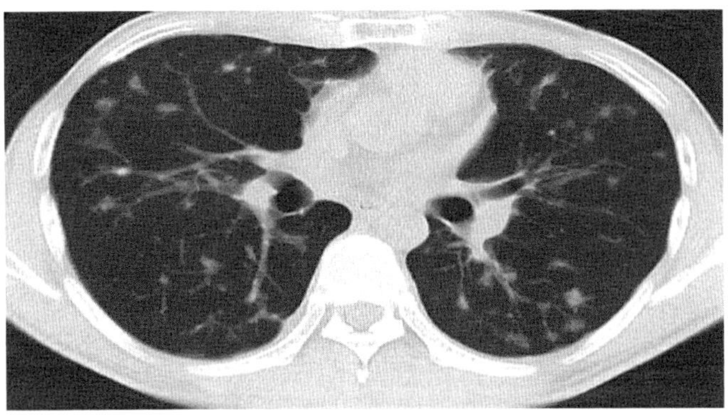

Fig. 5.36 A male patient aged 54 years with AIDS complicated by Kaposi's sarcoma. Both lungs were demonstrated with multiple irregular small nodular density and opacity, which were proved to be lung involvement by Kaposi's sarcoma

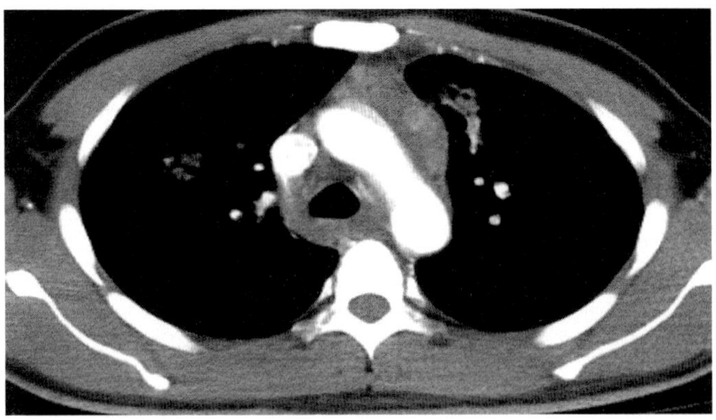

Fig. 5.37 A male patient aged 26 years with AIDS complicated by non-Hodgkin's lymphoma. The diagnosis was defined by pathological examination. The mediastinum was demonstrated with multiple lymphadenectasis that fused into mass, and the bronchus was shown to be compressed

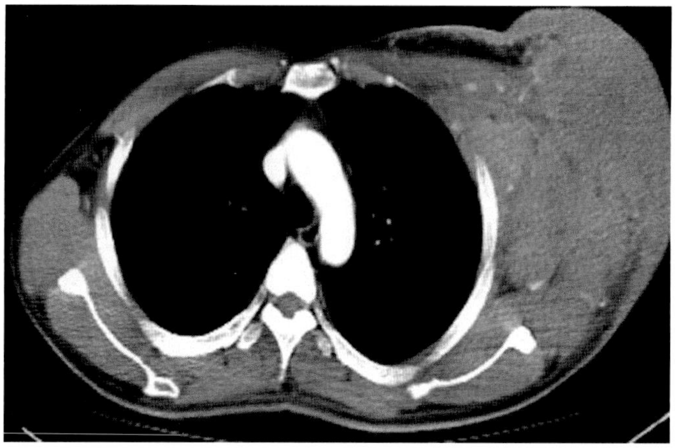

Fig. 5.38 A male patient aged 23 years with AIDS complicated by Burkitt's lymphoma. The left axillary fossa was shown with lymphadenectasis that fused into mass. The diagnosis was pathologically defined to be Burkitt's lymphoma

MRI commonly demonstrates the lesions at the frontal-parietal lobe and the white matter of the temporal lobe, with deep gray matter possibly involved. And about one third of the lesions are located at the posterior cranial fossa of the occipital lobe. It has been reported that the lesions are commonly located at the white matter or interface of gray and white matters where JC virus-infected B-lymphocytes tend to stagnate due to the abundant blood supply. The lesions are displayed with hypointense T1WI signal and hyperintense T2WI signal but no space-occupying effect. However, the lesions tend to be integrated. MR imaging typically demonstrates the lesions with large area of hypointense T1WI signal at the parietal-occipital lobe and hyperintense T2WI signal and well-defined fan-shaped lateral margin of subcortical white matter. In some cases, the lesions are demonstrated as ring shaped, with central hypointense T2WI signal and peripheral hyperintense signal (Fig. 5.56).

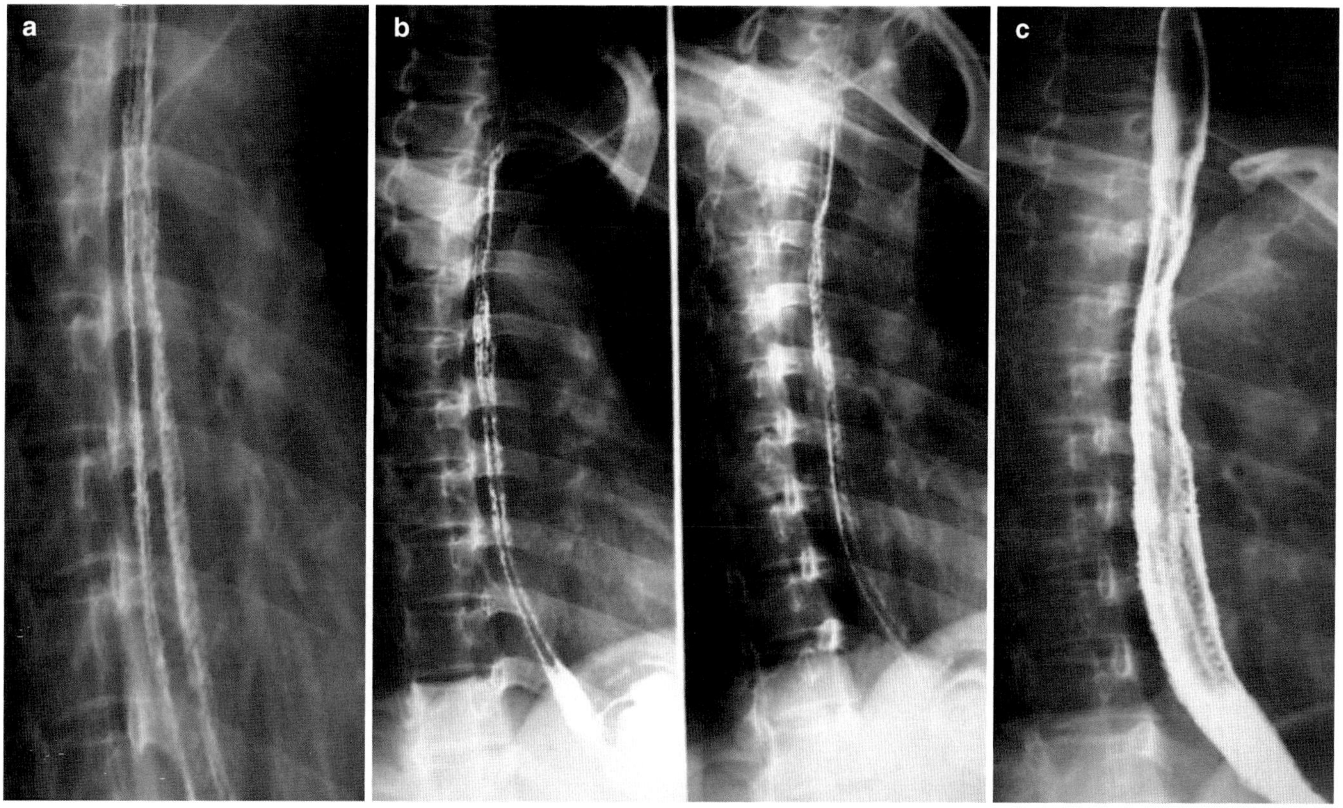

Fig. 5.39 (**a–c**) AIDS complicated by esophageal candidiasis. The esophagus was shown by fMRI with brushlike sign

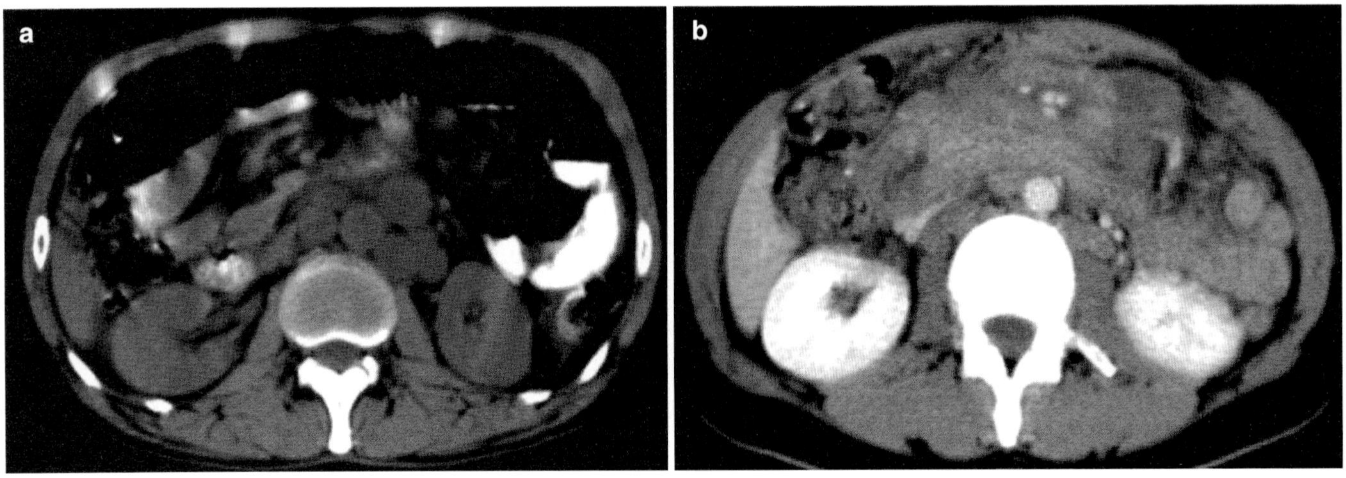

Fig. 5.40 (**a**, **b**) A female patient aged 40 years with AIDS complicated by *Penicillium marneffei* infection. The patient was shown with retroperitoneal lymphadenectasis as well as intestinal canal and mesentery adhesion

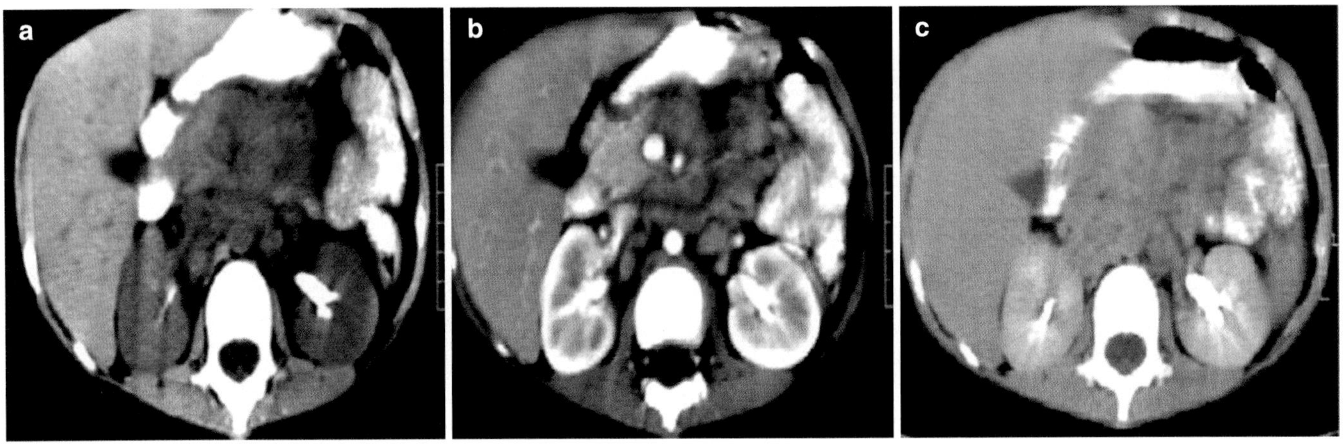

Fig. 5.41 (**a–c**) A boy aged 8 years with complaints of recurrent cough and weight loss for 6 months. His PPD was negative (–) and his CD4 T-cell count was 39/uL. By biopsy of axillary lymph nodes, the diagnosis was defined to be lymphoid tuberculosis. CT scan indicated abdominal lymphadenectasis

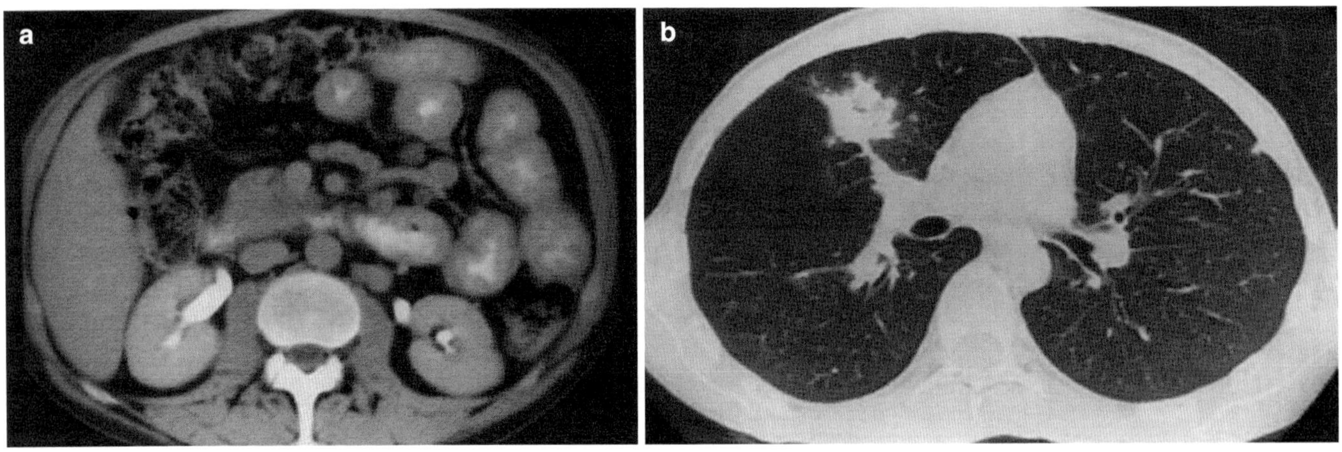

Fig. 5.42 (**a**, **b**) A male patient aged 27 years.(**b**) Contrast CT showed extensive thickening of the jejunal wall and multiple low-density nodules at the mesentery and retroperitoneum, indicating lymphoid tuberculosis. (**b**) Chest CT showed nodules and cavities at the right upper lung

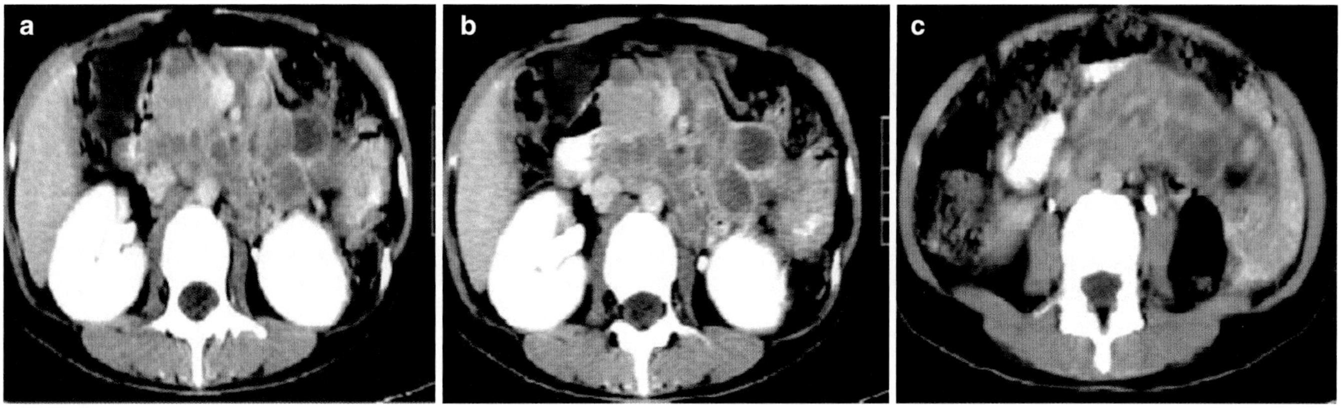

Fig. 5.43 (**a–c**) A female patient aged 25 years with AIDS (stage IV, class C, grade 3) complicated by abdominal lymphoid tuberculosis

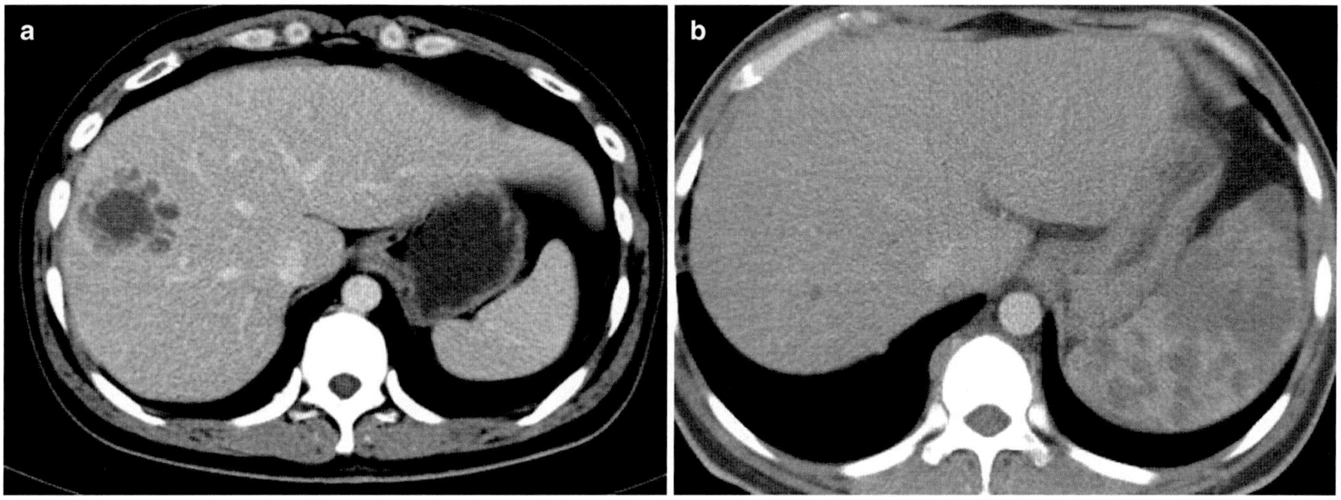

Fig. 5.44 (**a**, **b**) (**a**) A male patient aged 38 years with AIDS complicated by liver tuberculosis. CT scan showed the liver with multilocular liver abscess. (**b**) A male patient aged 54 years with AIDS complicated by spleen tuberculosis. Contrast CT scan showed the liver with low-density lesion and the surrounding enhancement

5.7.3.3 Neoplasm

Lymphoma

Primary central nervous system lymphoma (PCNSL) is neoplasm of lymphatic tissue, which is typically non-Hodgkin's lymphoma.

By CT plain scan, the lesions are demonstrated with obvious changes and the neoplasm is characterized by rapid growth and central necrosis. In patients with AIDS, the lesion is commonly demonstrated with low density and mostly shows ring-shaped enhancement but rarely homogeneous or heterogeneous enhancement by contrast imaging. MRI displays hypointense or isointense T1WI signal of the lesion, isointense or hyperintense T2WI signal of the parenchymal part, and hyperintense T2WI signal of the necrotic part. Contrast imaging showed heterogeneous enhancement of the lesion. Compared to the size of neoplasm, the surrounding edema is relatively much slight. And the lesion is commonly singular and rarely multiple, which is commonly located under the ependyma and pia mater. The infiltrated lesion around the ventricle can be shown as characteristic ventricle embedded sign, commonly with corpus callosum involved. Compared to lymphoma in patients with normal immunity, lymphoma complicating AIDS is more invasive, with much shorter period of time to double its size (about 2 weeks) (Fig. 5.57).

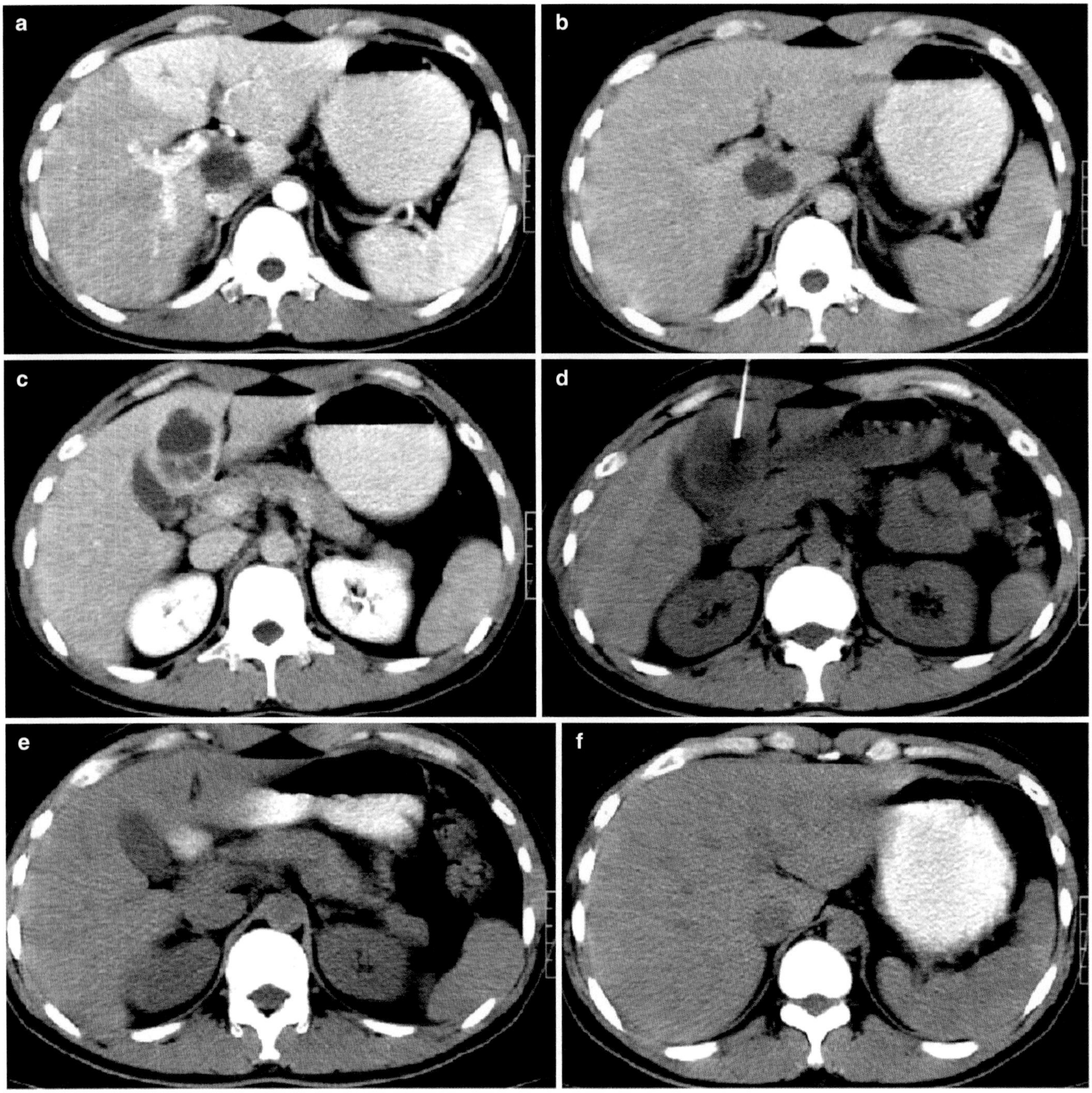

Fig. 5.45 (**a–f**) A male patient aged 28 years with AIDS complicated by liver abscess. He was detected to be HIV positive (+) but PPD negative (−) and his CD4 T-cell count was 388/ul. The 3 indicators for tuberculosis were negative (-). (**a–d**) CT scan revealed multiple abscesses in the liver. Pathological examination of the fluid collected by puncture demonstrated tissue necrosis, many neutrophil granulocytes, and acid-fast staining negative (-). By culture of pus, no fungi were detected. (**e**, **f**) Reexamination after anti-infection therapy for 1 month revealed almost absorption of the lesions

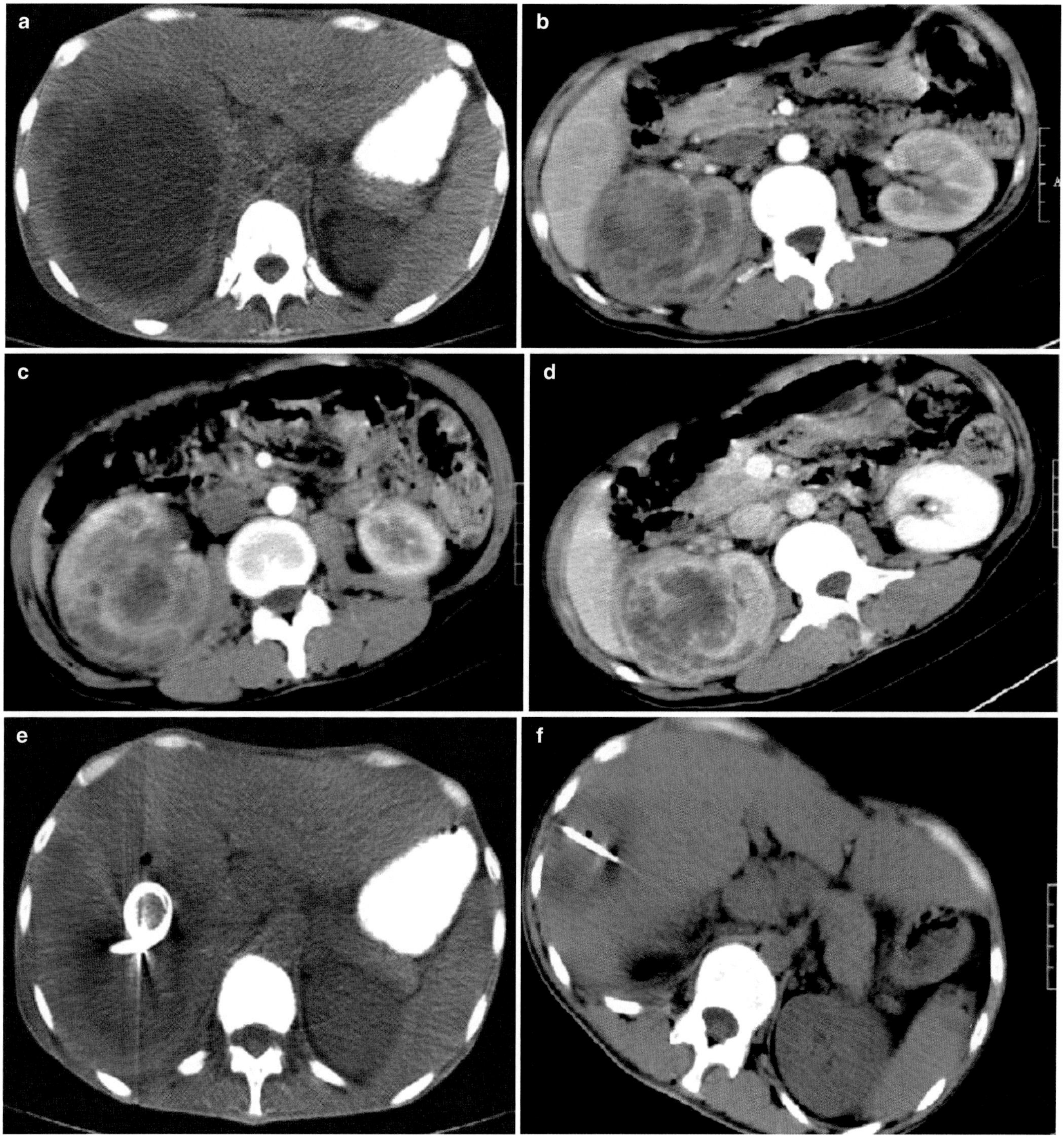

Fig. 5.46 (**a–f**) A male patient aged 36 years with AIDS complicated by liver and kidney aspergillus infection. His CD4 T-cell count was 2/uL. By biopsy after kidney puncture and percutaneous puncture of liver abscess for tube placement and drainage 3 times, the diagnosis was defined. (**a–d**) Before treatment, the liver was displayed with round-like low density and opacity with a diameter of 5 cm. (**e, f**) By CT-guided percutaneous tube placement for drainage, 500 ml dark brown pus was collected. And the lesion was shown with shrinkage

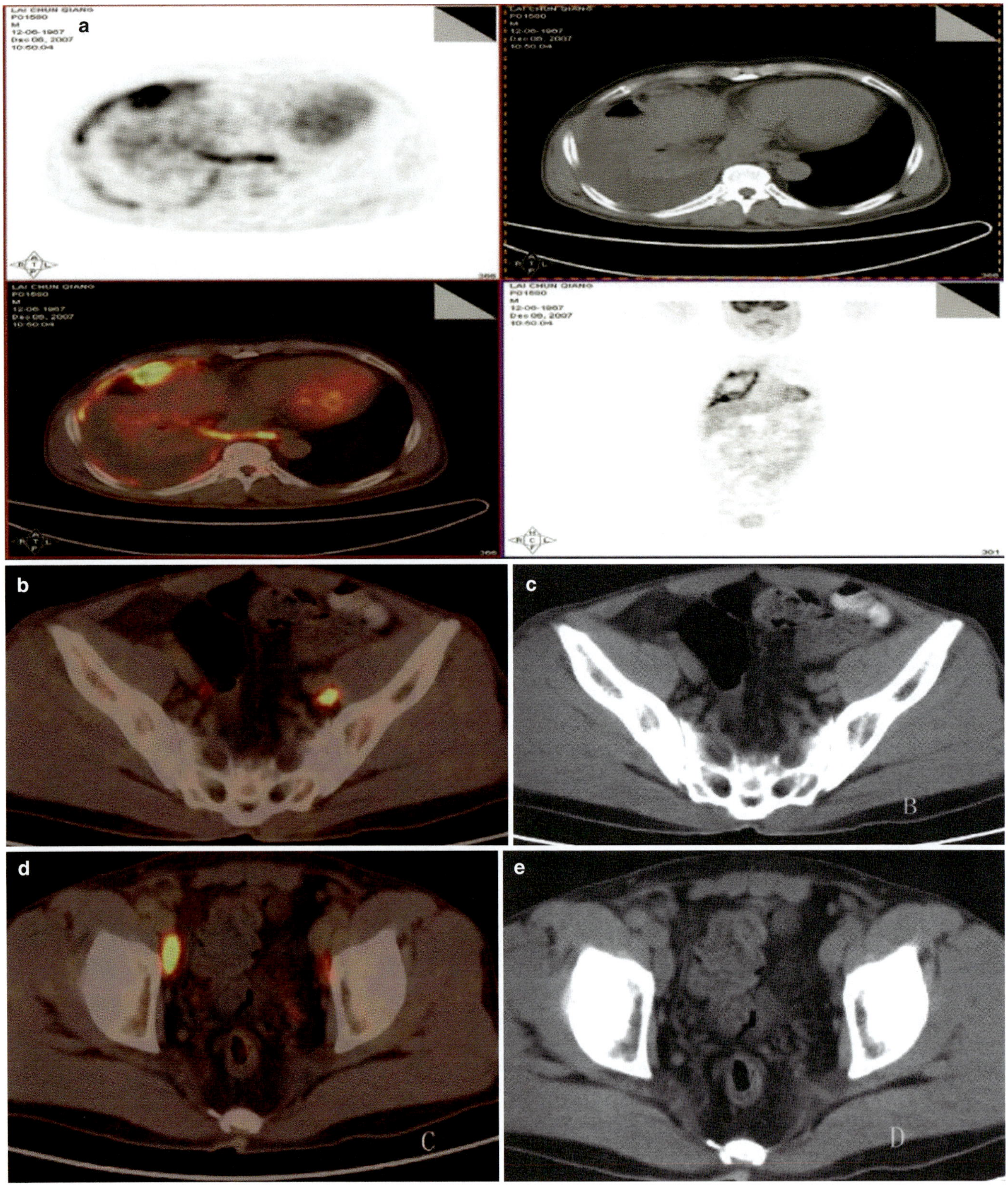

Fig. 5.47 (**a**–**e**) A homosexual male patient aged 44 years with pathological diagnosis of Kaposi's sarcoma. (**a**, **b**) PET/CT showed round nuclein aggregation at the liver capsule and adjacent to left iliacus in the pelvis. (**c**) CT scan showed increased density and opacity at the corresponding soft tissue. (**d**) Perivascular round nuclein aggregation was shown to be located lateral to right iliacus in the pelvis. (**e**) CT scan showed high density and opacity at the corresponding soft tissue

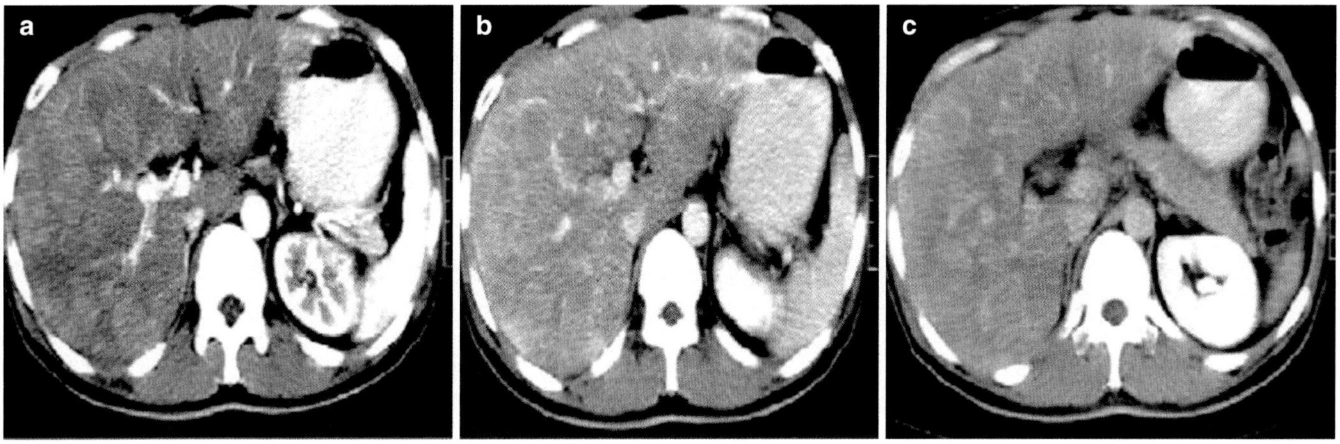

Fig. 5.48 (**a**–**c**) A male patient aged 38 years with AIDS (stage IV) complicated by non-Hodgkin lymphoma. His CD4 T-cell count was 19/ul, and the diagnosis was defined based on pathological examination. The liver was demonstrated with multiple masses opacity, which was slightly enhanced at the arterial phase and was better defined at the portal venous phase

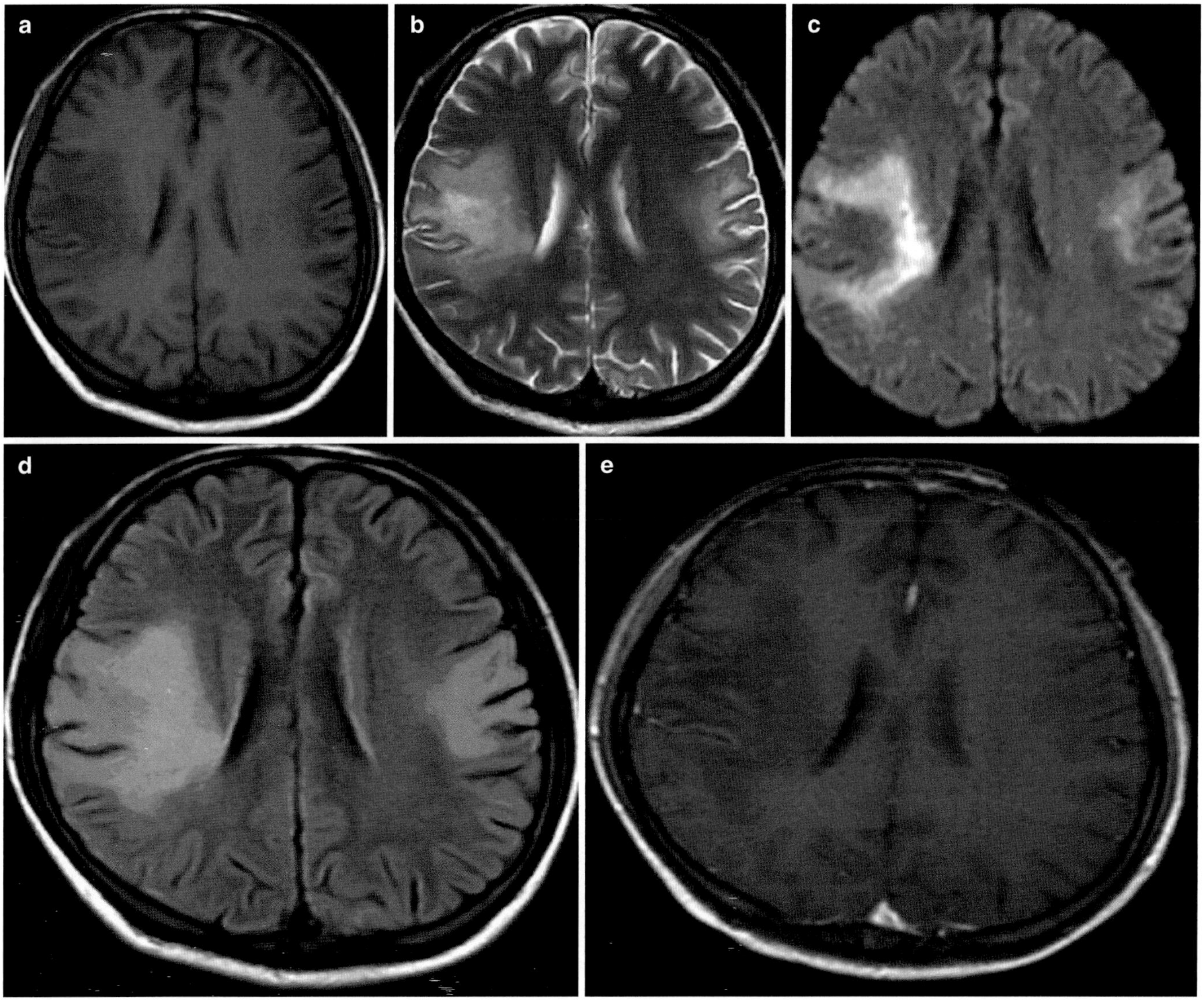

Fig. 5.49 (**a**–**e**) A male patient aged 36 years with HIV-associated encephalopathy. (**a**) MRI T1 showed bilateral cerebral hemispheres with hypointense signal at the temporal-parietal lobe and demyelination. (**b**) T2 showed bilateral cerebral hemispheres with hyperintense signal at the temporal-parietal lobe. (**c**) Diffusion imaging displayed irregular hyper-intense signal. (**d**) Water suppression imaging showed bilateral cerebral hemispheres with hyperintense signal at the temporal-parietal lobe. (**e**) Contrast MRI showed no obvious enhancement of the lesions

Kaposi's Sarcoma

In patients with AIDS, Kaposi's sarcoma may be disseminated to involve almost all the systems and tissues but rarely intracranial tissues. Its intracranial involvement can be radiologically shown as nonspecific enhancing mass. By brain CT or MR imaging, the scalp and nasopharynx may be demonstrated to be involved. Maxillofacially involved Kaposi's sarcoma commonly originates from subcutaneous

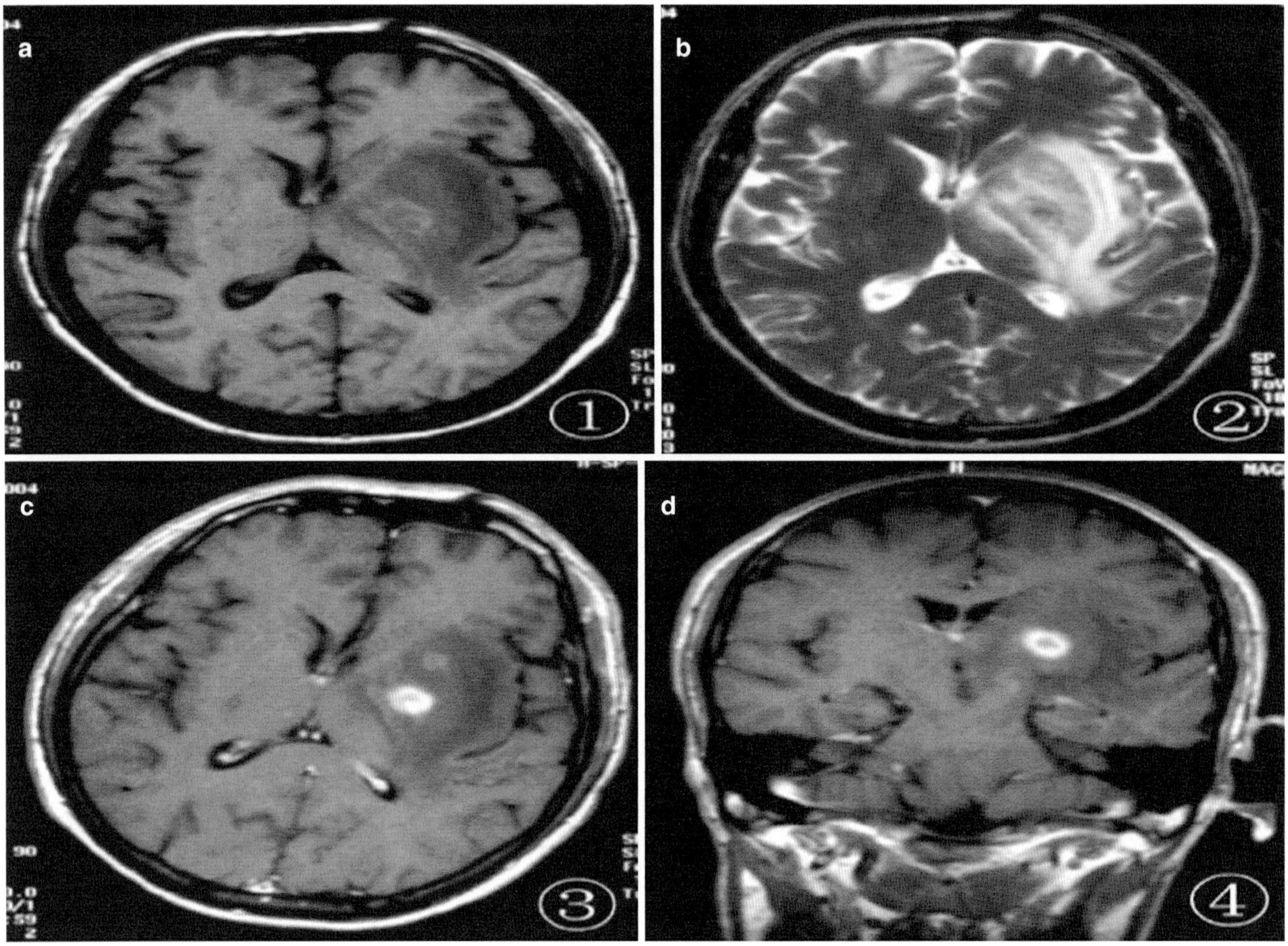

Fig. 5.50 (**a**–**h**) A male patient aged 31 years with AIDS complicated by toxoplasma encephalopathy. (**a**–**d**) Head MRI showed lesion at the left basal ganglia, with hypointense T1WI signal accompanied by surrounding edema and inhomogeneous hyperintense T2WI signal accompanied by better defined surrounding edema and axially compressed ventricle. Contrast imaging demonstrated ring-shaped enhancement of the lesion (A-T1WI, B-T2WI, C-contrast axial T1WI, D-contrast coronal T1WI). (**e**–**h**) Reexamination by head MRI after 26 days anti-Toxoplasma *gondii* treatment, the lesion at the left basal ganglia was shown with obvious shrinkage, almost no surrounding edema, and morphologically normal ventricle (E-T1WI, F-T2WI, G-contrast axial T1WI, H-contrast coronal T1WI)

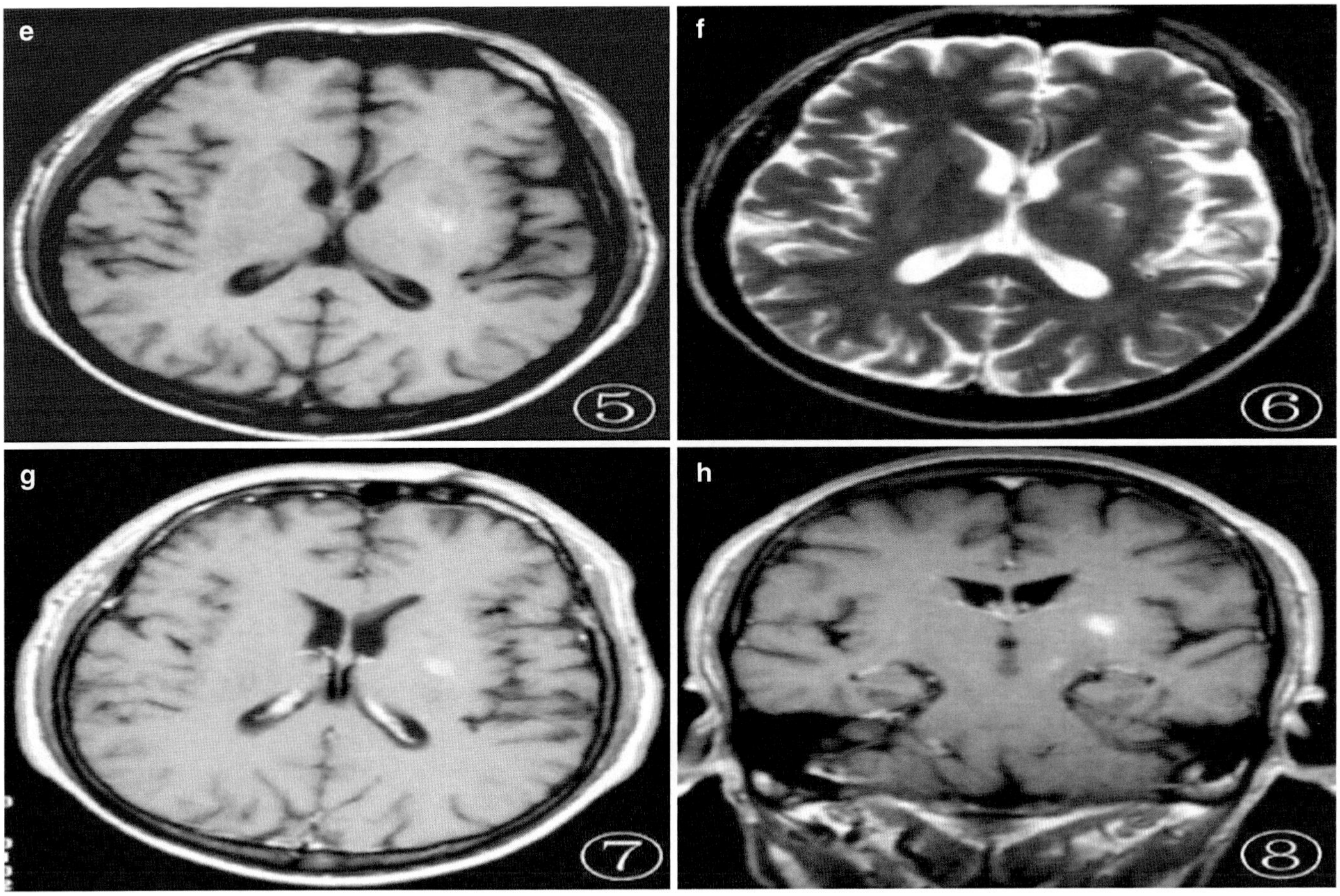

Fig. 5.50 (continued)

soft tissue, followed by its expanding to the maxillary bones or submaxillary bones including tooth root. Kaposi's sarcoma originating primarily from maxillary bones or submaxillary bones is rare. Maxillofacially involved Kaposi's sarcoma is demonstrated as mass with soft tissue density and the involved bones are demonstrated with bone destruction or defect but no marginal sclerosis. By contrast scan or imaging, the lesion is obviously enhanced. PET displayed the lesion to be hypermetabolic (Fig. 5.58).

In patients with AIDS, the lesions in central neural system are diverse. Different complications may occur at different stages of AIDS, and several complications may even coexist, which present challenge to their diagnosis and differential diagnosis. Specific diagnosis is commonly defined based on histopathological biopsy. However, CT and MRI play important roles in detecting and diagnosing the complications of central nervous system as well as predicting their prognosis.

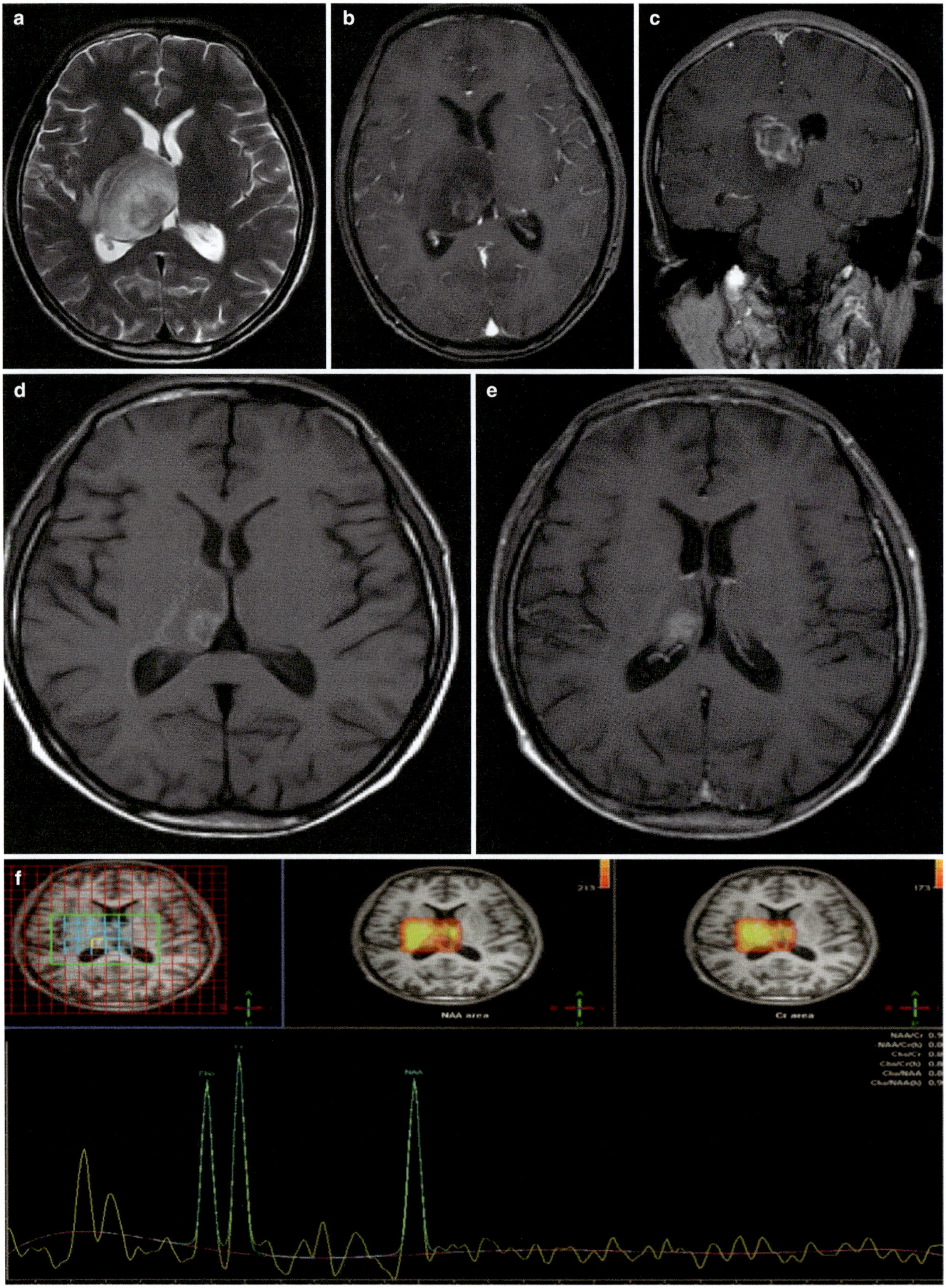
a
b
c
d
e
f
NAA area
Cr area
Cho
NAA

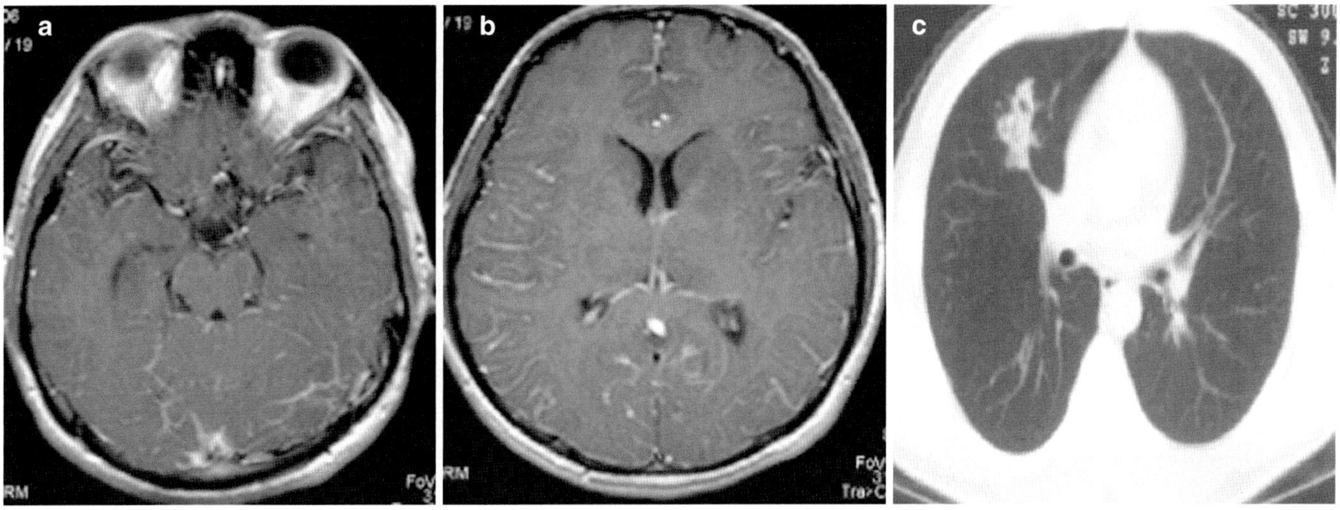

Fig. 5.52 (**a**, **b**, **c**) A male patient aged 36 years with AIDS complicated by cryptococcal encephalitis. (**a**, **b**), Enhancement of cerebral gyrus and meninges was displayed. (**c**) Lung infection was displayed

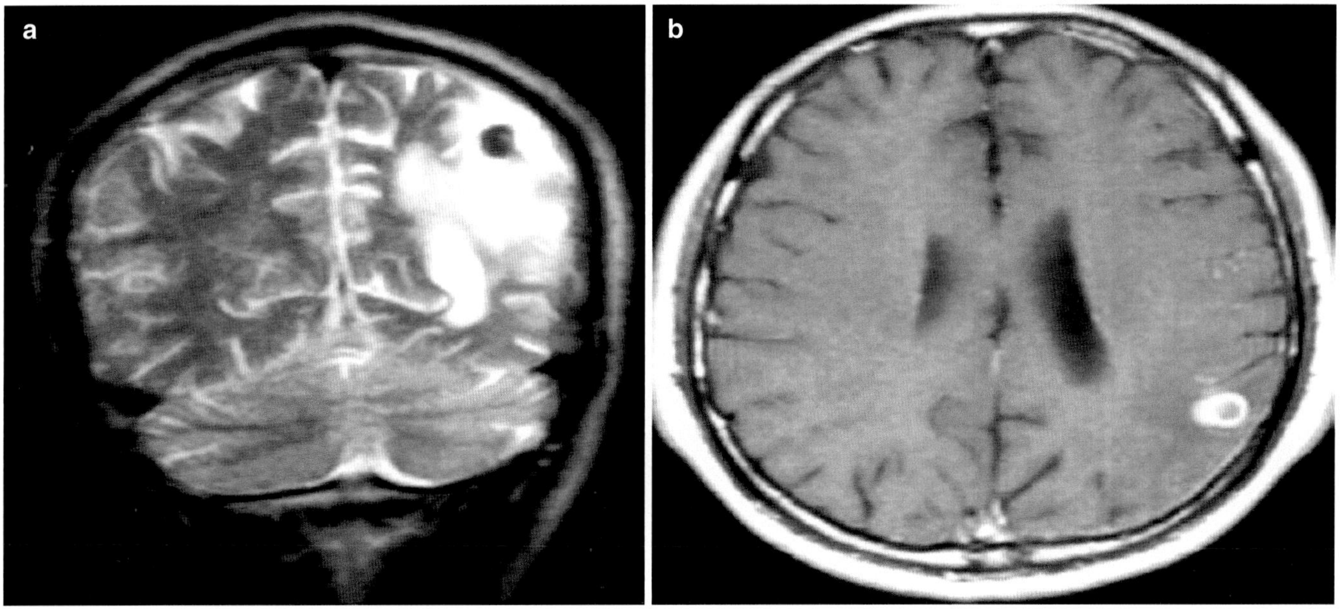

Fig. 5.53 (**a**, **b**) A case of AIDS complicated by cryptococcal encephalitis. Contrast MRI showed nodular ring-shaped enhancement of the lesion, with extensive surrounding edema

Fig. 5.51 (**a**–**f**) A male patient aged 29 years with AIDS complicated by toxoplasma encephalopathy. His CD4 T-cell count was 9 /uL.(**a**–**c**) The right thalamus was shown with space-occupying lesion, with mixed T2 signal, hypointense central signal and hyperintense peripheral signal, and surrounding edema. Contrast imaging displayed ring-shaped enhancement within the lesion but no obvious enhancement of the surrounding edema. (**d**, **e**) Reexamination after treatment demonstrated obvious shrinkage of the lesion at the right thalamus, but still ring-shaped enhancement by contrast imaging. (**f**) MRS showed Cho/Cr ratio of 0.85, NAA/Cr ratio of 0.97, and NAA/(Cho+Cr) ratio of 0.88

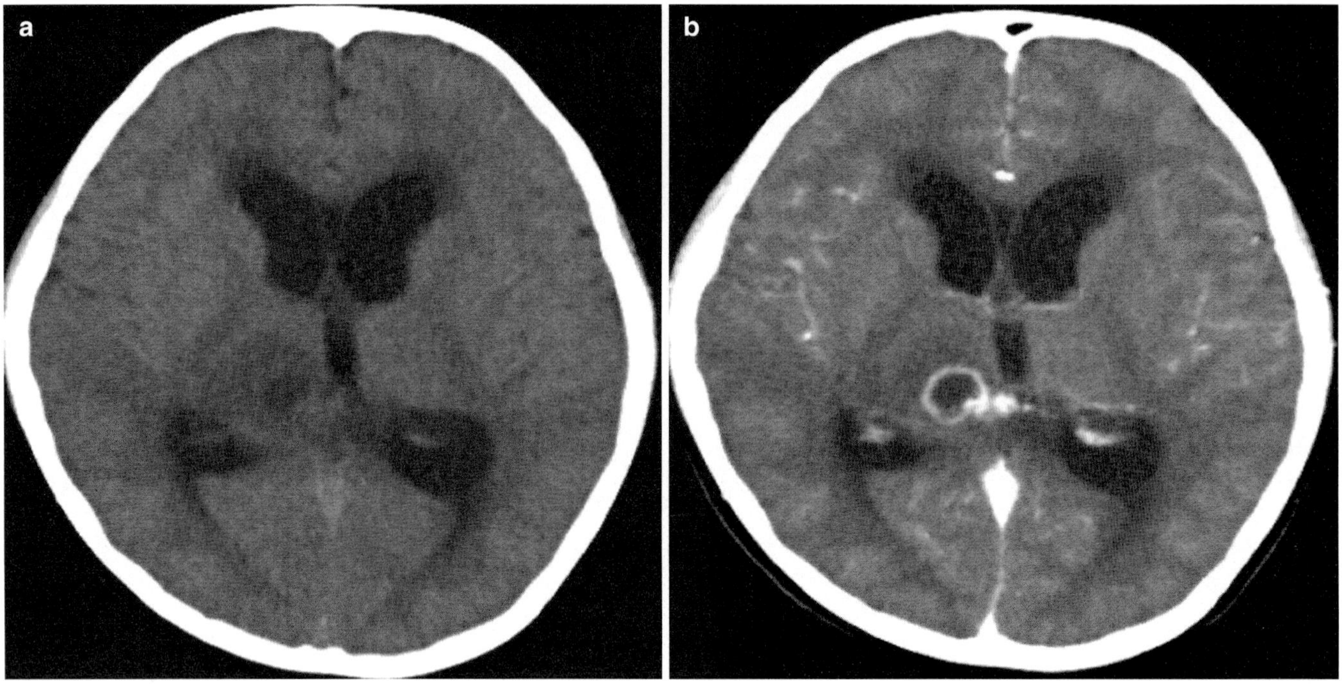

Fig. 5.54 (**a**, **b**) A boy aged 12 years with AIDS complicated by tuberculous encephalitis. CT scan showed intracranial lesion. Contrast scan displayed ring-shaped enhancement of the lesion, which was defined to be tuberculosis infection

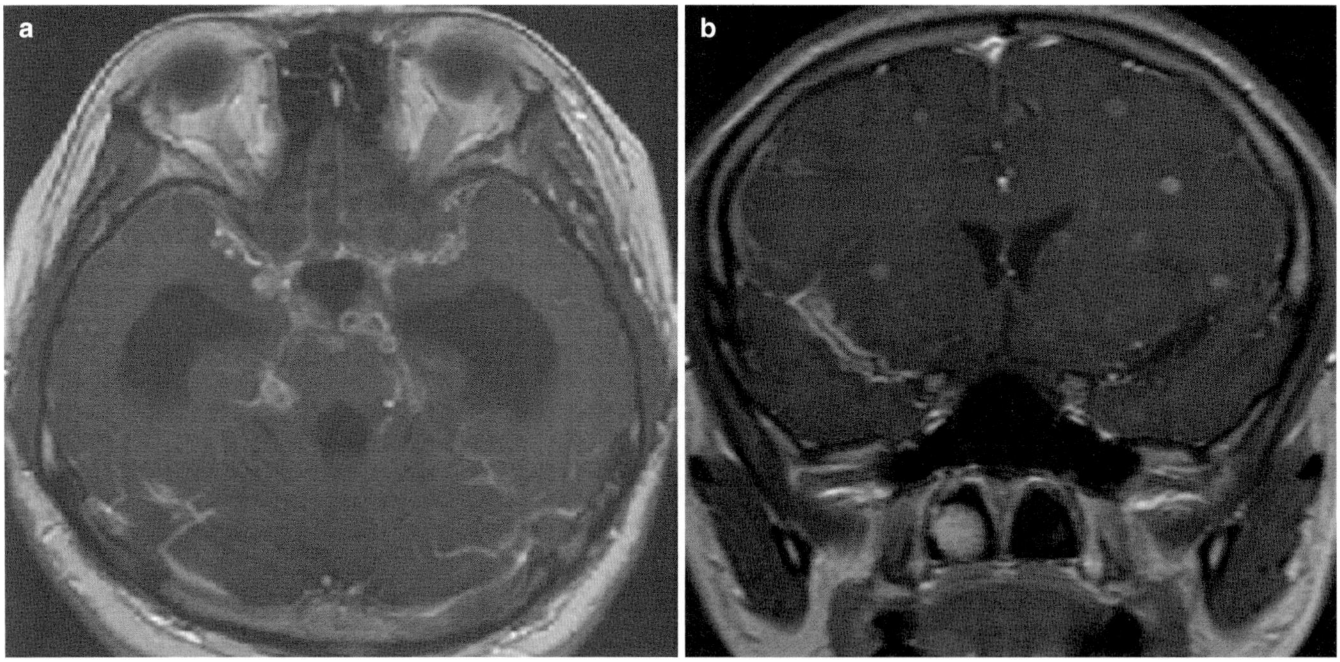

Fig. 5.55 (**a**, **b**) A male patient aged 47 years with AIDS complicated by tuberculous meningitis.(**a**) Gd-DTPA contrast T1WI showed extensive irregular linear enhancement of the meninges at the basal cistern, multiple ring-shaped enhanced nodules, and obviously expanded lateral ventricle. (**b**) Gd-DTPA coronal contrast T1WI showed obvious enhancement of the meninges at the lateral fissure cistern and accompanying multiple ring-shaped enhanced nodules in the brain parenchyma

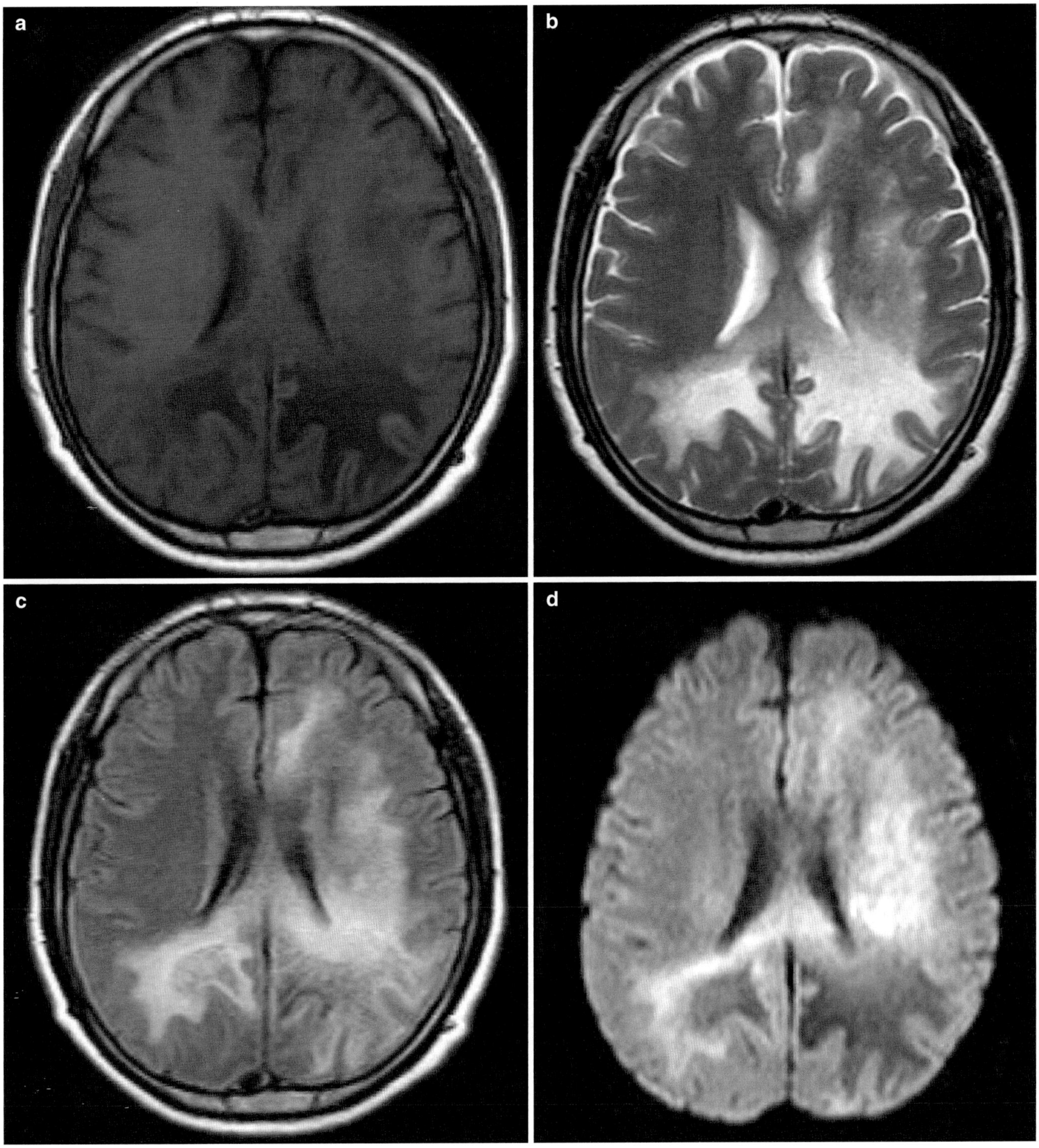

Fig. 5.56 (**a–e**) A male patient aged 30 years with AIDS (stage IV) complicated by progressive multifocal leukoencephalopathy. He was detected to be HIV positive. By cerebrospinal fluid culture and urine culture, JC virus was detected positive. (**a**) T1WI sequence of cranial MRI displayed large flake of hypointense signal in the white matter surrounding the body of bilateral lateral ventricles, especially obvious at the left side. (**b**) T2WI sequence showed hyperintense signal of the lesion. (**c–d**) FLAIR and DWI sequences displayed hyperintense signal. (**e**) Contrast MRI demonstrated the lesion with no enhancement

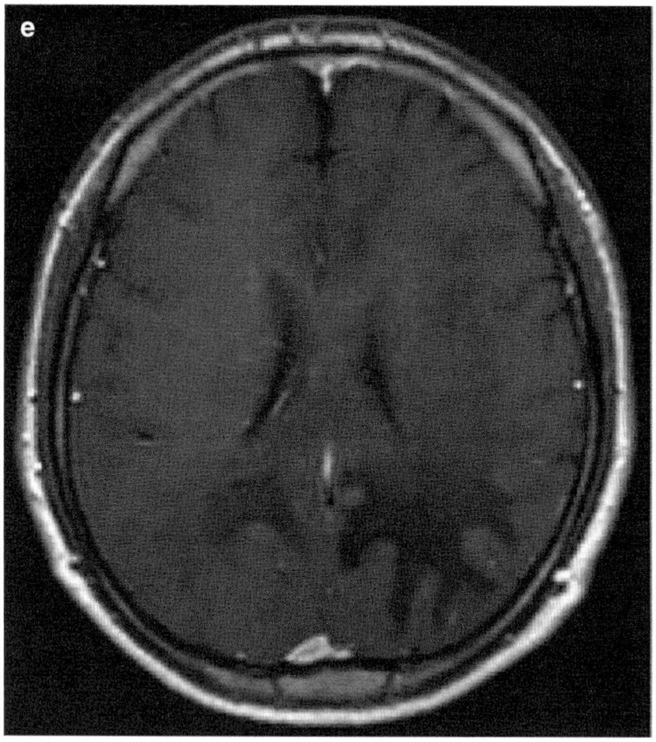

Fig. 5.56 (continued)

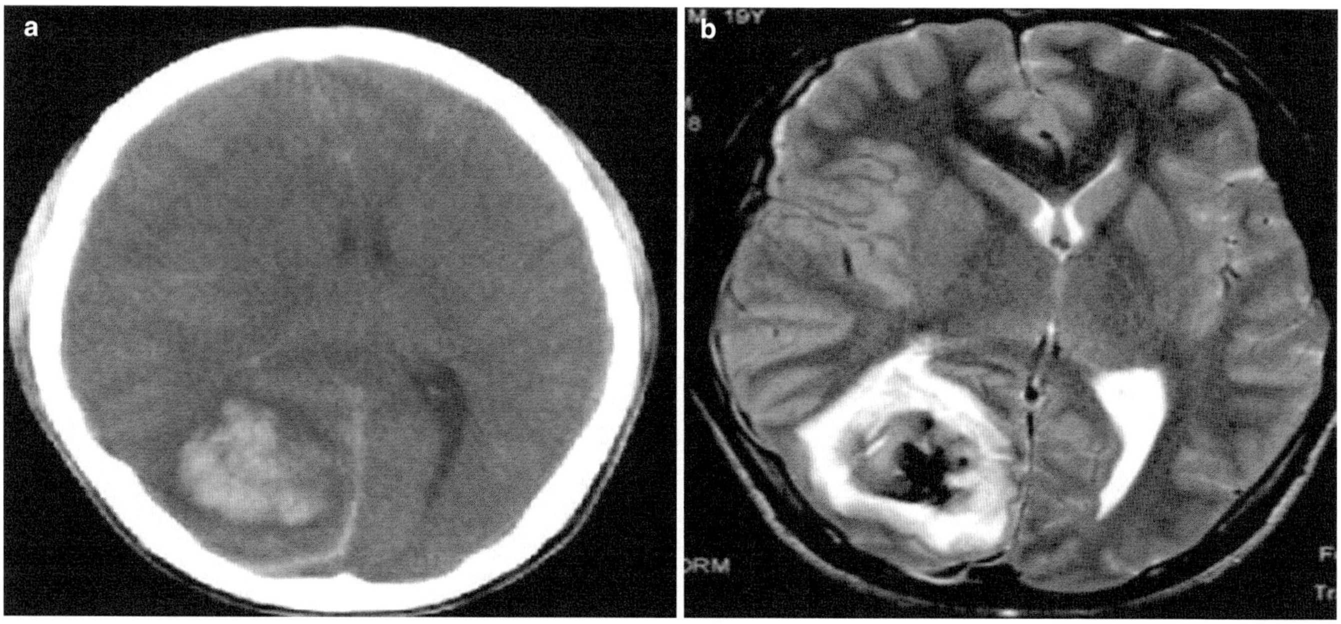

Fig. 5.57 (**a**, **b**) (**a**) Head CT showed irregular high density and opacity in the right temporal-occipital lobe, with small nodular low density and opacity inside. (**b**) MRI showed ring-shaped hyperintense T2WI signal and central hypointense signal, indicating lymphoma with hemorrhage

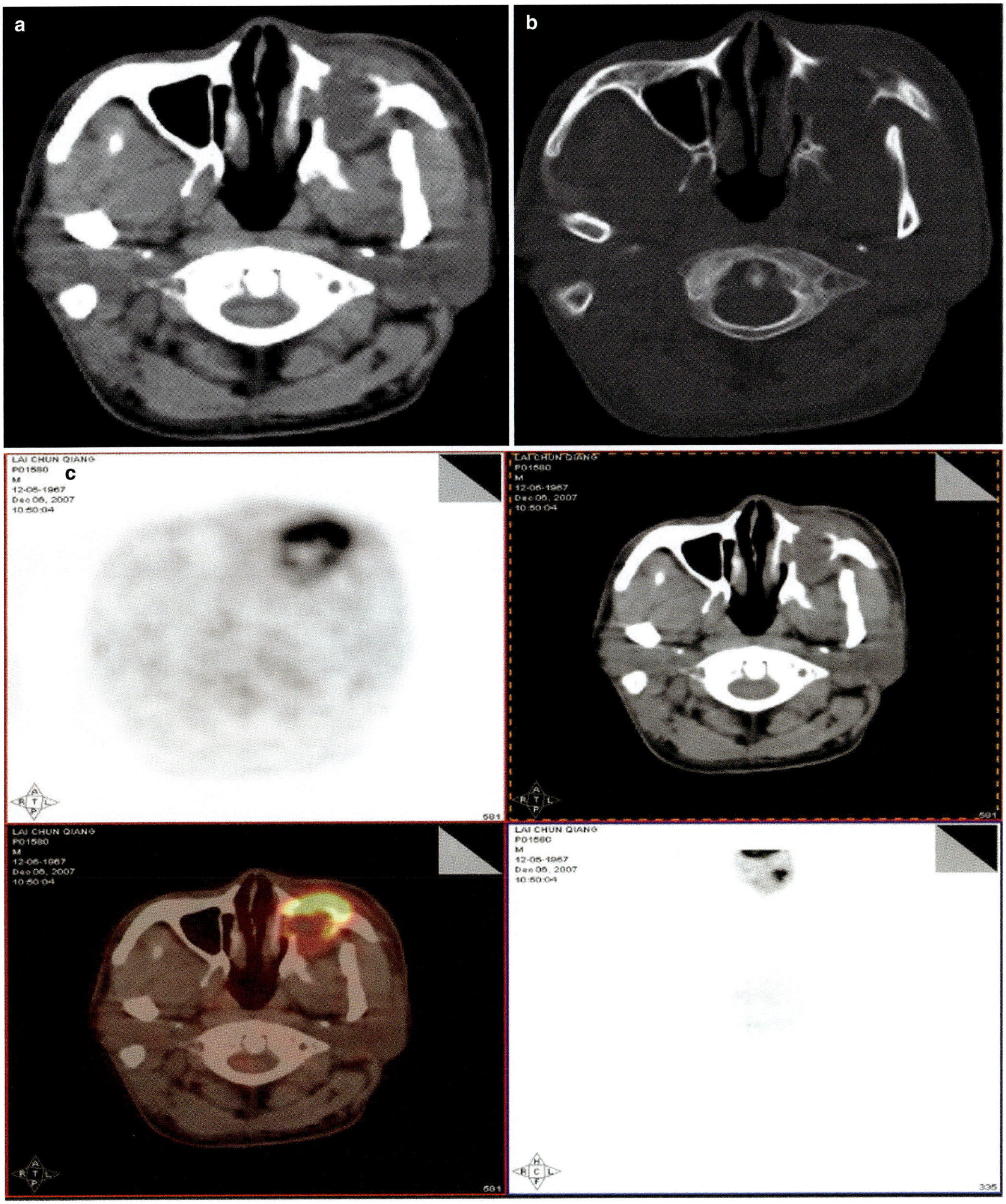

Fig. 5.58 (**a–c**) A male patient aged 44 years with AIDS complicated by Kaposi's sarcoma. (**a**, **b**) The left maxillary sinus was shown with a space-occupying lesion, with bone destruction and soft tissue density mass. (**c**) PET/CT showed nuclein aggregation in the mass, which was pathologically defined to be Kaposi's sarcoma

Further Reading

1. Ayouba A, Souquieres S, Njinku B, et al. HIV-1 group N among HIV-1-seropositive individuals in Cameroon. AIDS. 2000;14(16):2623–5.
2. TakebE Y, Kusagawa S, Motomura K. Molecular epidemiology of HIV: tracking AIDS pandemic. Pediatr Int. 2004;46(2):236–44.
3. Lu L, Jia M, Ma Y, et al. The changing face of HIV in China. Nature. 2008;455(7213):609–11.
4. Wang L, Wang N, Wang L, et al. The 2007 estimates for people at risk for and living with HIV in China: progress and challenges. J Acquir Immune Defic Syndr. 2009;5O(4):414–8.
5. Yue-ming L, Yang F-e, Xi-he N. Clinical manifestations and imaging diagnosis of HIV/AIDS associated pneumocystis carinii pneumonia. Chin J Nosoconmiol. 2005;15(2):1376–9.
6. Bartha I, Simon P, Muller V. Has HIV evolved to induce immune pathogenesis? Trends Immunol. 2008;29(7):322–8.
7. Sodora DL, Silvestri G, et al. Immune activation and AIDS pathogenesis. AIDS. 2008;22(4):439–46.
8. Catherinot E, Lanternier F, Bougnoux ME, et al. Pneumocystis jirovecі pneumonia. Infect Dis Clin North Am. 2010;24(1):107–38.
9. Murchan EM, Redelman-Sidi G, Patel M, et al. Esophageal actinomycosis in a fifty-three-year-old man with HIV: case report and review of the literature. AIDS Patient Care STDS. 2010;24(20):73–8.
10. Epeldegui M, Vendrame E, Martinez-Maza O, et al. HIV-associated immune dysfunction and viral infection: role in the pathogenesis of AIDS-related lymphoma. Immunol Res. 2010;48(1–3):72–83.
11. Aouizerat BE, Pearce CL, Miaskowski C, et al. The search for host genetic factors of HIV/AIDS pathogenesis in the post-genome Era: progress to date and new avenues for discovery. Curr HIV/AIDS Rep. 2011;8(1):38–44.
12. Wonderlich ER, Kader M, Wijewardana V, et al. Dissecting the role of dendritic cells in simian immunodeficiency virus infection and AIDS. Immunol Res. 2011;50(2–3):228–34.
13. Huysentruyt LC, McGrath MS. The role of macrophages in the development and progression of AIDS-related non-Hodgkin lymphoma. J Leukoc Biol. 2010;87(4):627–32.
14. Lu P-x, Bo-ping Z. Chest clinical radiology of HIV/AIDS. Beijing: Science Press; 2012.
15. Magrath I. Epidemiology: clues to the pathogenesis of Burkitt lymphoma. Br J Haematol. 2012;156(6):744–56.
16. Liu Y, Yu W-y, Lu P-x, et al. AIDS complicated by tuberculosis of mesentric lymph nodes: diagnosis and treatment for 11 cases. Chin J Tuberc Respir Dis. 2009;32(11):835–7.
17. Cao J, McNevin J, Malhotra U, et al. Evolution of CD8+ T cell immunity and viral escape following acute HIV-1 infection. J Immunol. 2003;17(7):3837–46.
18. Camere E. Unchecked thrombin is bad news for troubled arteries. J Clin Invest. 2007;117(6):1486–9.
19. Mohamed MA, Lentz MR, Lee V, et al. Factor analysis of proton MR spectroscopic imaging data in HIV infection: metabolite -derived factors help identify infection and dementia. Radiology. 2010;254(2):577–86.
20. Legoff J, Bouhlal H, Gresenguet G, et al. Real-time PCR quantification of genital shedding of herpes simplex virus(HSV) and human immunodeficiency virus (HIV) in women coinfected with HSV and HIV. J Clin Microbiol. 2006;44(2):423–32.
21. Lu P-x, Yu W-k, Zhu W-k, et al. Radiological demonstrations of AIDS complicated by pulmonary tuberculosis and their relationship with CD4+ T lymphocytes. Chin J Tuberc Respir Dis. 2005;28(1):13–6.
22. Lu P-x, Yang G-d, Jin-qing L, et al. Imaging diagnosis of AIDS complicated by Pneumocystis Carinii pneumonia. Chin J Medical Radiol. 2003;11(3):166–8.
23. Lentz MR, Kim WK, Lee V, et al. Changes in MRS neuronal markers and T cell phenotypes observed during early HIV infection. Neurology. 2009;72(17):1465–72.
24. Lu ZW-k, Pu-xuan LX-h, et al. AIDS complicated by pulmonary tuberculosis: comparative study of CT and pathologic findings. Radiologic Practice. 2011;26(09):931–3.
25. Da-wei Z, Chun-wang Y, Li-jie Z, et al. Radiological demonstrations of AIDS complicated by tuberculosis of hilar/mediastinal lymph node. Chin J Radiol. 2005;39(7):772–5.
26. Lu P-x, Deng Y-y, Shui-teng L, et al. Typing of AIDS complicated by Pneumocystis Carinii Pneumonia based on its radiological demonstrations. Radiologic Practice. 2009;24(9):948–51.
27. Lu YG-d, Pu-xuan ZN-y, et al. Imaging diagnosis of pulmonary cryptococcosis in patients with AIDS. Chin J Medical Imaging Technology. 2009;25(9):1581–3.
28. Ke Z, Ma D-q, Fu-jing L, et al. Clinical diagnosis and treatment of AIDS complicated by tuberculosis. Chin J Tuberc Respir Dis. 2001;24(11):682–4.
29. Jin-xin L, Xiao-ping T, Song-feng J, et al. Chest radiology of penicilliosis marneffei in patients with AIDS. Chin J Radiol. 2007;41(3):239–42.
30. Lu YW-y, Pu-xuan ZW-k, et al. Clinical and radiological manifestations of AIDS complicated by disseminated penicillium marneffei infection. Chin J Clinical Medical Imaging. 2007;7(6):434–7.
31. Wen-yan S, Hong-jun L. AIDS complicated by pulmonary cytomegalovirus infection: comparative study of radiology and pathology. Radiologic Practic. 2010;25(1):44–6.
32. Yang G-d, Lu P-x. Radiological diagnosis of AIDS complicated by candidal esophagitis and its differential diagnosis. Modern Medical Radiology. 2012;21(05):278–80.
33. Lu YG-d, Pu-xuan QJ, et al. AIDS complicated by candidal esophagitis: comparative study of X-ray radiology and gastroscopy. Radiologic Practic. 2009;24(09):939–42.
34. Fan S-f, Gu W-z. Radiology of AIDS (II). Journal of Clinical Radiology. 2001;20(4):297–301.
35. Reeders JW, Yee J, Gore RM, et al. Gastrointestinal infection in the immunocompromised (AIDS) patient. Eur Radiol. 2004;14(Suppl 3 N):E84–102.
36. Yang J. Radiological diagnosis of AIDS complicated by abdominal diseases. Radiologic Practic. 2009;24(10):1056–60.
37. Da-wei Z, Tong Z, Wang W, et al. Radiological finings of AIDS complicated by abdominal diseases. Chin J Radiol. 2007;41(3):254–8.
38. Cota GF, Assad EC, Christo PP, et al. Ventriculitis: a rare case of primary cerebral toxoplasmosis in AIDS patient and literature review. Braz J Infect Dis. 2008;12(1):101–4.
39. Chaudhari VV, Yim CM, Hathout H, et al. Atypical imaging appearance of toxoplasmosis in an HIV patient as a butterfly lesion. J Magn Reson Imaging. 2009;30(4):873–5.
40. Smith HD, Gupta S. Ring-enhancing brain lesion in a man with acquired immunodeficiency syndrome. Am J Med. 2006;119(3):246–7.
41. De Silva T, Raychaughuri M, Poulton M, et al. Ventriculitis and hydrocephalus: an unusual presentation of toxoplasmosis in an adult with human immunodeficiency virus. J Neurol Neurosurg Psychiatry. 2005;76(8):1074.
42. Ozgiriary E, Oner K, Ovul I. HIV related toxoplasmic encephalitis mimicking multiple metastasis: case report. Turk Neurosurg. 2007;7(3):207–10.
43. Li Q, You C, Liu Q, et al. Central nervous system cryptococcoma in immunocompetent patients: a short review illustrated by a new case. Acta Neurochir. 2010;152(1):129–36.
44. Offiah CE, Turnbull IW. The imaging appearances of intracranial CNS infections in adult HIV and AIDS patients. Clin Radiol. 2006;61(5):393–401.
45. Huang H, Lu P-x. Radiological findings of AIDS complicated by progressive multi-focal leukoencephalopathy and its differential diagnosis. Chin J Medical Imaging Technology. 2009;25(7):103–5.

46. Huang H, Deng Y-y, Lu P-x. Radiological findings of AIDS complicated by toxoplasma encephalopathy. Chin J Magnetic Resonance Imaging. 2010;1(5):353–8.
47. Masur H. Prevention of pneumocystis carinii pneumonia. Rev Infect Dis. 1989;11 Suppl 7:S1664–8.
48. Lu ZW-k, Pu-xuan HX-r, et al. Percutaneous interventional therapy for AIDS complications. Chin J Interv Imaging Therapeutics. 2009;6(6):552–4.
49. Zhu W-k, Huang X-r, Lu P-x, et al. CT-guided percutaneous lung puncture and biopsy for the diagnosis of AIDS complications. Radiologic Practice. 2009;24(10):1064–6.
50. Diprose P, Deakin CD, Smedley J. Ignorance of post-exposure prophylaxis guidelines following HIV needlestick injury may increase the risk of seroconversion. Br J Anaesth. 2000;84(6):767–70.
51. Kreuter A, Wieland U. Human papillomavirus-associated diseases in HIV-infected men who have sex with men. Curr Opin Infect Dis. 2009;22(2):109–14.
52. Trottier H, Burchell AN. Epidemiology of mucosal human papillomavirus infection and associated diseases. Public Health Genomics. 2009;12(5–6):291–307.
53. D'Ambrogio A, Yerly S, Sahli R, et al. Human papilloma virus type and recurrence rate after surgical clearance of anal condylomata acuminata. Sex Transm Dis. 2009;36(9):536–40.
54. Granich RM, Gilks CF, Dye C, et al. Universal voluntary HIV testing with immediate antiretroviral therapy as a strategy for elimination of HIV transmission: a mathematical model. Lancet. 2009;373(657):48–57.

6 Viral Hepatitis

Wu Shi-Pin, Bo-Ping Zhou, Liu Ying-Xia, Chong Yu-Tian, Xu Cheng, He Qing, Dong Chang-Feng, Huang Ting, Yang Gen-Dong, Wang Yi-Xiang, Wang Zhao-Qin, Zhang Xiang-Mei, Yuan Hong, Zeng Zheng, and Wang Jun-Qing

6.1 General Introduction

Virus hepatitis is a group of systemic infectious diseases induced by various types of hepatitis virus, predominantly with liver damages. Based on the pathogen, virus hepatitis can be categorized into five types: hepatitis A, hepatitis B, hepatitis C, hepatitis D, and hepatitis E. Hepatitis A and hepatitis E are transmitted mainly via fecal-mouth route which are mainly manifested as acute infections. Hepatitis B, hepatitis C, and hepatitis D are transmitted mainly via extra-gastrointestinal routes, commonly manifested as chronic infection, and the condition rarely develops into hepatic cirrhosis and even hepatocellular carcinoma.

Wu Shi-Pin (✉)
Department of Infection, Shenzhen People's Hospital Guangdong, Shenzhen, China
e-mail: wupoem@126.com

Bo-Ping Zhou
Department of Infection, Shenzhen Third People's Hospital Guangdong, Shenzhen, China
e-mail: zhoubp@hotmail.com

Liu Ying-Xia • Xu Cheng • He Qing • Dong Chang-Feng
Huang Ting • Yang Gen-Dong • Wang Zhao-Qin
Zhang Xiang-Mei • Yuan Hong • Zeng Zheng
The Shenzhen No.3 People's Hospital, Guangdong College, Shenzhen, China

Chong Yu-Tian
The Third Affiliated Hospital Zhongshan University, Shi Pai, Guangzhou, China

Wang Yi-Xiang • Wang Jun-Qing
The Chinese University of Hong Kong, Prince of Wales Hospital, Hong Kong, China

6.2 Etiology

6.2.1 Hepatitis A Virus (HAV)

In 1993, HAV was categorized into the genus of *Hepadnaviridae* and the family of *Picornaviridae*. The genome of HAV is linear single-stranded positive chain with about 7487 bases and genome-encoded single reading frame and is a polyprotein translating 2227 amino acids. HAV has only one serotype.

The virus is non-capsulated spherical in regular icosahedron whose diameter is about 27 nm. HAV-specific antigen is on its capsid.

HAV possesses stronger resistance to external environment. Its infectivity still remains at a temperature of −20 °C for several years. It is tolerant to 20 % of ether, acid, chloroform, and chlorine ions. But it can be completely inactivated at a temperature of 100 °C within 1 min.

6.2.2 Hepatitis B Virus (HBV)

Hepatitis B virus is categorized into the genus of *Hepadnaviridae* and the family of *Orthohepadnavirus*. HBV has a strong resistance in external environment and is tolerant to heat, low temperature, dryness, ultraviolet rays, and common chemical disinfectants of moderate concentration. It remains stable at a temperature of −20 °C for 20 years. However, it can be deprived of its infectivity at 100 °C within 10 min or 65 °C within 10 h.

6.2.3 Hepatitis C Virus (HCV)

HCV is categorized into the genus of *Hepacivirus* and the family of *Flaviviridae*. HCV is a capsulated spheric RNA virus particle whose diameter is about 55–65 nm. Its nucleocapsid is a three-dimensionally symmetric icosahedron that

P.-X. Lu, B.-P. Zhou (eds.), *Diagnostic Imaging of Emerging Infectious Diseases*, DOI 10.1007/978-94-017-7363-8_6

is encapsulating a genome consisted of about 9500 nucleotides in length.

HCV is sensitive to chloroform, fat solvent, and other common disinfectants. And the virus can be inactivated at a temperature of 37 °C within 96 h, 60 °C within 10 h, and 100 °C within 5 min.

6.2.4 Hepatitis D Virus (HDV)

HDV is a member of the delta virus genus and *Arenaviridae* family. It is a defective RNA virus, which is spherical with a diameter of 35 ~ 37 nm. The outer layer of HDV particle composed of lipid bilayers and HBsAg, which encapsulate ribonucleoprotein body composed of viral genome RNA and delta hepatitis antigen. HDV genome is a single-stranded circular closed negative strand RNA, with a length of about 1674 ~ 1683 bases. HDAg is the only protein encoded by HDV. Currently, HDV is classified into eight dominant genotypes whose differences of nucleotide sequence from each other are above 40 %.

HDV is sensitive to any disinfectant, such as the formaldehyde solution, fat solvent, and chloroform. However, it is tolerant to heat.

6.2.5 Hepatitis E Virus (HEV)

HEV is categorized into the genus of *Hepevirus* and the family of *Hepatitis*. It is a symmetric icosahedrons sphere with no envelope whose diameter is 27 ~ 38 nm and a mean of 32 ~ 34 nm. It can be either solid or hollow. Its genome is single positive-stranded RNA with a length of 7.5 kb to encode 2400 ~ 2533 amino acids. Its genome encoding area is composed of three open reading frames. And HEV has only one serotype.

HEV is sensitive to high concentration of salt, cesium chloride, and chloroform. But it is relatively stable in alkaline environment.

6.3 Epidemiology

6.3.1 Hepatitis A

6.3.1.1 Source of Infection

The patients at the acute stage and those with subclinical infection are the main sources of hepatitis A infection. During 2 weeks before the onset of jaundice, the stool and blood possess the infectivity that persists for about 3 weeks. Due to lack of typical symptoms, the cases of acute nonicteric hepatitis have more epidemiological significance.

6.3.1.2 Route of Transmission

Hepatitis A is mainly transmitted via the fecal-oral route, commonly along with contaminated food or drinking water. Especially, intake of uncooked fishery food is more likely to cause hepatitis A. In the developing countries or regions, the water-borne transmission is an important factor causing endemic prevalence of hepatitis A. Daily-life contact is another important route of infecting hepatitis A.

6.3.1.3 Susceptible Population

Human is generally susceptible to HAV. Those with a medical history of hepatitis A or those with a history of asymptomatic infection can acquire persistent immunity.

6.3.2 Hepatitis B

6.3.2.1 Source of Infection

The patients with acute or chronic hepatitis B as well as asymptomatic persons carrying HBV are the source of infection. Those asymptomatic persons carrying HBV virus are highly possible to spread the infection.

6.3.2.2 Route of Transmission

Hepatitis B virus is mainly transmitted via parenteral route. Data revealed that 40–50 % of HBsAg carriers in China are infected via vertical mother-to-child transmission.

Contact to blood or body fluid contaminated by hepatitis B virus plays an important role in its transmission. Hepatitis B virus can also be iatrogenically transmitted via transfusion of blood or blood products, surgical procedure, injection, and other needle stab.

In patients with hepatitis B or those carrying HBsAg, HBV can be detected in their saliva, seminal fluid, and vaginal secretions. Therefore, sexual contact is also an important route spreading HBV.

Close contact among family members may cause aggregative infection of HBV in the family.

6.3.2.3 Population Susceptibility

Human is generally susceptible to hepatitis B virus. Anti-HB positive after HBV infection indicates acquired long-lasting specific immunity against the same serotype of HBV.

6.3.3 Hepatitis C

6.3.3.1 Source of Infection

The patients with acute or chronic hepatitis C are the main source of its infection. The asymptomatic patients with HCV infection are of great significance in spreading the infection due to the unawareness of the disease.

6.3.3.2 Route of Transmission

HCV is mainly transmitted via blood or blood products. Intravenous drug abuse is currently the most common route spreading HCV, especially in the developed countries.

Generally, the infection rate of HCV in infants of HCV-positive mother is lower than 6 %.

HCV can be excreted along with saliva, seminal fluid, and vaginal secretions. Therefore, sexual contact is also an important route of transmission. The anti-HCV positive rate in family members of an infected patient is higher than the infection rate in general population, being about 5.1–5.2 %.

Medical staff with a history of contact to blood or body fluid of patient can be infected. The anti-HCV positive rate in patients receiving hemodialysis is positively related to the duration and frequency of dialysis. The risk factors spreading HCV also include some therapeutic behaviors such as surgical procedure, acupuncture and needle stab, repeated use of syringe and needle, use of medical instrument without strict sterilization, and endoscopy.

6.3.3.3 Susceptible Population

Human is generally susceptible to HCV infection.

6.3.4 Hepatitis D

6.3.4.1 Source of Infection

The sources of HDV infection mainly include the patients with acute or chronic hepatitis D and chronic HDV/HBV carriers.

6.3.4.2 Route of Transmission

The routes of HDV transmission resemble to those of HBV transmission.

6.3.4.3 Susceptible Population

HDV infection commonly overlaps or concurs with HBV infection, but predominantly HDV infection. The high risk population of HDV infection is patients with chronic hepatitis B.

6.3.5 Hepatitis E

6.3.5.1 Source of Infection

The main source of HEV infection is the patients at the terminal latency and the early acute stage of HEV infection.

6.3.5.2 Route of Transmission

The contaminated water source by feces can cause outbreak of hepatitis E. Outbreak of hepatitis E has been also reported to be caused by contaminated food.

The anti-HEV positive rate is higher in populations of intravenous drug abuser, blood supplier, patient receiving hemodialysis, and those with frequent contact to blood, which indicates blood-borne transmission of HEV.

6.3.5.3 Susceptible Population

Any age group of population can be infected by HEV, but higher incidence rate is found in young and middle-aged adults. The incidence rate is relatively low in children and the elderly. And the incidence rate in males is higher than that in females.

6.4 Pathogenesis and Pathological Changes

6.4.1 Pathogenesis

The mechanism underlying the occurrence of viral hepatitis is complex. The disease spectrum is extensive, which is related to the virus itself, immunity of human body, as well as the interaction between them.

6.4.1.1 The Direct Damage to Hepatocyte by Virus

The virus replicates itself in the hepatocytes to cause structural and functional changes of the liver cells. These changes further interfere the synthesis of hepatocyte protein, leading to degeneration and necrosis of the liver cells.

6.4.1.2 Impaired Immunity Caused by Virus Infection

The patients with viral hepatitis may produce antibody of the corresponding virus to form immune complex, which could induce acute and chronic liver damage. In addition, the immune complex may also deposit in extrahepatic tissue to induce various extrahepatic lesions of viral hepatitis.

The virus antigen is processed by the antigen-presenting cells (APC) to be presented to the epitope of CD4+ T lymphocyte and CD8+ T lymphocyte. Therefore, these two types of lymphocytes with corresponding receptor are activated and expressed. The activated T lymphocytes aggregate around the virus-infected target cell to fight against the virus with various ways.

6.4.1.3 Effects of Apoptosis

The Fas system contributes a lot in immune-mediated cell apoptosis. Firstly, the effect cells, assisted by T-cell receptors, recognize the histocompatible complex carrying the sensitizing antigen target cells and are activated to express Fas L. Therefore, they turn into cytotoxic T cells whose Fas L specifically binds to the target cell-expressed Fas to conduct signal of apoptosis. The apoptosis procedures are then activated in the target cells to eliminate the virus-infected liver cells.

6.4.1.4 The Effects of Cytokine

Various cytokines constitute a network of balance and a disturbed balance can trigger a series of pathological changes. The tumor necrosis factor (IFN-α) is an important cell regulation factor produced by the mononuclear macrophage system. It is capable of promoting expression of HLA-I, II antigens on the surface of hepatocyte to directly kill the virus-infected liver cells. Meanwhile, it can also induce and activate immune cell to impair the liver cells.

6.4.2 Pathological Changes

Viral hepatitis is a type of inflammatory disease predominantly with degeneration. Specifically, the pathological changes mainly include hepatocyte degeneration and necrosis accompanied by inflammatory cell infiltration as well as regeneration of the interstitial cells and liver cells.

6.4.2.1 Hepatitis A

Hepatitis A is histologically change of acute hepatitis, with three characteristic findings: (1) Bile stasis at the liver cells around the central vein is obvious, but with slight liver cell damage or inflammation. (2) Necrosis of the liver cells around the portal area is accompanied by dense mononuclear cell infiltration at the portal area including a large quantity of plasmocytes. (3) The necrotic and inflammatory lesions around the portal area are more obvious than the lesions around lobular central vein.

6.4.2.2 Hepatitis B

Acute Hepatitis B

The pathological changes of acute hepatitis B include:

1. Intralobular pathological changes

   The whole hepatic lobule is demonstrated with loosened and balloon-like plasma in the liver cells. Some other liver cells are demonstrated with shrinkage, acidophilic plasma, and karyopyknosis, which are known as acidophilic degeneration. It commonly scatters in the hepatic lobule (Fig. 6.1). In the hepatic sinus, acidophilic body or apoptotic body is common, and spots of focally necrotic liver cells are common.

2. Changes at the portal area

   The portal inflammation is mostly slight or moderate, with inflammatory cell infiltration. The infiltrated cells are predominantly small lymphocytes and commonly small quantities of neutrophilic granulocytes and eosinophilic granulocytes.

Chronic Hepatitis B

The Parenchymal Lesions

1. Periportal changes: interface inflammation

   Except for slightest chronic hepatitis, the inflammatory infiltration in the cases of other chronic hepatitis extends from the portal area into the neighboring parenchyma. The liver cells around the portal area are then damaged to show interface inflammation. In addition, fibrous septum may extend out of the portal area.

2. Lobular lesions

   Different degrees of hepatocellular damages and inflammatory response occur in deep liver parenchyma, which is known as lobular lesions or lobular hepatitis. Lobular lesions are commonly manifested as spots of focally necrotic hepatocyte (Fig. 6.2). However, fused necrosis and bridging necrosis may also be observable. In addition, ground-glass-like liver cells (Fig. 6.3) as well as small round or oval adenoid cluster formed by liver cells, hepatocellular rosette, can also be observable.

Changes at the Portal Area

In most small portal areas, different degrees of lymphocytic infiltration can be observed, commonly with a small quantity of plasmocytes but rarely neutrophilic granulocytes. The portal area is commonly enlarged with accompanying different degrees of fibrosis. The bile ducts within hepatic lobule may be damaged, sometimes with observable bile ductule proliferation.

Based on the inflammation of the portal area and the interface as well as intralobular inflammatory activeness and fibrotic degree, the inflammatory activeness is graded as G0 ~ 4 and fibrosis is staged as S0 ~ 4 (Figs. 6.4, 6.5, 6.6, and 6.7). Chronic hepatitis can be defined as mild, moderate, and severe based on inflammatory activeness.

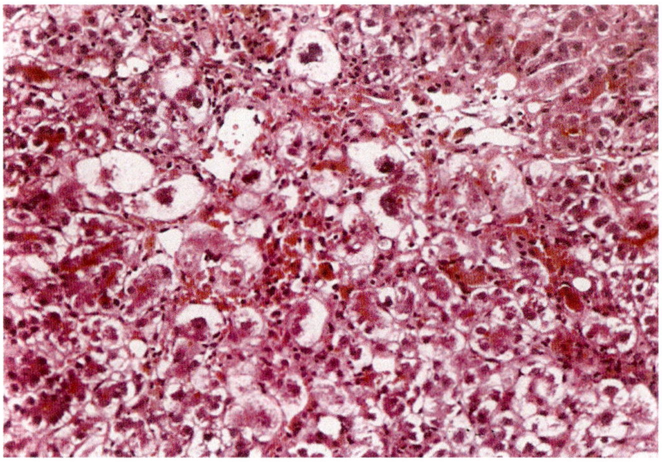

Fig. 6.1 Acute hepatitis, with balloon-like change and acidophilic change of the hepatocytic plasm as well as spots of focally necrotic hepatocytes. H&E, ×200

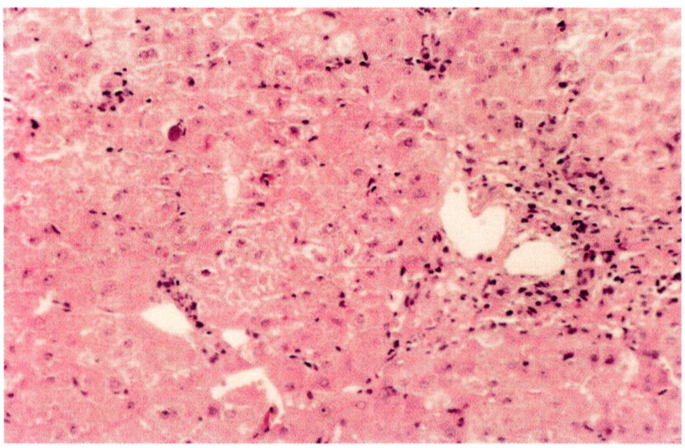

Fig. 6.2 Intralobular multiple spots of focally hepatocyte necrosis. H&E × 100

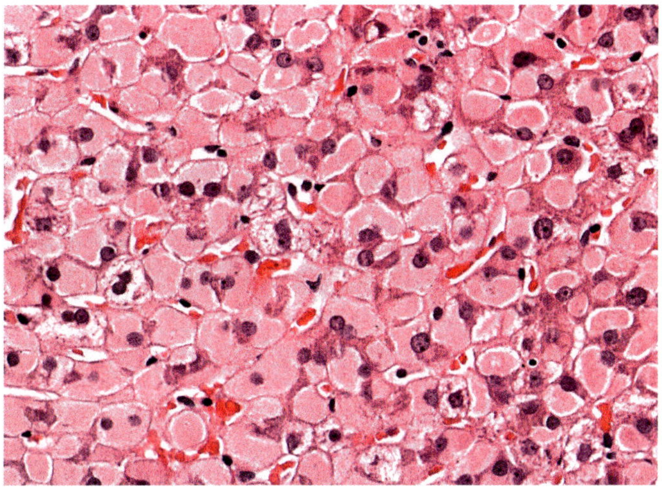

Fig. 6.3 Ground-glass-like hepatocytes. H&E×400

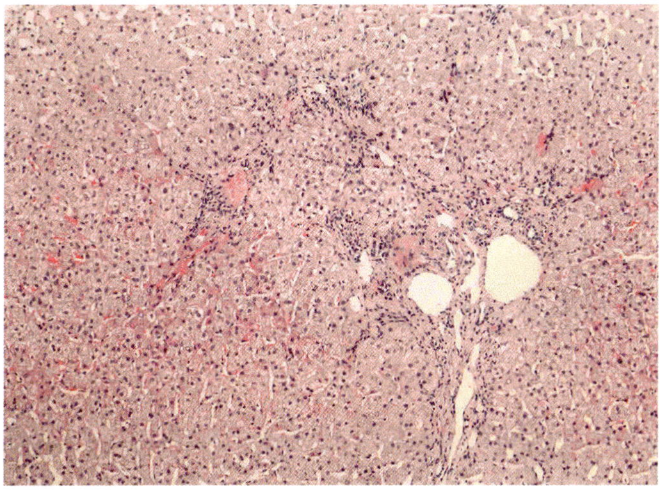

Fig. 6.4 Enlarged portal area with interface inflammation and the inflammatory activeness graded as G2. H&E×100

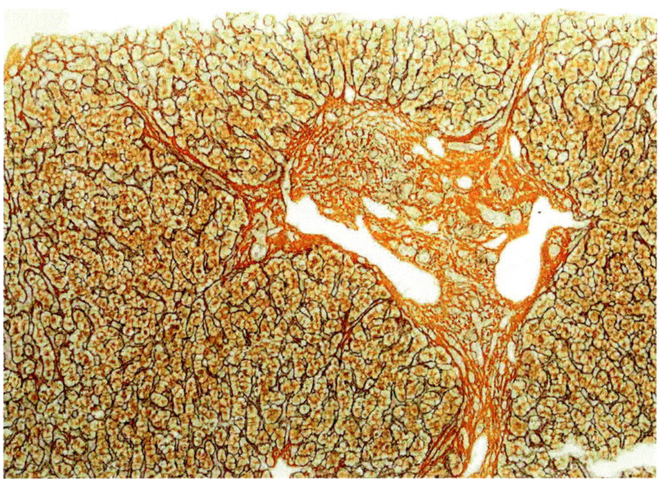

Fig. 6.5 Fibrosis at the portal area with accompanying formation of septum and fibrosis staged as S2. Reticular fiber×200

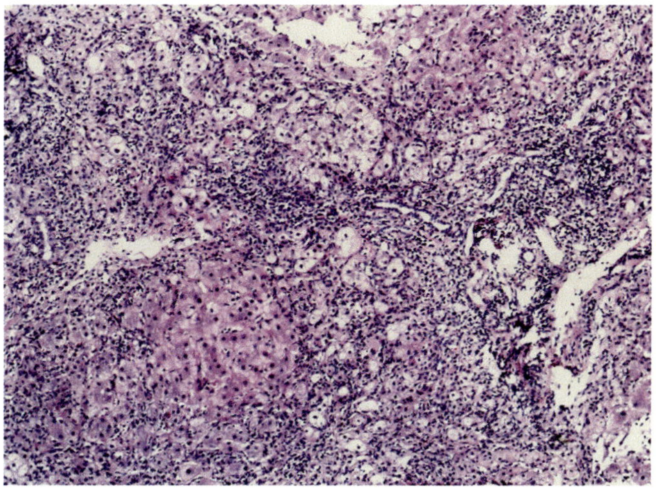

Fig. 6.6 Extremely enlarged portal area with severe interface inflammation and the inflammation activeness graded as G4. H&E×100

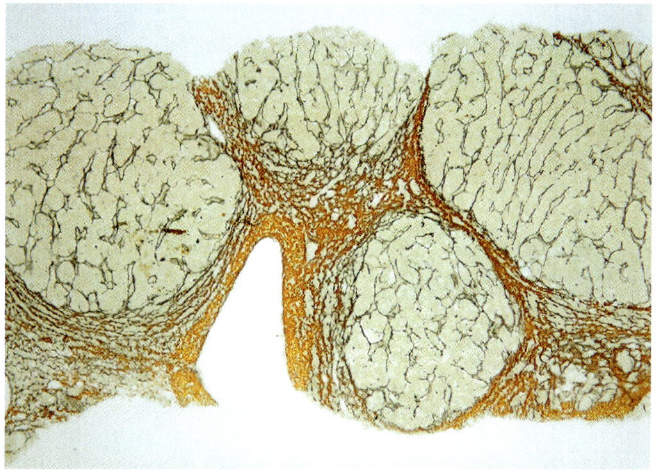

Fig. 6.7 Early stage of liver cirrhosis with formation of pseudolobule. Gorden & Sweets, ×100

Detection of HBV at Liver Tissue Section

By immunohistochemistry, the expression of HBsAg, HBcAg, Pre-sl, HBeAg, and HB×Ag in hepatocytes can be detected (Figs. 6.8 and 6.9).

6.4.2.3 Pathology of Hepatitis C

The pathologic changes of hepatitis C resemble to those of other types of hepatitis, showing inflammation and necrosis of the liver cells as well as infiltration of lymphocytes. Hepatitis C commonly develops into chronic condition.

Acute Hepatitis C

Histologically, acute hepatitis C resembles to acute hepatitis induced by other types of hepatitis viruses. Under a light microscope, acidophilic degeneration of plasma is obvious with formation of apoptotic bodies, which commonly scatter

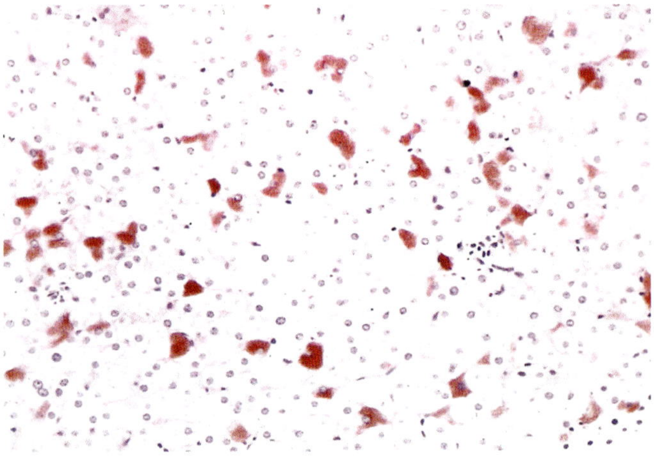

Fig. 6.8 Expression of HBsAg in hepatocyte as plasma and inclusion. Immunohistochemistry × 100

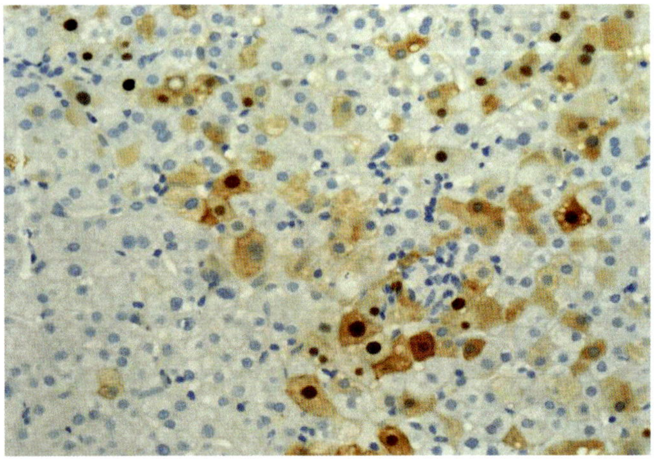

Fig. 6.9 Expression of HBcAg in hepatocyte as cytoplasm and nucleus. Immunohistochemistry × 400

near the central vein. The portal area and the hepatic lobule are shown with infiltration of lymphocytes, plasmocytes, and even neutrophilic and eosinophilic granulocytes. In some cases, the infiltration of lymphocytes within the hepatic sinus appears like strings of beads. In the cases with dense lymphocytes in the portal area, formation of lymphatic follicles can be observed.

Chronic Hepatitis C

Chronic hepatitis C is histologically characterized by: (1) aggregation of lymphocytes in the portal area (Fig. 6.10), (2) damages to the small bile ducts, (3) hepatocyte fat degeneration (Fig. 6.11), and (4) activation of the hepatic sinus cells.

Molecular Pathological Examination

In liver tissue, the detection rate of hepatitis C-related antigens is low and the percentage of hepatocytes with positive antigen is also low. HCAg is expressed as nucleus and plasma (Fig. 6.12). Due to highly variant genes of HCV, the positive

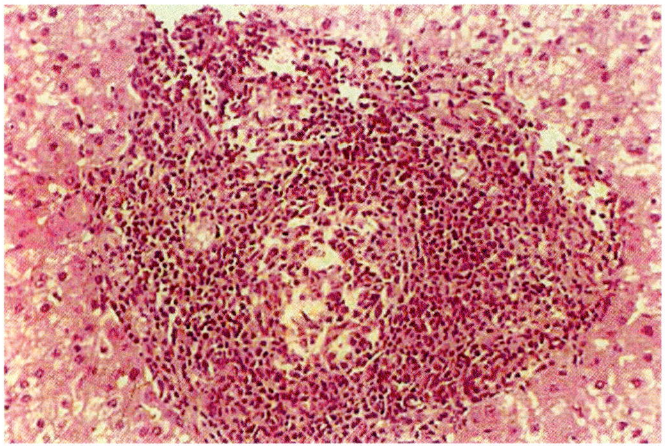

Fig. 6.10 Chronic hepatitis C with infiltration of dense lymphocytes in the portal area and formation of lymphatic follicles. H&E × 200

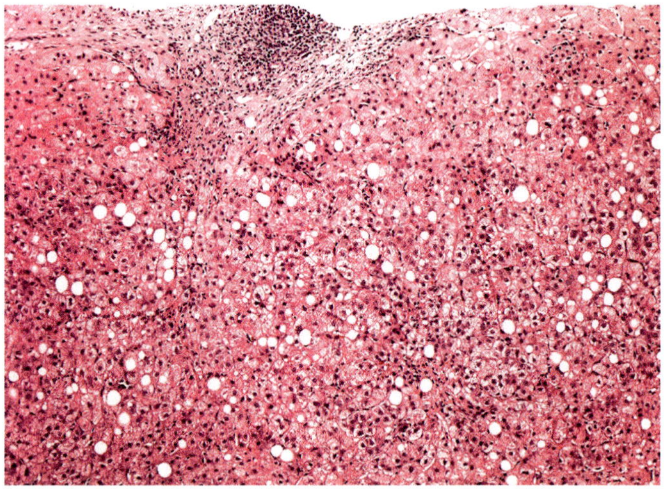

Fig. 6.11 Scattering distribution of fatty degenerated hepatocytes in the hepatic lobules. H&E × 200

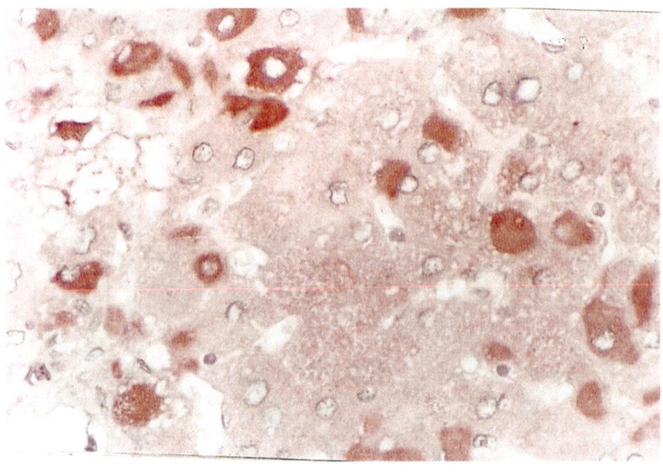

Fig. 6.12 Expression of HCV NS3Ag-positive signal in hepatocyte plasma. Immunohistochemistry × 400

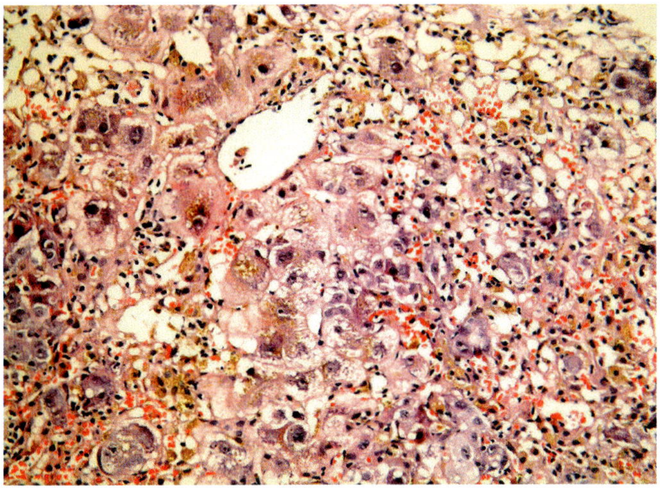

Fig. 6.13 Balloon-like change of intralobular hepatocyte, bile stasis, and inflammatory cell infiltration. H&E×400

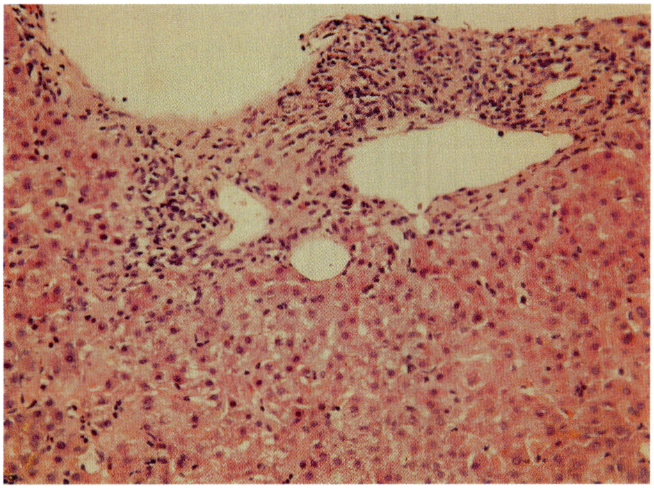

Fig. 6.14 Infiltration of predominant lymphocytes in the portal area, with observable plasmocytes. H&E×200

rates of HCV RNA in the liver tissue by in situ hybridization are commonly inconsistent.

6.4.2.4 Viral Hepatitis D

Simplex HDV infection is extremely rare. Histologically, acute and chronic hepatitis D resemble to that of other types of acute and chronic hepatitis, with the same modes of necrotic inflammation and fibrosis. In most cases, HDV and HBV infections are concurrent or overlapping, with more serious histological changes than simplex HBV infection. The histological changes include balloon-like changes, more hepatocytes with focally distributed acidophilic change fatty degeneration, more serious focal necrosis, fragment-like necrosis, bridging necrosis, and multilobular fusing necrosis. Severe interface inflammation is commonly serious.

6.4.2.5 Hepatitis E

The histologic changes of hepatitis E resemble to those of hepatitis A, with classical and bile-stasis changes of lobular hepatocytes in the cases of acute hepatitis. The classical pathological changes include spots of hepatocellular focal necrosis, formation of apoptotic body, balloon-like change, as well as infiltration of lymphocytes in hepatic lobule and the portal area (Fig. 6.13). Some of the bile-stasis-type lesions resemble to those of hepatitis A, with cholangiolar bile stasis and adenoid structural changes of the hepatocytes. However, the hepatocyte degeneration and necrosis are not so obvious as those in the cases of classical acute hepatitis. Although the infiltrated inflammatory cells are predominantly lymphocytes, large quantities of neutrophilic granulocyte and plasmocyte can be observed to infiltrate in the hepatic lobule and the portal area (Fig. 6.14). No fibrosis can be observed in the portal area. The inflammatory response of Kupffer cell proliferation in the hepatic lobule is mild. The hepatocytes are shown with fatty degeneration and bile stasis, and formation of bile thrombus in bile capillaries is common.

6.5 Clinical Diagnosis

The clinical diagnosis of viral hepatitis is mainly based on the epidemiological data, clinical manifestations, and laboratory tests.

6.5.1 Epidemiological Data

For the diagnosis of hepatitis A and hepatitis E, data about local prevalence of hepatitis should be collected and analyzed. In addition, the history of intaking possibly contaminated food should also be taken into account. And the history of vaccination preventing hepatitis A and E acts as reference for the diagnosis.

For the diagnosis of hepatitis B and C, the history of transfusion blood or blood products and the history of unsterilized injection should be reported. Other histories, such as history of vaccination preventing hepatitis B and history of family hepatitis B virus infection, especially history of HBsAg positive in mother of infant patient, facilitate the diagnosis of hepatitis B.

6.5.2 Etiological Diagnosis

6.5.2.1 Hepatitis A

Hepatitis A can be etiologically diagnosed based on the following finding: (1) serum anti-HAV IgM positive in patients with acute hepatitis, (2) at least four times increase of serum anti-HAV antibody titer at the acute and convalescent stages, (3) detected hepatitis A virus particle in the stool or detected hepatitis A virus antigen, and (4) detected hepatitis A virus RNA in serum or stool. Patients with any ONE positive finding of above conditions can be defined with recent infection of hepatitis A.

6.5.2.2 Hepatitis B

Chronic HBV infection can be categorized into the following conditions:

1. Chronic hepatitis B
   Based on HBeAg positive or negative, chronic hepatitis B can be categorized into HBeAg-positive chronic hepatitis B and HBeAg-negative chronic hepatitis B.
2. HBV carriers
   The chronic HBV carriers are defined to be HBsAg and HBV DNA positive as well as HBeA or anti-HBe positive. Within 1 year, follow-ups show serum ALT and AST levels to be within normal range for at least consecutive three times, with negative findings by biopsy of liver tissue.
   The nonactive HBsAg carriers are defined to be serum HBsAg positive, HBeAg negative, anti-HBe positive or negative, and HBV DNA lower than the lowest limit. Within 1 year, consecutive follow-ups show at least three times of ALT level within the normal range. Histological examination of the liver tissue demonstrates the Knodell hepatitis activity index (HAI) to be lower than four or qualitatively mild condition by other semiquantitative scoring systems.
3. Latent chronic hepatitis B
   Latent chronic hepatitis B refers to the condition of serum HBsAg negative but serum/liver tissue HBV DNA positive with clinical manifestations of chronic hepatitis B. In addition to HBV DNA positive, the patients may also show serum anti-HBs, anti-HBe, and/or anti-HBc positive. However, in about 20 % patients with latent chronic hepatitis B, HBV DNA is positive, but all other serological indicators are negative.

6.5.2.3 Hepatitis C

In patients with both HCV RNA and anti-HCV positive, the diagnosis of hepatitis C can be defined. Anti-HCV negative but HCV RNA positive can be detected in patients receiving hemodialysis or intense immunosuppressive therapy.

6.5.2.4 Hepatitis D

The patients with current HBV infection and serum HDV antigen or HDV antibody IgM or high titer of serum HDV antibody IgG or serum HDV RNA positive can be diagnosed with hepatitis D. Otherwise, the patients with current HBV infection and intrahepatic HDV antigen or HDV RNA positive can be diagnosed with hepatitis D.

6.5.2.5 Hepatitis E

The diagnosis of hepatitis E can be defined based on detected anti-HEV IgG and/or IgM antibodies. In the cases with high titer of anti-HEV IgG during the acute stage, or with a change from low titer to high titer along with the progress of the condition, or with a change from high titer to low titer and even negative, the diagnosis of acute HEV infection can be made.

6.6 Imaging Diagnosis of Hepatitis and Its Related Diseases

6.6.1 Ultrasound

6.6.1.1 Ultrasound of Severe Viral Hepatitis

In the cases of severe viral hepatitis, the ultrasonic demonstrations are characteristic, including:

1. Shrinkage of the liver with abnormal shape and unsmooth liver capsule or with folds.
2. Echo from the hepatic parenchyma is reticular, patchy, or granular due to interlace scattering large masses of necrosis and residual liver tissues, which is known as maplike liver or worm-bitten-like liver (Fig. 6.15).
3. When the supporting framework collapses due to large masses of necrosis, the portal vein may be twisted to shift its primary position. Such a sign demonstrated at the early stage or to be serious indicates a poor prognosis.

6.6.1.2 Ultrasonic Changes of the Common Conditions Complicating Viral Hepatitis Portal Hypertension

1. The luminal diameter of the trunk of portal vein ≥14 mm indicates occurrence of portal hypertension. In the cases with complicating dilation of superior mesenteric vein and splenic vein as well as splenomegaly, the diagnosis of portal hypertension can be defined.

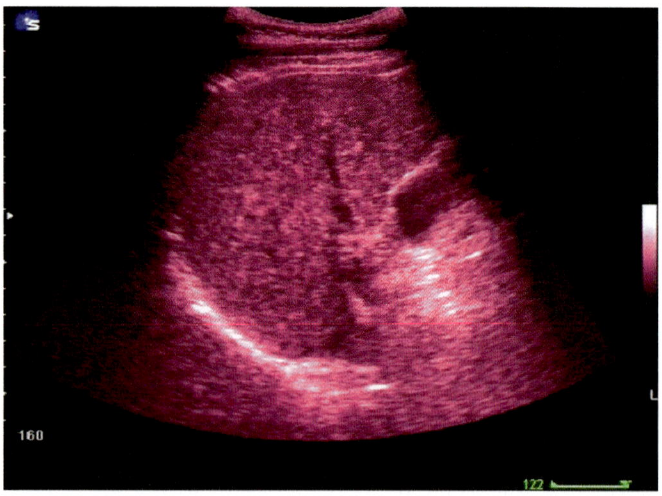

Fig. 6.15 Severe hepatitis. Echo from the liver parenchyma is worm-bitten-like due to the scattering large masses of necrosis

2. Decreased blood flow rate in the portal vein (<14 ~ 15 cm/s) or the blood flow directing away from the liver indicates occurrence of portal hypertension.
3. Formation of portosystemic collateral circulation with luminal diameter of the coronary vein >5 mm indicates the occurrence of portal hypertension. The reopening of adult umbilical vein is demonstrated as extending duct-like non-echo structure from sagittal part of the portal vein toward the abdominal wall, with portal-vein-like blood flow signal inside.

Pleural Effusion and Ascites

Pleural effusion is ultrasonographically demonstrated as crescent-shaped or large flaky liquid dark area at the inferior thoracic cavity. Ascites is ultrasonographically demonstrated as flaky irregular liquid dark area at the inferior abdominal cavity, anterior liver, interspace between the liver and kidney, as well as interspace between the spleen and kidney.

6.6.1.3 Viral Hepatitis and Liver Cirrhosis

Direct Signs

1. The liver section is morphologically abnormal, with disproportional liver lobes. The volume of liver is diffusively enlarged (at the early stage) or shrunk (at the advanced stage), with obvious shrinkage of the posterior segment of the right liver lobe. The lateral segment of the left liver lobe and the caudate lobe is commonly demonstrated with proliferation and swelling.
2. The surface of the liver is unsmooth, with wavelike, serration-like, or humplike change.
3. The echo from liver parenchyma is disordered, with unevenly distributed intrahepatic light spots. The echo is thickened and enhanced, possibly with reticular and poorly defined patches of changes. Repeated hepatocellular destruction and regeneration can be demonstrated as low-echo or high-echo nodules with three-dimensional profile.
4. The intrahepatic tubal system is demonstrated with no abnormality at the early stage. At the advanced stage, the lumen of hepatic vein is thinner or uneven, possibly with compressed vascular wall. The hepatic vein is twisted, stiff, or even absent. The hepatic artery may be compensatorily widened, and the minor branches of intrahepatic portal vein are twisted and thinner, with enhanced echo from the vascular wall. The trunk of portal vein as well as its secondary- and third-graded branches is widened, sometimes with portal thrombus and portal sponge degeneration.

Indirect Signs

1. Spleen

   The spleen is displayed with enhanced echo from its parenchyma, with a thickness of ≥40 mm and a length of ≥120 mm. Even megalosplenia may be shown. The splenic vein is dilated and tortuous. In the cases with obviously dilated splenic vein, the splenic hilum can be demonstrated as a honeycomb-like no-echo area, with splenic vein engorgement. The lumen of the splenic vein may exceed 9 mm and may even larger than the lumen of portal vein.
2. Formation of ascites

   Ascites is commonly demonstrated as liquid no-echo area with favorable sonolucency. A small quantity of ascites is commonly found anterior or peripheral to the liver and sometimes can be observed at the lower abdomen. Occasionally, a small quantity of ascites is confined anterior to the liver, at the hepatorenal recess, or at the lower abdomen.
3. Portal hypertension

   Portal hypertension may be demonstrated as:
   (a) increased luminal diameter of the portal vein, with the luminal diameter of the portal venous trunk mostly being ≥14 mm. The luminal diameter does not change along with respiration. Colored Doppler ultrasound shows decreased velocity of the blood flow in the portal vein, possibly with bidirectional blood flow or reverse directional blood flow, the velocity of blood flow in the portal vein mostly within 15 cm/s.
   (b) Splenomegaly.
   (c) Open collateral circulation, including open umbilical vein and dilated coronary vein (the left gastric vein).
4. Thinner hepatic vein

   In patients with liver cirrhosis, the hepatic vein can be demonstrated to be twisted, thinner, or poorly defined. The normal three-phase oscillogram of the hepatic vein may be absent, which may be related to decreased adaptability of the hepatic vein induced by liver parenchyma fibrosis around the hepatic vein and its fatty degeneration.
5. Short-circuit formation of the hepatic artery and vein

   By ultrasonography, the hepatic artery and vein are demonstrated with shortened filling period, mostly less than 12 s.

6.6.1.4 Primary Liver Cancer

Ultrasonic Typing of HCC and the Direct Signs

The typing of HCC by ultrasound resembles to its pathological typing, including the huge-mass type, the nodular type, and the diffuse type.

The Huge-Mass Type

A huge solid mass in the liver parenchyma can be demonstrated, with a diameter of >10 cm. The mass is mostly found at the right liver lobe, rarely with an exophytic growth. It has vascularized pedicle attached to the liver.

The mass mostly grows in a spherically expanding manner, with well-defined but irregular boundary (Fig. 6.16). In rare cases, the mass has an infiltration-like growth in the liver parenchyma, with poorly defined boundary. In the

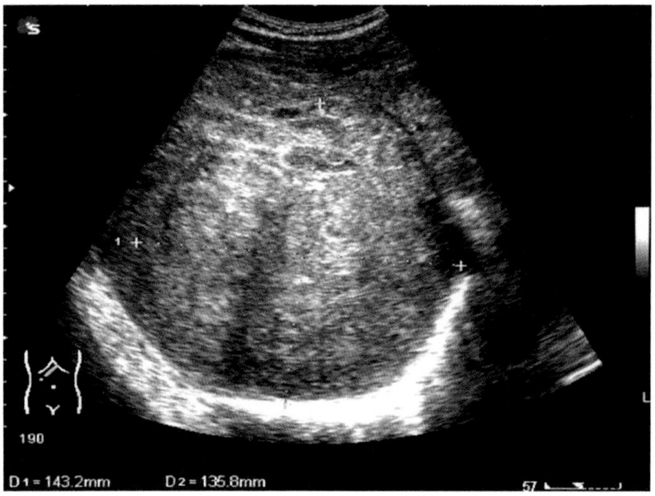

Fig. 6.16 The huge-mass type HCC. A mass in size of 14.3 cm × 13.5 cm was demonstrated at the right liver lobe in expansive growth, with well-defined but irregular boundary

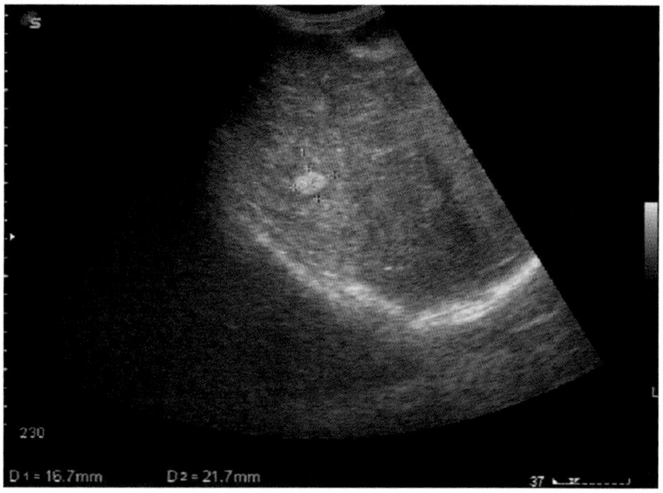

Fig. 6.17 The nodular type of HCC. It was demonstrated with oval-shaped hyperintense echo nodule in the liver parenchyma, which had well-defined boundary and peripheral light acoustic halo

cases with isointense echo of the mass, the diagnosis can be missed.

In most cases, the mass has hyperintense echo, which is thick and uneven. Within the hyperintense echo, heterogenous hypointense echo is mostly present with necrotic liquefied cavities at the center.

Around the mass, small nodules are sometimes demonstrated with a diameter of 1–2 cm.

At marginal mass, hypointense acoustic halo is demonstrated, which is thin with poorly defined external boundary but well-defined internal boundary.

The typical sign of rapid-in-rapid-out of the contrast agent can be demonstrated by ultrasonography.

The Nodular Type

The nodules in the liver parenchyma are relatively small, whose diameter is commonly <5 cm. The lesion is mostly singular but rarely multiple.

Within the nodules, the echo is commonly heterogenous, which may be hypointense, isointense, hyperintense, or mixed intense (Fig. 6.17).

The nodules are commonly round or oval, with well-defined boundary.

The nodules with hyperintense echo are demonstrated with lateral acoustic shadow. However, the nodules with isointense or hypointense echo may be demonstrated with slightly enhanced posterior echo.

By colored Doppler, the nodules are demonstrated with inner or peripheral arterial blood flow signal.

By ultrasonography, the typical sign of rapid-in-rapid-out of the contrast agent can be demonstrated.

6.6.2 CT Scan

6.6.2.1 Hepatocirrhosis After Viral Hepatitis by CT Scan

In China, the most common hepatocirrhosis includes hepatocirrhosis after viral hepatitis and schistosomiasis hepatocirrhosis.

Direct Signs (Fig. 6.18)

1. Change of liver size

   Extensive fatty degeneration at the early stage causes enlargement of the liver. However, at the advanced stage, the liver shrinks with disproportional liver lobes (especially transverse diameter ratio of the caudal lobe to the right lobe). The right lobe is commonly demonstrated with atrophy and the caudal lobe with compensatory enlargement. The left lobe is normal or shrinks or has its lateral segment enlarged.
2. Change of liver shape

   The nodules protrude to cause unsmooth lateral margin of the liver. In addition, the protrusion of nodules also causes protrusion of the primarily sunk medial margin, with widened liver fissures.
3. Change of liver density

   The density of liver is made decreased due to fatty degeneration. However, in some cases, focally decreased density is not a sign to distinguish hepatocirrhosis from when the fat changed, but the localized decrease of the density sometimes is hard to make it be differentiated from the primary hepatocellular carcinoma or secondary liver cancer.

   The liver was demonstrated with shrinkage, disproportional liver lobes, and unsmooth lateral margin. Plain scan

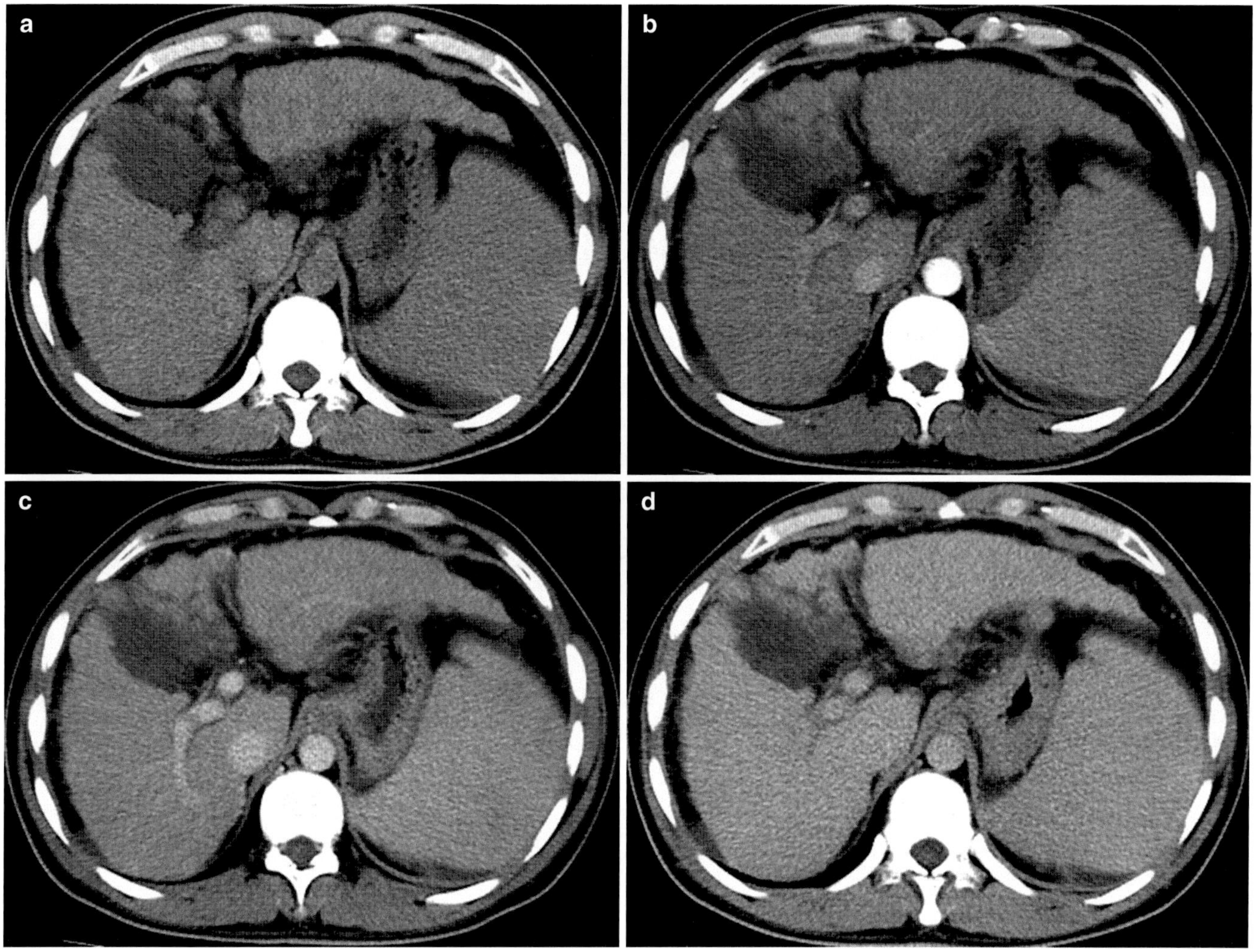

Fig. 6.18 Direct signs of hepatocirrhosis after viral hepatitis. (**a**) Plain scan; (**b**) arterial phase; (**c**) portal venous phase; (**d**) delayed phase

of the liver parenchyma demonstrated nodules with even density. Contrast scan displayed the equal density of the nodules with the surrounding liver parenchyma. By dynamic observation, the nodules were shown with no growth; the spleen was enlarged and thickened; and a small quantity of ascites was displayed.

Indirect Signs (Fig. 6.19)

1. Enlarged spleen

   It is an important indirect sign indicating cirrhosis of the liver. However, not all the cases of liver cirrhosis show the sign of splenomegaly.
2. Portal hypertension

   The diameter of the portal vein is increased and the splenic vein shows varicose. Thick and twisted vascular sign is demonstrated in the vicinity of splenic hilum. The veins at the gastric fundus and inferior segment of the esophagus are twisted and varicose, appearing like earthworm and grape cluster.

   The liver was demonstrated with shrinkage and the spleen was large and thick. The luminal diameter of the portal vein was increased and the splenic vein was thick and twisted.
3. Widened liver fissure and shift of the liver hilum
4. Ascites

   The distance between the liver and abdominal wall is increased, with waterlike density strip of opacity.

Regenerated Nodules of Liver Cirrhosis

By plain CT scan, typical regenerated nodule of liver cirrhosis is demonstrated with abnormal shape of the liver, unsmooth liver surface, disproportional liver lobes, and equal-density or low-density nodule in the liver. Occasionally, the nodular density is relatively high. By contrast scan, the density of regenerated nodule after liver cirrhosis is equal to its surrounding liver parenchyma. By dynamic observation, the regenerated nodule is shown with no growth.

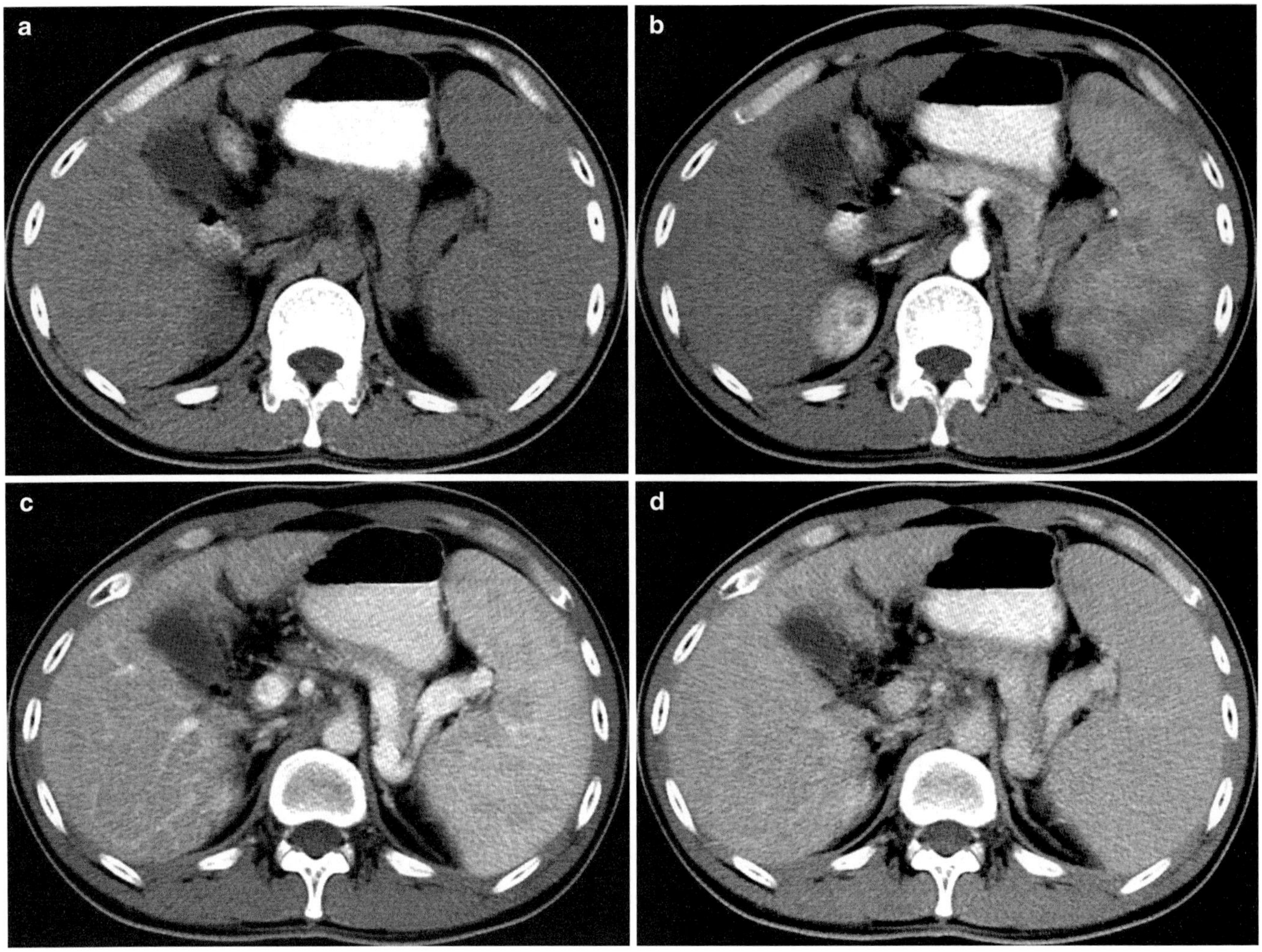

Fig. 6.19 Indirect signs of liver cirrhosis after viral hepatitis. (**a**) Plain scan; (**b**) arterial phase; (**c**) portal phase; (**d**) delayed phase

Differential Diagnosis from Schistosomiasis Cirrhosis

Patients with schistosomiasis cirrhosis commonly have a history of living in the epidemic area. By CT scan, the intrahepatic calcification is demonstrated as interlaced linear calcification (Fig. 6.20). These calcification lesions divide the liver into small areas with different shapes and sizes, which appear like a map. Under the liver capsule, the calcification is demonstrated as fine linear or wide strip. Otherwise, the calcification lesions may aggregate into mass like with marginal irregularity. In the liver, crablike calcification may be demonstrated, with calcifications aggregated into mass at the center and strips of opacity protruding out of the center. The calcification is commonly located at the right lobe, followed by the quadrate lobe and the caudal lobe. The calcification is the most rarely located at the left lobe. The degree of calcification is more serious at the right lobe than that at the other lobes and is more serious at the vicinity of the liver than that at the central liver. At the area closer to the liver surface, the calcification is more obvious. In rare cases, extensive calcification can be

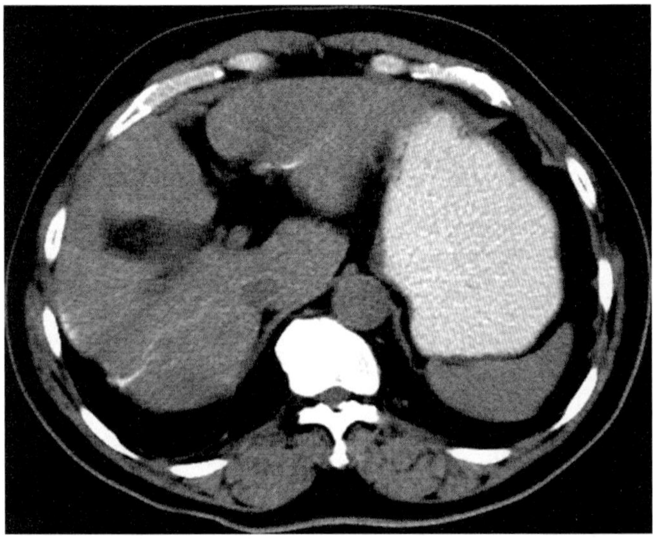

Fig. 6.20 Schistosomiasis hepatocirrhosis. Plain scan demonstrated shrinkage of the liver, disproportional liver lobes, and unsmooth lateral margin of the liver. Linear calcification was displayed under the liver capsule or in the liver, which separated the liver into small areas

demonstrated in the whole liver. Extrahepatic calcification is demonstrated as spots or semi-archlike calcification at the portal venous wall. Even calcification of the whole portal venous wall is demonstrated. Sometimes, strip of calcification at the splenic vein and arch shape calcification at the colon wall can be demonstrated.

CT Signs of Liver Cirrhosis Complicated by Hepatocellular Carcinoma: Fig. 6.21
Liver cirrhosis occurring based on viral hepatitis may be complicated by primary hepatocellular carcinoma whose incidence rate is about 30–50 %. Pathological studies have demonstrated that large nodule-type liver cirrhosis or liver cirrhosis after viral hepatitis is more likely to be complicated by primary hepatocellular carcinoma. Therefore, for patients with chronic liver cirrhosis, cancer lesions should be attentively detected during CT scan. In the cases of liver cirrhosis complicated by primary hepatocellular carcinoma, CT signs for liver cirrhosis include changes of liver density, size, and shape as well as regenerated nodule of liver cirrhosis. The CT signs for complicated hepatocellular carcinoma are also typical, especially the huge mass type and the nodular type, including low-density masses in different sizes. Some large masses can be demonstrated with even lower density area of central necrosis. The neoplasm is encapsulated. After injection of contrast agent, obvious or irregular enhancement of the neoplasm is demonstrated.

Plain CT scan displayed shrinkage of the liver, widened liver fissure, and wavelike liver margin. The posterior segment of the right lobe was shown with a slightly low-density nodule in size of about 2.7 × 3.1 cm. At the arterial phase, the

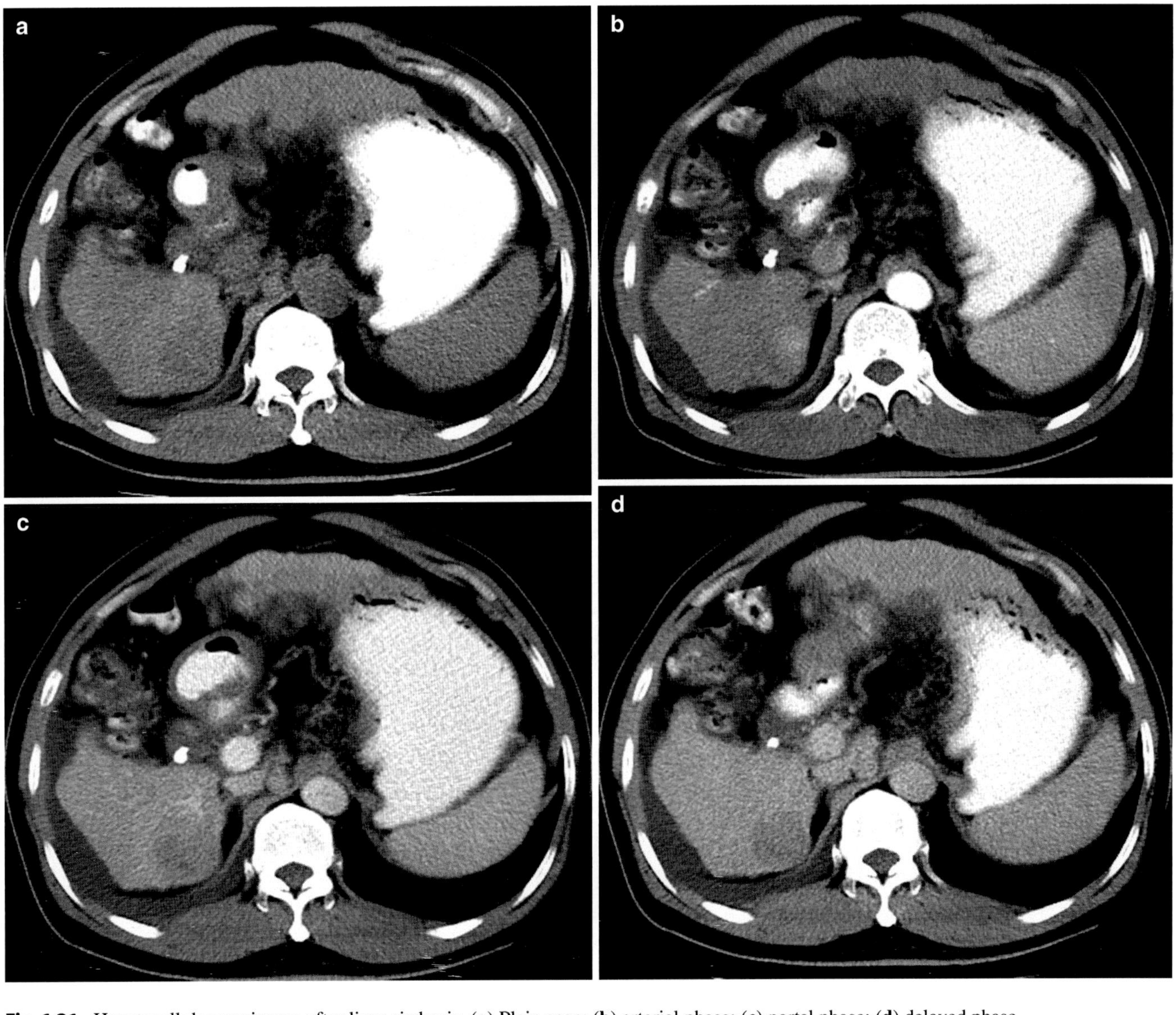

Fig. 6.21 Hepatocellular carcinoma after liver cirrhosis. (**a**) Plain scan; (**b**) arterial phase; (**c**) portal phase; (**d**) delayed phase

nodule was rapidly and heterogeneously enhanced. At the portal and delayed phases, the enhancement was demonstrated to be decreased, with less enhancement than surrounding liver parenchyma. A small quantity of ascites was displayed.

6.6.2.2 CT Signs of Primary Liver Cancer

The malignancies of liver mainly include hepatocellular carcinoma, cholangiocellular carcinoma (intrahepatic biliary cancer), bile duct cystadenocarcinoma, mixed hepatocellular and cholangiocellular carcinoma, hepatoblastoma, and undifferentiated cancer.

Hepatocellular carcinoma (HCC) is the most common cellular carcinoma in primary liver cancer. In China, the incidence rate of liver cirrhosis complicating HCC is about 90 %, which is commonly manifested as portal hypertension and large nodular liver cirrhosis. HCC can be categorized into three types: the huge-mass type, the nodular type, and the diffusive type (Figs. 6.22 and 6.23).

Direct Signs of HCC

CT Plain Scan

Density CT plain scan can hardly display the nodular lesion with a diameter within 1 cm. In most cases of liver cancer, plain scan only demonstrates low-density lesion in the hepatic area, or rarely equal-density or high-density lesion. It is related to the differentiation of HCC and its components as well as the background of the liver. The density may be homogeneous or heterogeneous. Within lesion with heterogeneous density, even lower-density area can be demonstrated due to tissue necrosis and liquefaction, with central or marginal tumor nodule. In some rare lesions, high-density lesion of hemorrhage or calcification can be displayed.

Morphology

Most lesions are round or oval and rare lesions are lobulated or irregular. Most lesions of neoplasm are demonstrated with poorly defined boundary. And lesions with expansive growth

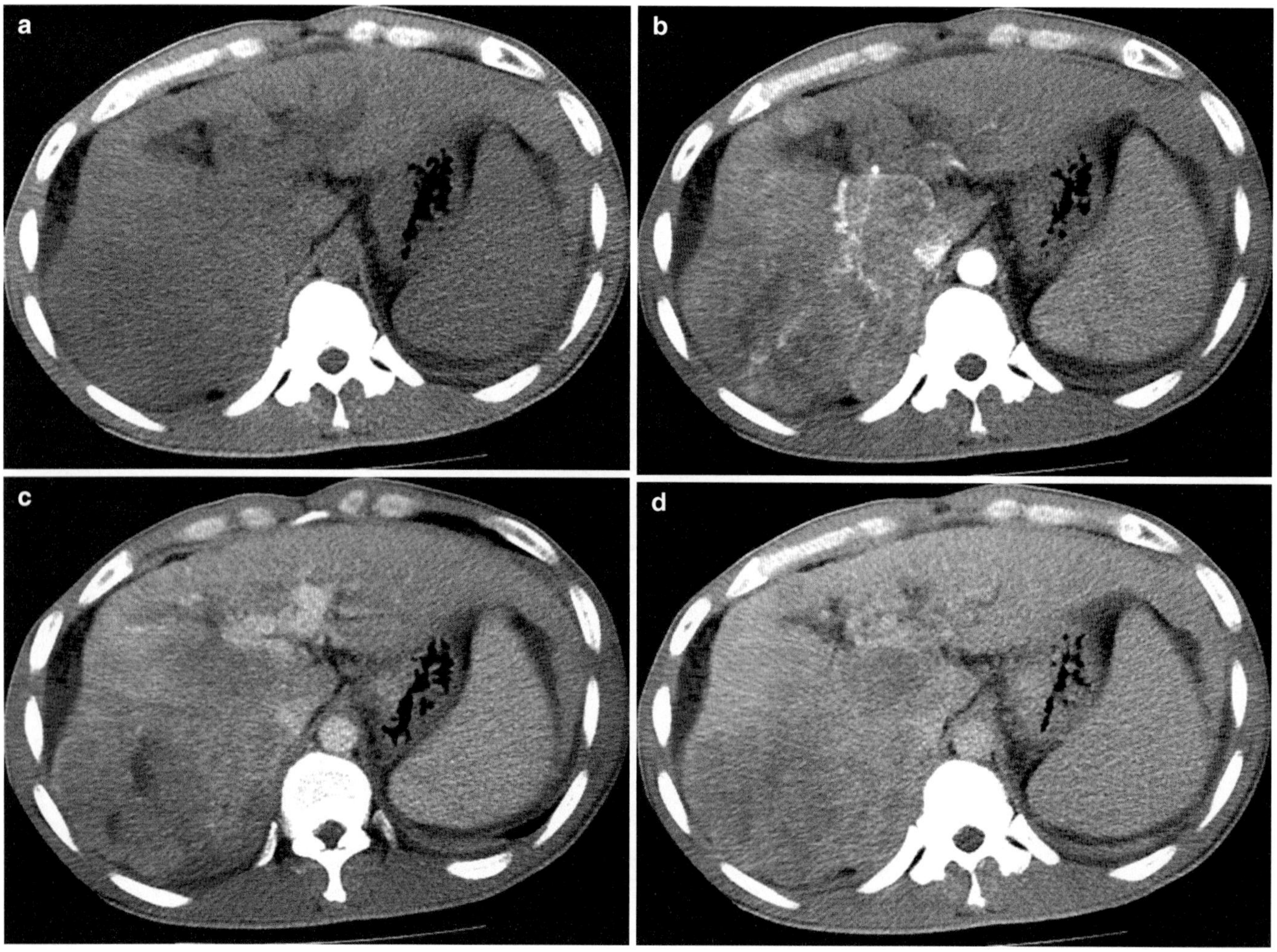

Fig. 6.22 Huge-mass type of liver cancer. (**a**) Plain scan; (**b**) the arterial phase; (**c**) the portal vein phase; (**d**) the delayed phase

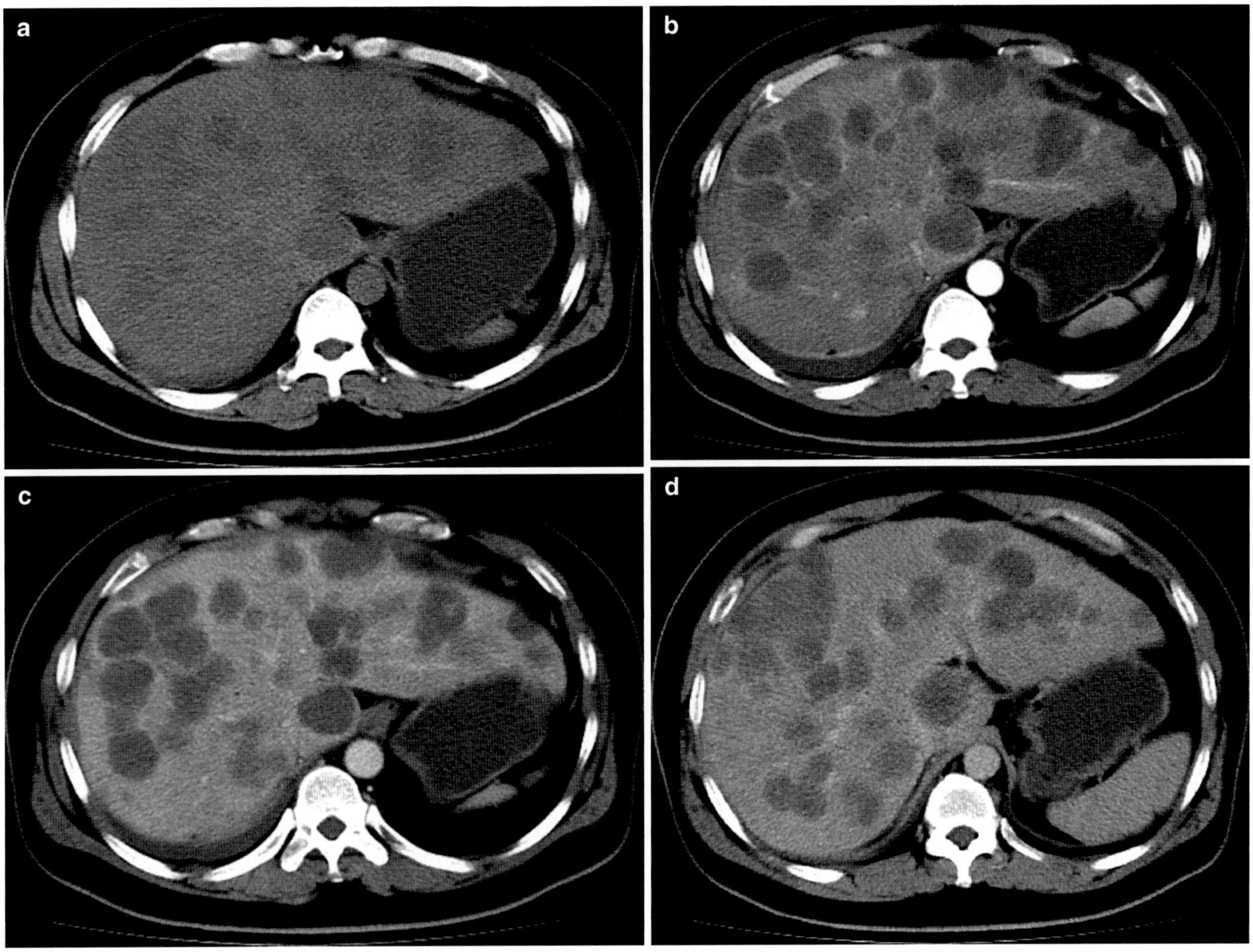

Fig. 6.23 Diffuse type of hepatocellular carcinoma. (**a**) Plain scan; (**b**) the arterial phase; (**c**) the portal vein phase; (**d**) the delayed phase

are demonstrated with ring-shaped transparent area, which is known as the halo ring sign. It is a characteristic CT sign of primary liver cancer, which is mostly singular but rarely multiple.

Contrast CT Scan The dynamic circulation of the contrast agent within the liver can be staged into three phases: the arterial phase, the portal vein phase, and the equilibrium phase.

The Arterial Phase The arterial phase is actually the contrast phase of the abdominal aorta and its major branches, with uncontrasted portal vein and inferior vena cava. The liver parenchyma is only slightly enhanced with increasingly stronger enhancement. Due to the main blood supply from the hepatic artery, the lesion of HCC shows immediate enhancement at the arterial phase, with rapid increase of its CT value to the peak to exceed that of the liver parenchyma. The peak value lasts only for a short period of time, with following rapid decrease.

The Portal Vein Phase During the phase, the contrast agent gradually distributes from intravascular to extravascular tissue, with peak enhancement of the liver parenchyma that is close to the density of HCC. The first equal-density cross of the liver parenchyma and HCC occurs.

The Equilibrium Phase The extravascular distribution of the contrast agent remains with equilibrium, with absent intrahepatic vascular opacity. When the CT value of the HCC decreases and that of the liver parenchyma increases, the lesion is demonstrated with low density. In 2–3 min, the CT value of liver parenchyma begins to decrease to be close to the density of lesion again, with recurrence of equal-density cross. In general, the contrast of liver cancer with abundant blood supply to normal liver parenchyma experiences three procedures from high density to equal density and following low density. The whole course is transient, with characteristic sign of rapid-increase-rapid-decrease.

Plain scan displayed the right liver lobe with huge mass with heterogeneous and slightly low density. The mass was heterogeneously enhanced at the arterial phase, with more neovascular shadow. At the portal vein phase and the delayed phase, the mass showed decreased enhancement with more heterogeneous density. The right branch of the portal vein was demonstrated with cancer embolus and filling defect.

The liver was displayed with increased size. Plain scan of the liver parenchyma demonstrated multiple round-like poorly defined nodular lesions with slightly low density. Contrast scan showed marginal enhancement of the lesion, with slight inner enhancement. However, the inner density of the lesion was lower than that of the surrounding normal liver tissue. By contrast scan, the cancer lesions were better defined and the branch of portal vein was demonstrated with filling defect.

The small lesions of cancer are mostly homogeneously enhanced, while the large lesions of cancer are mostly heterogeneously enhanced. Their density may be higher or lower than or equal to the normal liver tissue. The morphology of the cancer lesion by CT scan shows its growth manner. In the cases with the cancer nodule in infiltrative growth, CT scan shows its irregular shape. In the cases with the cancer nodule in expansive growth with central liquefaction and necrosis, CT scan shows central low density of the lesion. By contrast scan, the cancer lesion of diffuse type is displayed with no obvious enhancement. For the cases of cancer lesion with lower density than the normal liver tissue, the cancer lesion can be better defined. The capsule of cancer lesion can be demonstrated with slightly high-density ring by contrast scan. In addition, contrast scan can demonstrate the lesion that is poorly defined by plain scan, especially some small satellite lesions.

Indirect Signs

1. Cancer embolus of portal vein

   Cancer embolus of portal vein commonly occurs at the portal vein adjacent to the cancer lesion, with the involved portal vein dilated.

   By plain scan, the density of cancer embolus is equal to or slightly lower than that of the blood in portal vein.

   By contrast scan, filling defect can be displayed in the portal vein.

   The involved portal vein is compensatorily dilated due to the existence of nourishing vessels, with visible enhancement of the vascular wall.

   Collateral circulation occurs in vicinity of the trunk and major branches. Around the gall bladder, grid-like collateral vascular shadow can be demonstrated.

   The wedge-shaped low-density shadow is demonstrated due to insufficient blood supply to the tissue caused by cancer embolus.
2. The cancer lesion in the vicinity of portal area or deep liver may cause shift of the liver hilum or hepatic vascular vessels.
3. In about 80 % cases of liver cancer, liver cirrhosis occurs to complicate the condition.

CT Signs of Small Hepatocellular Carcinoma: (Fig. 6.24)

The triphasic spiral CT is an important radiological modality for the diagnosis of small hepatocellular carcinoma. The scan at the hepatic arterial phase is of the most significant in detecting lesion because most of the lesions are enhanced at this phase, with homogeneous or heterogeneous high density. Meanwhile, the liver parenchyma is demonstrated with slight enhancement at this phase. Therefore, the lesion can be detected due to the large discrepancy of the densities between the lesion and the liver parenchyma. Theoretically, the liver parenchyma is demonstrated with obvious enhancement at the portal vein phase, while the cancer lesion is demonstrated with low density. The lesion is also detectable at this phase due to the discrepancy of the densities between the liver parenchyma and the cancer lesion.

Differential Diagnosis of HCC

1. Focal nodular proliferation of the liver (Fig. 6.25)

   It is a rarely occurring benign neoplasm in the liver, commonly with a diameter of less than 5 cm and well-defined boundary. By CT plain scan, the nodule is commonly demonstrated with equal or slightly low homogeneous density as well as smooth, intact, and well-defined boundary. By contrast scan, the lesion is demonstrated with high density at the early stage but with no enhancement of its central scar tissue, appearing as starlike or radiating low density. The patients usually report no history of liver cirrhosis.

   By plain scan, the lesion was displayed with equal density. However, it was demonstrated with high density at the arterial phase and with equal density at the portal vein and delayed phases. In typical cases, the central fibrous scar was shown with starlike lower density at the arterial phase, with delayed enhancement.
2. Liver abscess (Fig. 6.26)

   Plain scan shows round or round-like low-density area, with uneven density but well-defined boundary. Contrast scan demonstrates the lesion with ring-shaped enhancement or double-target sign. By contrast scan, the multilocular or honeycomb-like low-density area is demonstrated with obvious marginal and septal enhancement, with petal-like sign. Gas shadow in the lesion has diagnostic significance. And the differential diagnosis can be made in combination to the clinical manifestations.

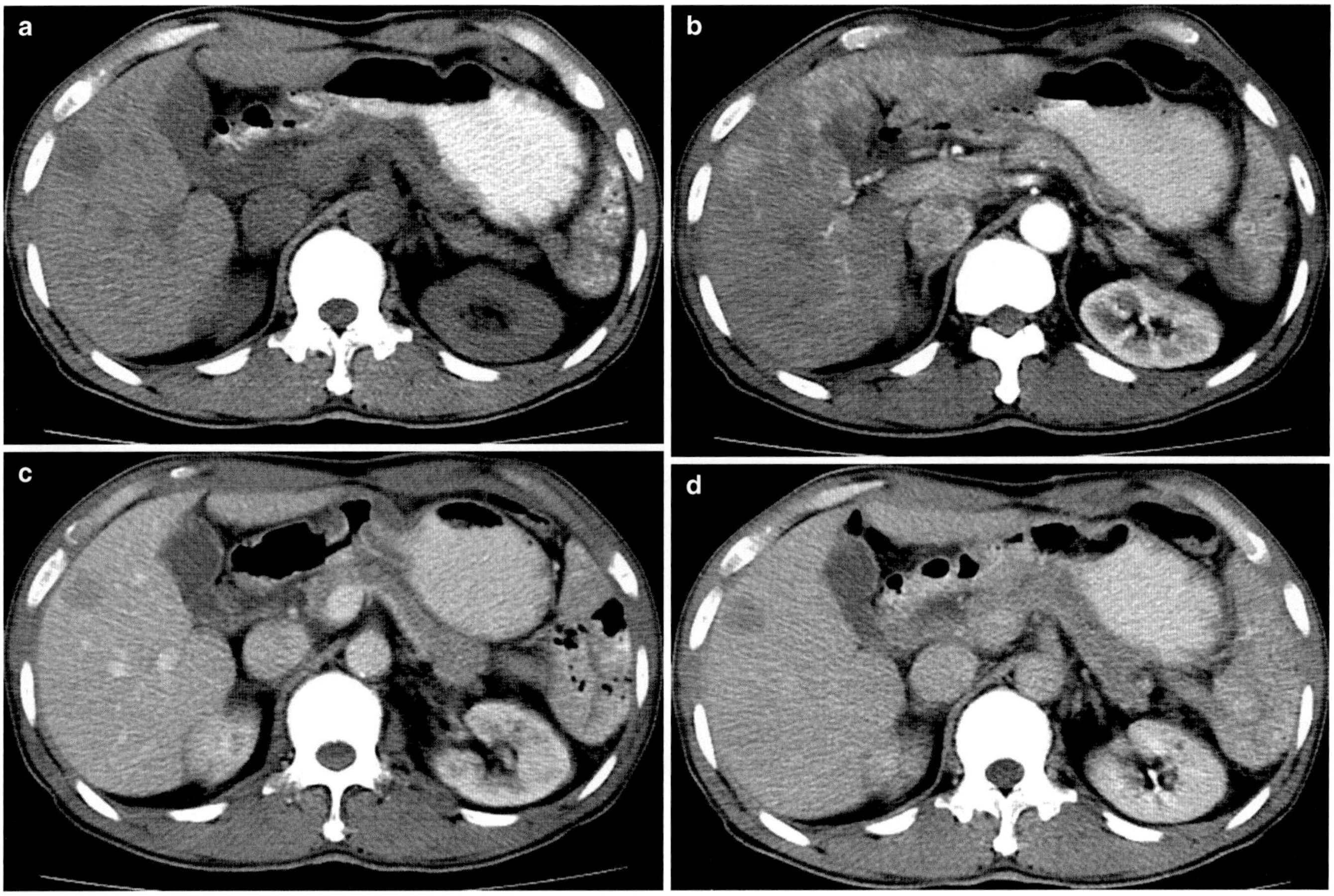

Fig. 6.24 Small hepatocellular carcinoma. (**a**) By plain scan, the right liver lobe was displayed with a round-like low-density lesion in diameter of 2.5 cm at the anterior segment. (**b**) Homogeneous and rapid enhancement of the lesion at the arterial phase. (**c**) Rapid decrease of the enhancement of the lesion at the portal vein phase. (**d**) The nodular lesion was still demonstrated in low density at 5 min of the delayed phase

The patient experienced high fever with obviously increased WBC count. By plain scan, the right liver lobe was displayed with irregular area in slightly low density adjacent to the portal area. By contrast scan, ring-shaped marginal enhancement was demonstrated, with no obvious enhancement at the inner liquefaction and necrosis. The bile duct at the portal area was shown to be compressed, which induced intrahepatic bile duct dilation.

6.6.3 MRI Demonstration

6.6.3.1 MRI Demonstration of Liver Cirrhosis After Viral Hepatitis

Direct Signs

1. Gross morphological change of the liver

   The shape of the liver is irregular, with increased or decreased volume. Shrinkage of the right liver lobe and enlargement of the caudal lobe commonly occur. The fibrous scar in the cases of liver cirrhosis causes shrinkage of the liver, while the nodule in the cases of liver cirrhosis or fatty degeneration and infiltration cause enlargement of partial or whole liver. Due to the imbalance size of liver parts, disproportional liver lobes and widened liver fissure are shown. The hepatic margin shows nodular protrusion, which can be slight or severe and is caused by nodules of liver cirrhosis. Due to direct three-dimensional imaging by MRI, it is more favorable in demonstrating morphological change of the liver than CT scan.

2. Regenerated nodule

   Regenerated nodule is formed by degeneration and necrosis of extensively proliferated collagen fiber septum at the advanced stage of liver cirrhosis and proliferated hepatocytes. Regenerated nodule can be categorized into small nodule type, large nodule type, and mixed nodule type. In the hepatocytes with nodular proliferation, there are cholestasis, fatty degeneration, bile pigment deposition, and hemosiderosis, which are demonstrated with characteristic MRI signals. The regenerated nodule can be demonstrated as intrahepatic nodules in different sizes, with the

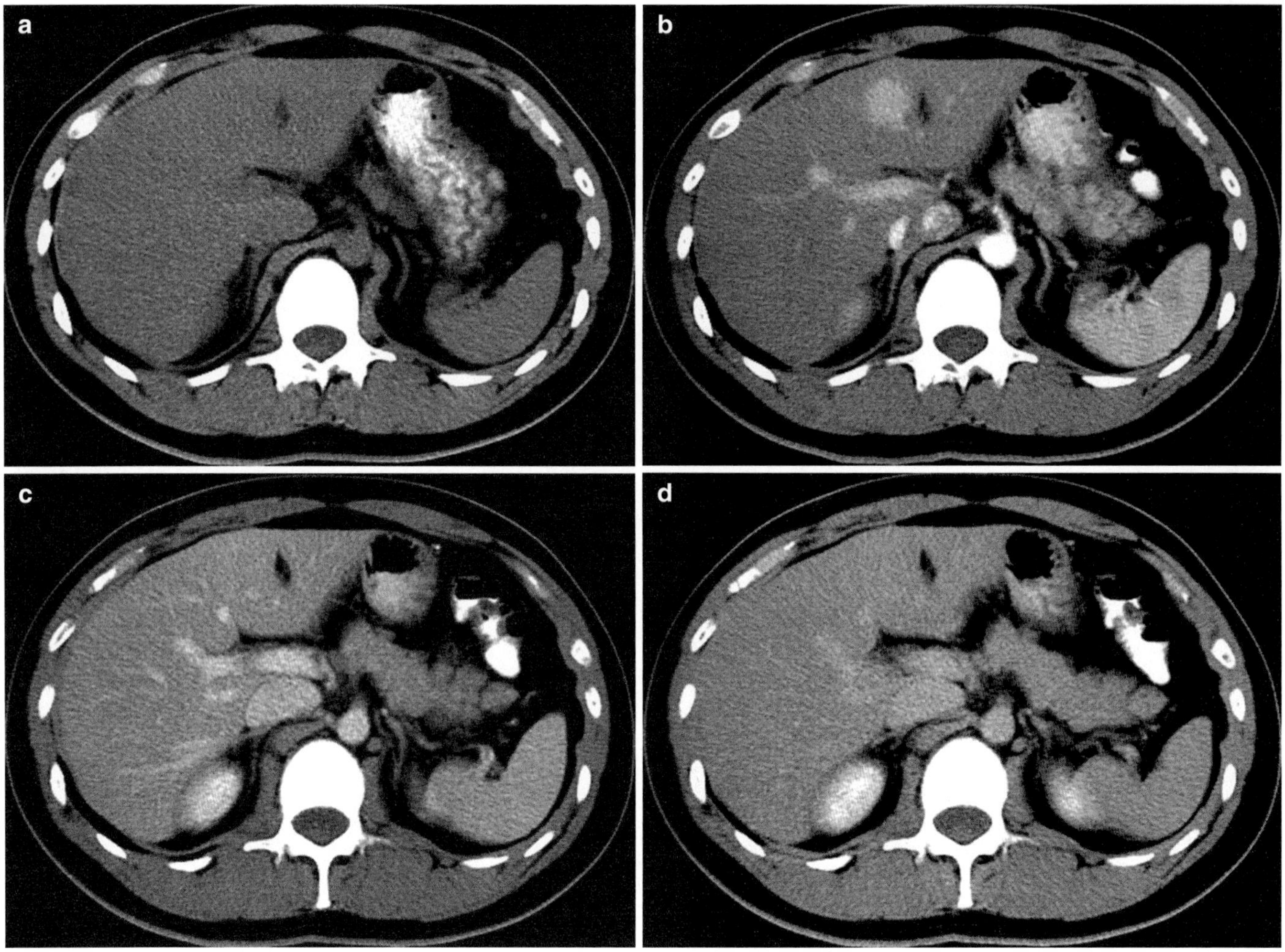

Fig. 6.25 Focal nodular proliferation of the liver. (**a**) Plain scan; (**b**) the arterial phase; (**c**) the portal vein phase; (**d**) the delayed phase

larger nodules possibly compressing the intrahepatic vascular vessels or intrahepatic bile ducts to curve or be deformed. The cirrhotic nodule is commonly demonstrated as isointense T1WI signal but rarely hyperintense T1WI signal due to increased content of triglyceride. The cirrhotic nodule is demonstrated as isointense and slightly hypointense T2WI signal, with homogeneous internal signal. The lesion is not encapsulated, with no obvious enhancement by contrast imaging. No abnormality can be demonstrated at the surrounding liver parenchyma (Fig. 6.27).

The cirrhotic nodule was demonstrated with isointense or slightly hyperintense T1WI signal, isointense or slightly hypointense T2WI signal, and homogeneous internal signal. The nodule was displayed with no capsule, with no obvious enhancement by contrast imaging. No abnormality was shown in the surrounding liver parenchyma.

The hypointense T2WI signal of the regenerated nodule is induced by hemosiderin deposition in the lesion or the hyperintense signal of the fibrous septum surrounding the nodule. Some other conditions, such as viral liver cirrhosis and alcoholic liver cirrhosis, may also induce increased iron content in the hepatocytes.

To detect and qualitatively define the regenerated nodule, MRI is more sensitive than CT and US. Particularly, the diffusively distributed small regenerated nodules are demonstrated as homogeneous miliary hyperintense T1WI signal, which can be defined by MRI. It is worth noting that in both literature and clinical practice, the nodule of liver cirrhosis has not been detected as hyperintense T2WI signal, which is of great importance for the diagnosis and differential diagnosis of liver cirrhosis.

Indirect Signs (Fig. 6.28)

1. Enlarged spleen (splenomegaly)

   It is the most common secondary change, whose diagnostic criteria are the same as that by CT scan. Due to hemosiderin deposition, the enlarged spleen is demonstrated with multiple spots of long T1 and short T2 signal.

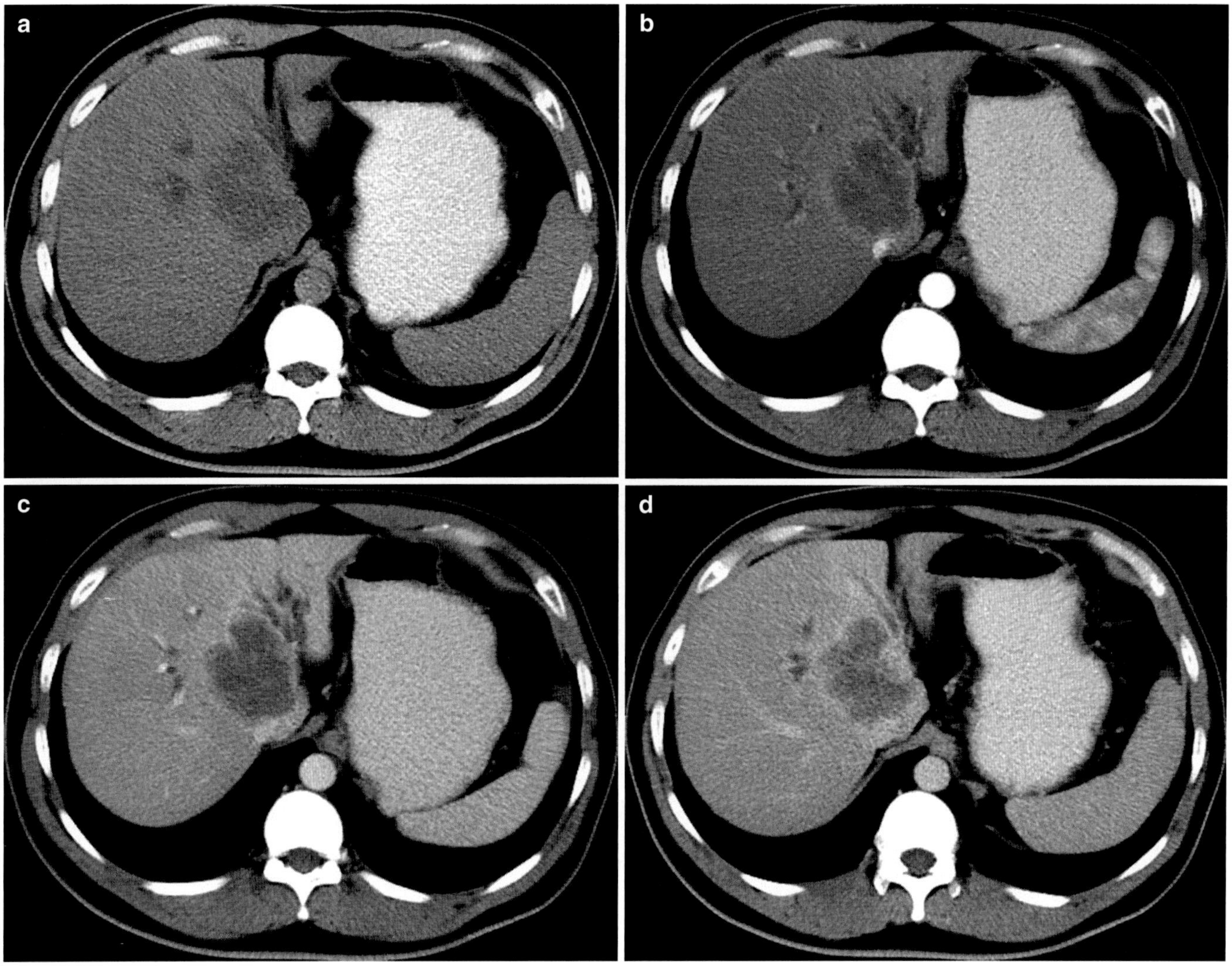

Fig. 6.26 Liver Abscess. (**a**) Plain scan; (**b**) the arterial phase; (**c**) the portal vein phase; (**d**) the delayed phase

2. Ascites

   Ascites is displayed as crescent-shaped long T1 and long T2 signal at the margin of the liver.

3. Signs of portal hypertension

   In the patients with portal hypertension, the portal vein is twisted and dilated, and the gastric short vein, the gastric coronary vein, and the esophageal vein show varicosity. These signs are of qualitative diagnostic value for liver cirrhosis. MRI shows images from any perspective, facilitating vascular imaging. Spin-echo sequence demonstrates special vascular void flowing, while the collateral circulation of the portal vein system is shown with nodular and cordlike flowing void signal. Their differentiation from surrounding soft tissue can be achieved with no use of the contrast agent.

   The liver was displayed with shrinkage of the volume, disproportional liver lobes, and widened liver fissure. The left liver lobe was demonstrated as beaver tail. And there were also enlarged spleen, a large quantity of ascites, and widened portal vein.

MRI Demonstrations of Liver Cirrhosis Complicated by HCC

In the patients with liver cirrhosis, those with the following MRI demonstrations should be suspected with canceration:

1. The cirrhotic nodule is demonstrated with hypo- or isointense T1WI signal, but mixed hyper- and isointense T2WI signals or hyperintense T2WI signal.
2. Irregular pseudomembrane is formed around the nodule, which is demonstrated with hypointense T1WI signal. The encapsulating membrane of the nodule is composed of coarse fibers, which are one of the important signs of primary hepatocellular carcinoma.
3. By contrast imaging, the nodule is demonstrated with patchy irregular slight enhancement or as slightly hypointense signal with no effect of enhancement. However, its encapsulating membrane is demonstrated with ring-shaped enhancement.

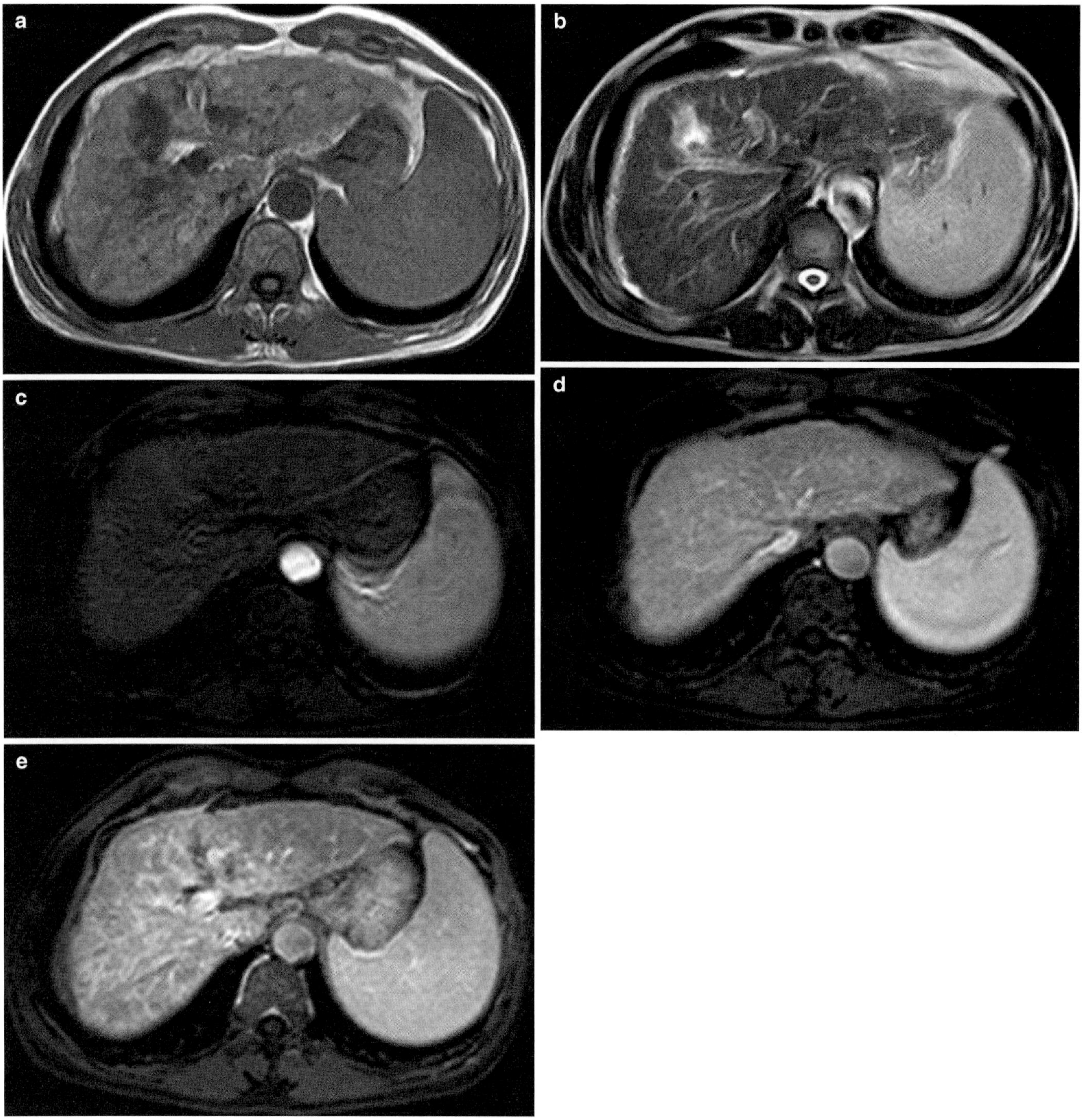

Fig. 6.27 Regenerated nodule of liver cirrhosis. (**a**) T_1WI; (**b**) T_2WI; (**c**) the arterial phase; (**d**) the portal vein phase; (**e**) the delayed phase

4. The cancer embolus forms in the portal vein, which is well defined by T1WI as widened portal vein and internal long strip isointense signal shadow.

In addition, MRI possesses multiple imaging parameters, which are sensitive to changes of water component and can favorably display hemorrhage, necrosis, and surrounding edema that complicate primary hepatocellular carcinoma. The necrotic lesion is demonstrated with long T1 and long T2 signals. The hemorrhagic lesion is displayed with short T1 and long T2 signals, while edema is shown with flake of slightly long T1 and slightly long or long T2 signal in the liver parenchyma around the neoplasm.

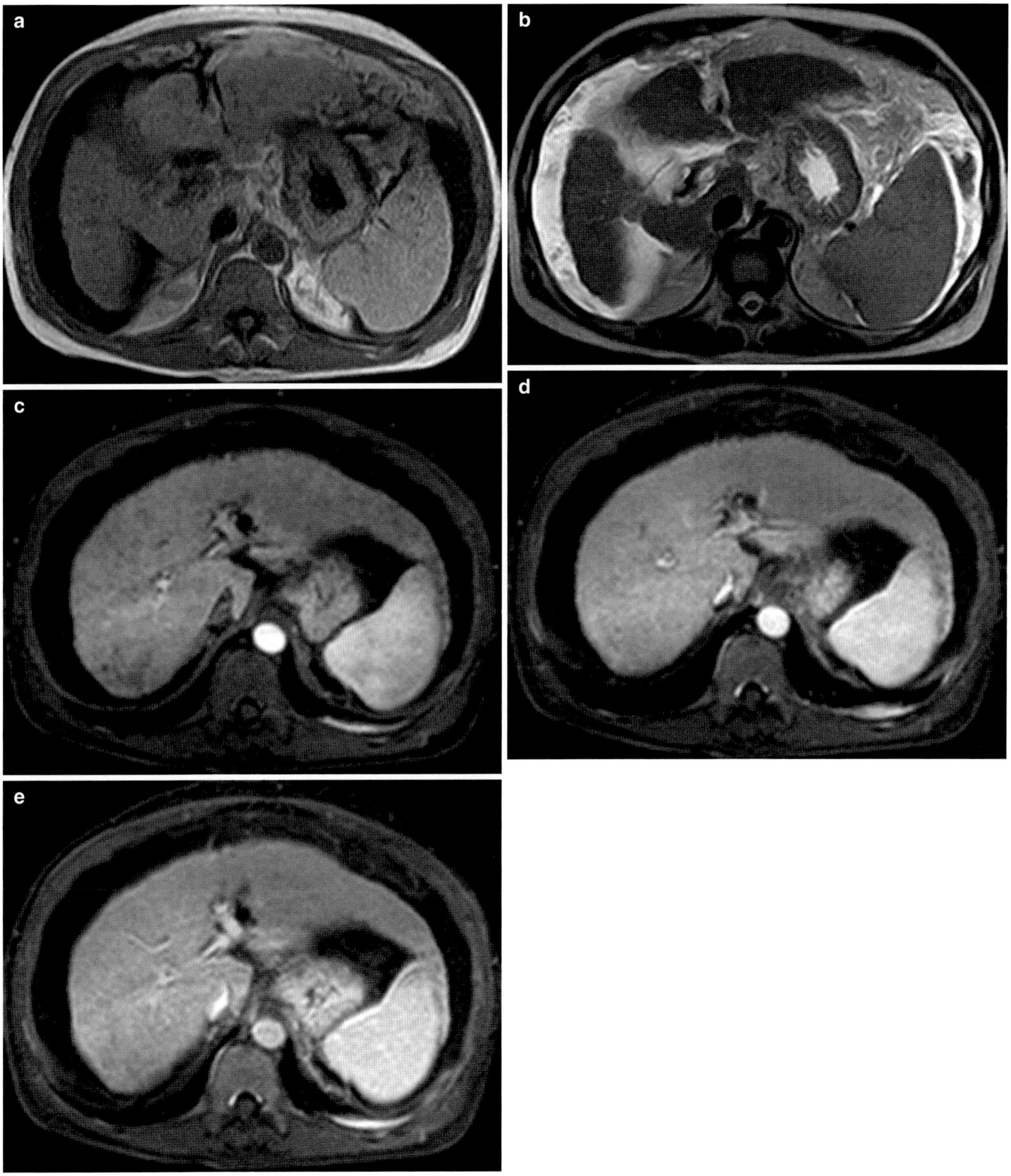

Fig. 6.28 Indirect signs of liver cirrhosis. (**a**) T1WI; (**b**) T2WI; (**c**) the arterial phase; (**d**) the portal vein phase; (**e**) the delayed phase

6.6.3.2 MRI Demonstrations of Primary Liver Cancer and Its Differential Diagnosis

Nodular Liver Cancer

The lesion has well-defined boundary with regular shape. Hemorrhage and necrosis are common, with obvious formation of encapsulating membrane. Most lesions are demonstrated with slightly long T1, slightly long T2 signal, whose intrahepatic metastasis and the formation of cancer embolus in the portal vein are rare (Fig. 6.29).

Plain imaging demonstrated a well-defined round-like nodular shadow at the interface of the left and right liver lobes, with slightly long T1 and T2 signals. The lesion was displayed with rapid enhancement at the arterial phase and with weakened enhancement at the portal vein and delayed phases whose signal was lower than that from the surrounding liver parenchyma.

Huge-Mass Type of Liver Cancer

The huge-mass type of liver cancer shows a growth of infiltration, with irregular shape. Its transverse diameter is generally larger than 3 cm with no obvious encapsulating membrane. Most lesions are subject to hemorrhage and necrosis and are demonstrated with slightly long T1 and T2 signals as well as mixed signals. Intrahepatic metastasis and formation of cancer embolus in the portal vein are common (Fig. 6.30).

By plain imaging, the right liver lobe was displayed with huge mass shadow of mixed long T1 and long T2 signals. The mass was demonstrated with irregular shape and internal necrosis. At the arterial phase, the solid mass was shown with rapid heterogeneous enhancement but weakened enhancement at the portal vein and delayed phases. The internal necrosis was displayed with no obvious enhancement. The signal of enhancement was shown to be mixed.

Diffuse Type of Liver Cancer

The lesion is poorly defined and has poorly defined boundary from the normal liver parenchyma. The boundary of the lesion is irregular, mostly with isointense signal. Formation of cancer thrombus in the portal vein is common. In some cases, it can be hardly differentiated from nodule of liver cirrhosis (Fig. 6.31).

The liver parenchyma was shown with multiple poorly defined nodules or masses, with blurry boundary from the normal liver parenchyma. The nodules or masses were shown with blurry boundary, with predominantly slightly long T1 slightly long T2 mixed signals. At the arterial phase, the nodules or masses were heterogeneously enhanced. Formation of cancer thrombus was detected in the portal vein, with filling defect.

Small Hepatocellular Carcinoma

Most of the lesions have regular shape, with well-defined boundary. In most cases, the encapsulating membrane of the lesion is intact. And most lesions are demonstrated with hypointense T1WI signal and hyperintense T2WI signal, with heterogeneous internal signal. No intrahepatic metastasis and formation of cancer thrombus in the portal vein can be detected.

Differential Diagnosis

Hepatic Angioma

By MRI, the lesion of hepatic angioma is well defined, with smooth and intact margin and homogeneous internal signal. The lesion is demonstrated with homogeneous hypointense T1WI signal. By proton density-weighted imaging or T2-weighted imaging, the lesion is displayed with homogeneous hyperintense signal. Along with the elongation of echo time, the signal is shown to be strengthened, with well-defined boundary. Additional proton density-weighted imaging is of great significance for the differential diagnosis.

Metastatic Liver Cancer (Fig. 6.32)

- The histological characteristics of primary neoplasm may affect the signal change of its intrahepatic metastatic lesion. In most cases with intrahepatic metastasis, T1WI demonstrates multiple metastatic lesions with hypointense signal and quite well-defined boundary. The signal intensity is homogeneous or heterogeneous and in rare cases, equal. In the cases with accompanying recent hemorrhage or metastatic lesions of melanoma and liposarcoma, the signal may be hyperintense. By T2WI, most of the metastatic lesion is shown with hyperintense signal, with poorly defined and irregular boundary. In some lesions, central necrosis is obvious, with target sign. By T1WI, the necrotic area is demonstrated with a round or irregular hypointense signal, which is shown with extremely hyperintense signal by T2WI. By T2WI, some metastatic lesions can be demonstrated to be surrounded by a ring of more hyperintense area in thickness of 2–10 mm, which is known as halo ring sign. It has been generally believed that the sign is related to edema around the neoplasm. However, some other scholars believe that the sign is induced by surrounding of hypointense necrosis by surviving tumor tissue or by necrosis of tissue around the neoplasm. In rare cases, the metastatic lesion may involve the blood vessels to cause cancer thrombus. By Gd-DTPA, contrast T1WI displays the metastatic lesion with heterogeneous or ring-shaped enhancement but occasionally with homogeneous enhancement. Imaging with 60 min delay occasionally demonstrates aggregation of contrast agent in the necrotic

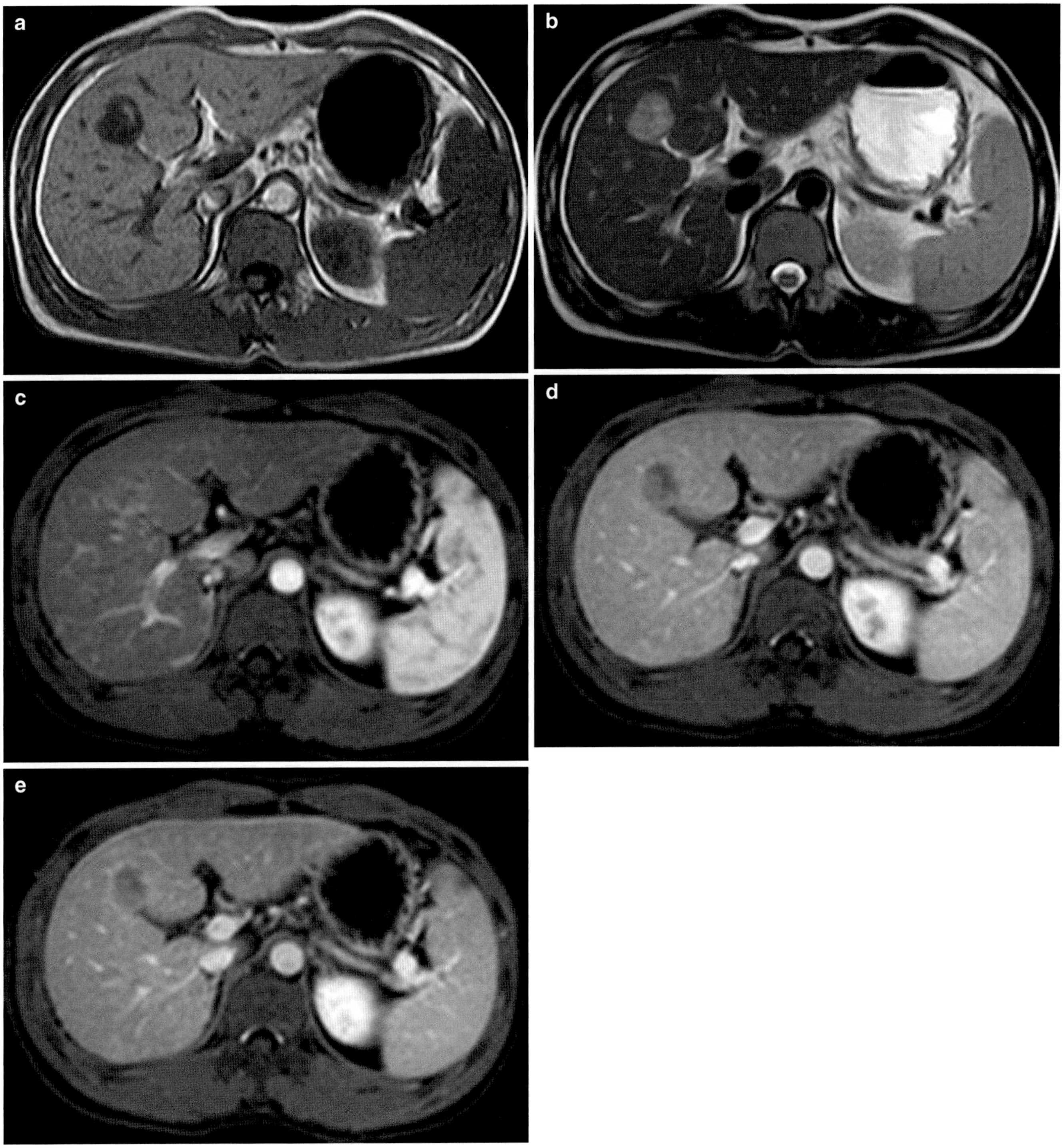

Fig. 6.29 Nodular liver cancer. (**a**) T_1WI; (**b**) T_2WI; (**c**) the arterial phase; (**d**) the portal vein phase; (**e**) the delayed phase

area, causing patchy hyperintense signal at the center of metastatic lesion.

The patient had a medical history of gastrointestinal malignancy. T1WI showed multiple mixed hypointense signal areas with well-defined or poorly defined boundaries. T2WI displayed mixed hyperintense signal and some lesions had central necrosis, with target sign.

6.6.4 PET/CT Demonstrations of HCC

6.6.4.1 Imaging Demonstrations of Primary Hepatocellular Carcinoma

^{18}F-FDG is currently the most commonly used tracer for PET/CT examination. ^{18}F-FDG can be uptaken in a large quantity by neoplasm in the liver. Under effect of hexose phosphatase, ^{18}F-FDG-6-phosphoric acid is produced, which

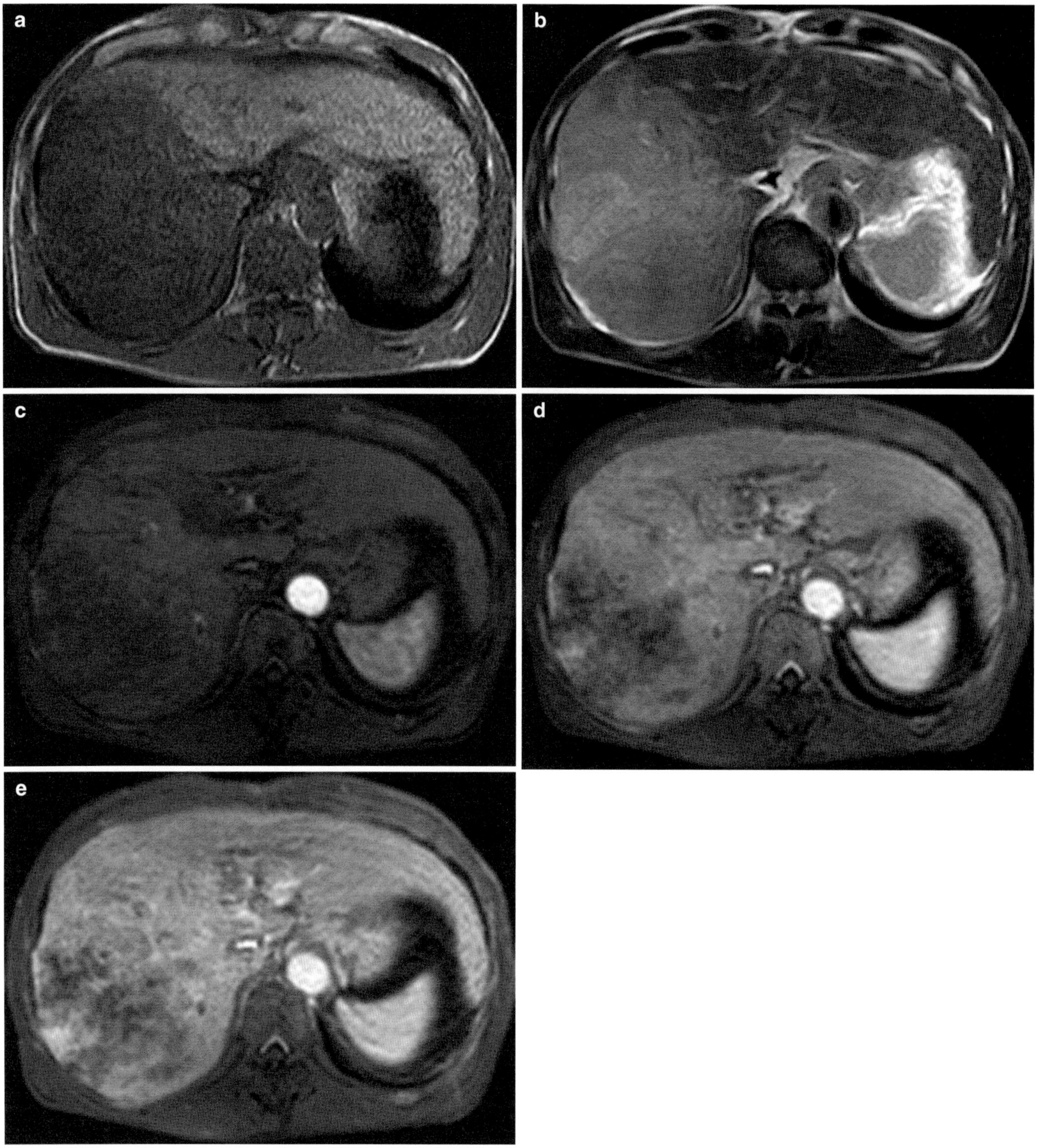

Fig. 6.30 Huge-mass type of liver cancer. (**a**) T_1WI; (**b**) T_2WI; (**c**) the arterial phase; (**d**) the portal vein phase; (**e**) the delayed phase

cannot further generate hexose diphosphate and is incapable of participating in the following aerobic and anaerobic metabolism. Therefore, ^{18}F-FDG-6-phosphoric acid remains in the tumor cells in a large quantity to induce radiologically hypermetabolic lesion (Fig. 6.33). Based on its SUV >3.5 and T/L >2.5 as the diagnostic criteria, the diagnosis can be made.

The left liver lobe was shown with hypermetabolic lesion in the medial segment, which had a SUVmax of 14.3. By biopsy, it was defined to be low-differentiated liver cancer.

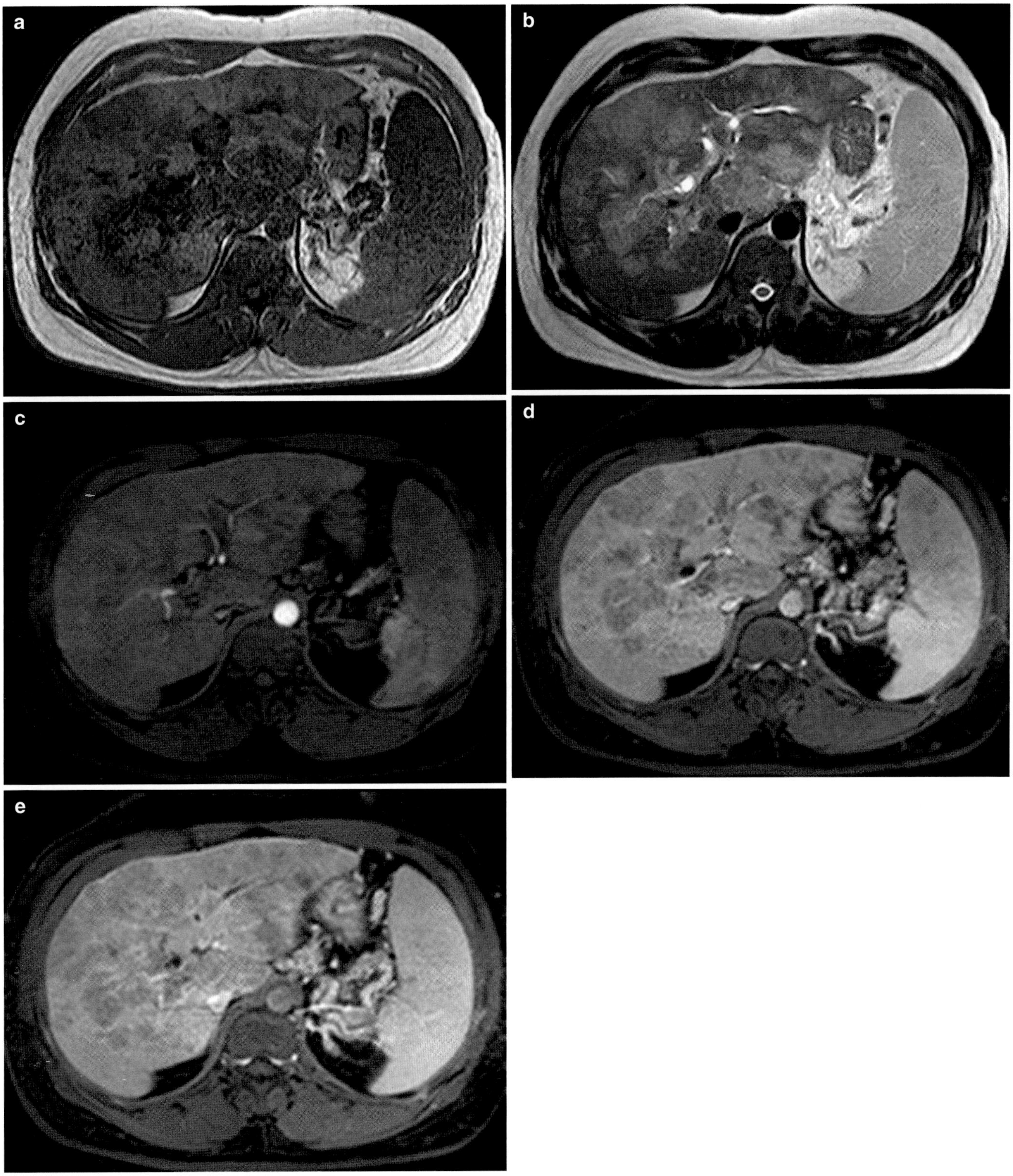

Fig. 6.31 Diffuse type of liver cancer. (**a**) T_1WI; (**b**) T_2WI; (**c**) the arterial phase; (**d**) thc portal vein phase; (**e**) the delayed phase

The uptake of ^{18}F-FDG is also dependent on its penetrating rate through cell membrane and the processes of intracellular phosphorylation and dephosphorylation. The uptake of glucose by tumor cells of primary liver cancer is special. The glucose-6-phosphatase in well-differentiated cellular carcinoma is highly active, which is histologically

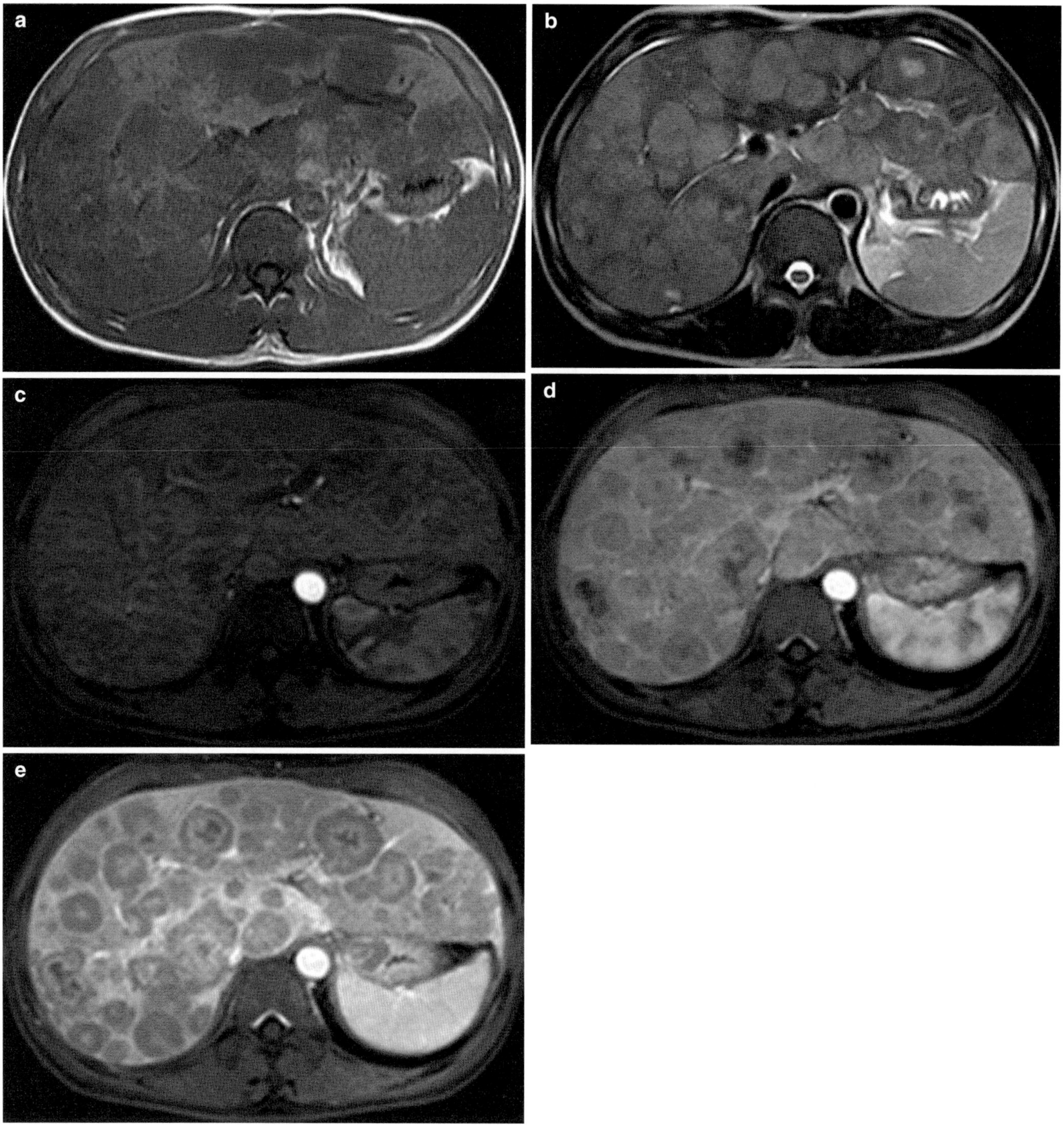

Fig. 6.32 Metastatic liver cancer. (**a**) T_1WI; (**b**) T_2WI; (**c**) the arterial phase; (**d**) the portal vein phase; (**e**) the delayed phase

closer to the normal hepatocyte than low differentiated type. Therefore, the uptake of ^{18}F-FDG by the well-differentiated type is less and sometimes undetectable, which causes false-negative diagnosis of well-differentiated type by ^{18}F-FDG PET.

Triphasic contrast CT has a high accuracy rate in the diagnosis of primary liver cancer, which has been reported to be 95 %. Therefore, it is the radiological modality of choice for the diagnosis of primary liver cancer. The combination of triphasic contrast CT with ^{18}F-FDG PET and the differentiation of hepatocellular carcinoma can be graded. Principally, the SUV and the ratio of T/L of low-differentiated liver cancer is higher than those of well-differentiated and moderately differentiated liver cancer.

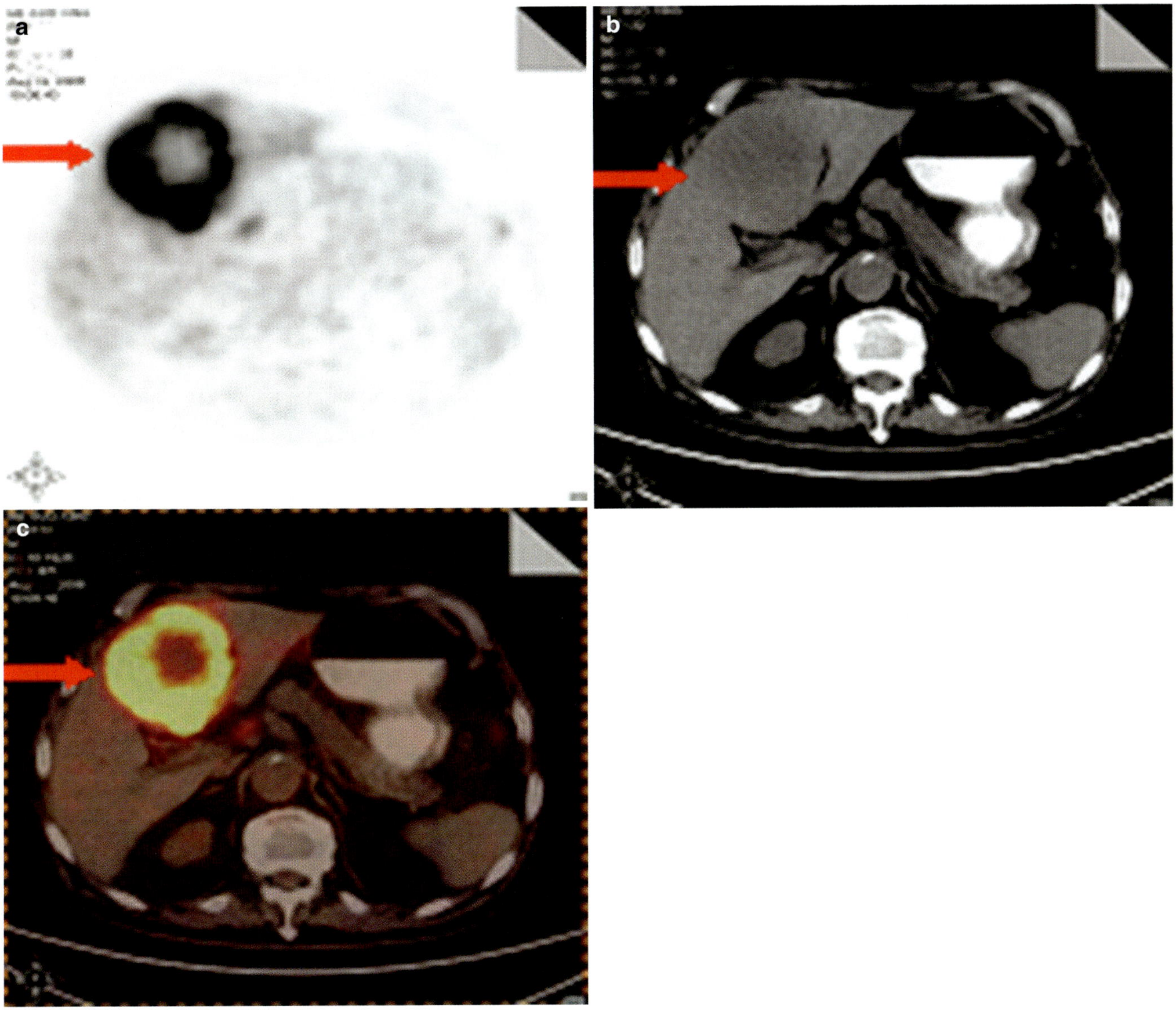

Fig. 6.33 Primary liver cancer. (**a**) PET image; (**b**) CT image; (**c**) PET/CT image

6.6.4.2 Imaging Demonstrations of Relapsed or Residual Liver Cancer

By commonly used radiological modalities, relapsed lesion of primary liver cancer, after treated by surgical removal, iodine oil embolization, and radiofrequency catheter ablation, can hardly be detected at the early stage. However, the relapsed and residual lesion can be detected by ^{18}F-FDG PET due to its superiority in functional molecular imaging.

6.6.4.3 Imaging Demonstrations of Remote Metastasis of Liver Cancer

Routine CT and MRI only serve local examination of the human body. In some cases, the detected lesion cannot be qualitatively defined. With no systemic examination, the therapeutic plan cannot be definitively stipulated. PET/CT is capable of examining the whole human body and therefore facilitates systemic assessment of the whole body. In addition, it facilitates accurate staging of cancer, which helps to stipulate the therapeutic plan (Fig. 6.34).

The left liver lobe was shown with mass-like hypermetabolism lesion, with SUXmax of 8.6. Meanwhile, osteolytic bone destruction was displayed in the T9 vertebrae, with increased metabolism and SUXmax of 4.6. Liver puncture for biopsy defined the diagnosis of low-differentiated hepatocellular carcinoma.

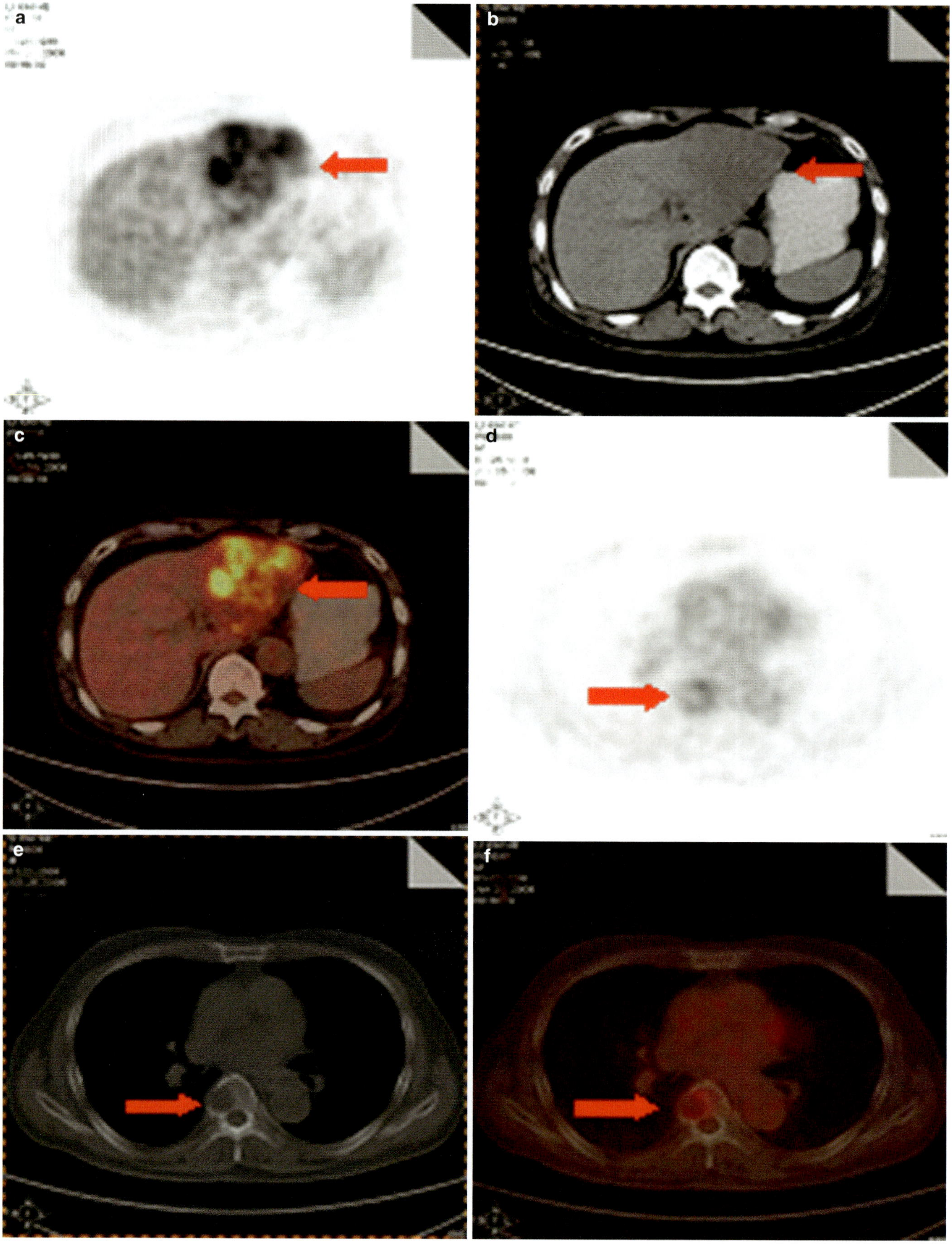

Fig. 6.34 Thoracic vertebral metastatic of primary liver cancer. (**a**) Liver PET; (**b**) liver CT; (**c**) liver PET/CT; (**d**) thoracic vertebra PET; (**e**) thoracic vertebra CT; (**f**) thoracic vertebra PET/CT

Further Reading

1. Vieth S, Manegold C, Drosten C, et al. Sequence and phylogenetic analysis of hepatitis B virus genotype G isolated in Germany. Virus Genes. 2002;24(2):153–6.
2. Arauz-Ruiz P, Norder H, Robertson BH, et al. Genotype H: a new Amerindian genotype of hepatitis B virus revealed in Central America. J Gen Virol. 2002;83(pt 8):2059–73.
3. Farci P, Shimoda A, Coiana A, et al. The outcome of acute hepatitis C predicted by the evolution of the viral quasispecies. Science. 2000;288(5464):339–44.
4. Stuyver L, De Gendt S, Van Geyt C, et al. A new genotype of hepatitis B virus: complete genome and phylogenetic relatedness. J Gen Virol. 2000;81(pt 1):67–74.
5. Amarapurkar D. Role of liver biopsy in management of chronic hepatitis B and chronic hepatitis C. Trop Gastroenterol. 2007;28(2):67–8.
6. Cholongitas E, Senzolo M, Standish R, et al. A systematic review of quality of liver biopsy specimens. Am J Clin Pathol. 2006;125(5):710–21.
7. Fiel MI. Pathology of chronic hepatitis B and chronic hepatitis C. Clin Liver Dis. 2010;14(4):555–75.
8. Goodman ZD. Grading and staging systems for inflammation and fibrosis in chronic liver diseases. J Hepatol. 2007;47(4):598–607.
9. Guido M, Rugge M. Liver biopsy sampling in chronic viral hepatitis. Semin Liver Dis. 2004;24(1):89–97.
10. Ishak KG. Pathologic features of chronic hepatitis. A review and update. Am J Clin Pathol. 2000;113(1):40–5.
11. Lok AS, McMahon BJ. Chronic hepatitis B. Hepatology. 2007;45(2):507–39.
12. Lefkowitch JH. Advances in hepatobiliary pathology: update for 2010. Clin Liver Dis. 2010;14(4):747–62.
13. Tsuang W, Subramanian R, Liu Q, et al. The need for liver biopsy in a patient with acute HCV infection. Nat Clin Pract Gastroenterol Hepatol. 2008;5(1):54–7.
14. Iloeje UH, Yang HI, Su J, et al. Predicting cirrhosis risk based on the level of circulating hepatitis B viral load. Gastroenterology. 2006;130(3):678–86.
15. Arase Y, Suzuki F, Suzuki Y, et al. Sustained virology response reduces incidence of onset of type 2 diabetes in chronic hepatitis C. Hepatology. 2009;49(3):739–44.
16. Buster EH, Flink HJ, Cakaloglu Y, et al. Sustained HbeAg and HBsAg loss after long-term follow-up of HbeAg positive patients treated with peginterferon alpha-2b. Gastroenterology. 2008;135(2):459–67.
17. Lok AS, McMahon BJ. Chronic hepatitis B. Hepatology. 2001;34(6):1225–41.
18. Kim HC, Yang DM, Jin W. The various manifestations of ruptured hepatocellular carcinoma: CT imaging finding. Abdom Imaging. 2008;33(6):633–42.
19. Xu PJ, Yan FH, Wang JH, et al. Added value of breath hold diffusion-weighted MRI in detection of small hepatocellular carcinoma lesions compared with dynamic contrast-enhanced MRI alone using receiver operating characteristic curve analysis. J Magn Reson Imaging. 2009;29(2):341–9.
20. Kim YK, Han YM, Kim CS. Comparison of diffuse hepatocellular carcinoma and intrahepatic cholangiocarcinoma using sequentially acquired gadolinium-enhanced and Resovist-enhanced MRI. Eur J Radiol. 2009;70(1):94–100.
21. Keeffe EB, Dieterich DT, Han SH, et al. A treatment algorithm for the management of chronic hepatitis B virus infection in the United States: an update. Clin Gastroenterol Hepatol. 2006;4(8):936–62.
22. Marcellin P, Chang TT, Lim SG, et al. Long-term efficacy and safety of adefovir dipivoxil for the treatment of hepatitis B e antigen-positive chronic hepatitis B. Hepatology. 2008;48(3):750–8.
23. Hadziyannis SJ, Tassopoulos NC, Heathcote EJ, et al. Long-term therapy with adefovir dipivoxil for HBeAg-negative chronic hepatitis B for up to 5 years. Gastroenterology. 2006;131(6):1743–51.
24. Hadziyannis SJ, Tassopoulos NC, Heathcote EJ, et al. Adefovir dipivoxil for the treatment of hepatitis B e antigen-negative chronic hepatitis B. N Engl J Med. 2003;348(9):800–7.
25. Chang TT, Gish RG, de Man R, et al. A comparison of entecavir and lamivudine for HBeAg-positive chronic hepatitis B. N Engl J Med. 2006;354(10):1001–10.
26. Lai CL, Shouval D, Lok AS, et al. Entecavir versus lamivudine for patients with HBeAg-negative chronic hepatitis B. N Engl J Med. 2006;354(10):1011–20.
27. Liaw YF, Gane E, Leung N, et al. 2-Year GLOBE trial results: telbivudine is superior to lamivudine in patients with chronic hepatitis B. Gastroenterology. 2009;136(2):486–95.
28. Lai CL, Gane E, Liaw YF, et al. Telbivudine versus lamivudine in patients with chronic hepatitis B. N Engl J Med. 2007;357(25):2576–88.
29. Marcellin P, Heathcote EJ, Buti M, et al. Tenofovir disoproxil fumarate versus adefovir dipivoxil for chronic hepatitis B. N Engl J Med. 2008;359(23):2442–55.
30. Ghany MG, Nelson DR, Strader DB, et al. An update on treatment of genotype 1 chronic hepatitis C virus infection: 2011 practice guideline by the American Association for the Study of Liver Diseases. Hepatology. 2011;54(4):1433–44.
31. Chen YC, Chu CM, Yeh CT, et al. Natural course following the onset of cirrhosis in patients with chronic hepatitis B: a long-term follow-up study. Hepatol Int. 2007;1(1):267–73.
32. Yang Gen-dong, Lu Pu-xuan, Zhou Bo-ping, et al. Hemochromatosis with excessive iron deposition in the liver: report of 1 case. Chin J Hepatol. 2006;8(14):634.
33. Wang Cheng-lin, Zhou Kang-rong. CT and MRI diagnosis of hepatopathy. Beijing: People's Health Publishing House; 2007.
34. Zhou Bo-ping, Chong Yu-tian. Viral hepatitis. Beijing: People's Health Publishing House; 2011.
35. Lang Zhen-wei. Hepatocytic apoptosis and pathology of viral hepatitis. Chin J Hepatol. 1999;7:116.

7 Hand-Foot-and-Mouth Disease

Yuan Jing, Huang Wen-Xian, Zeng Hong-Wu, Li Jian-Ming, Ou Shan-Xing, Gou Ji-zhou, Yang Guang, Zheng Guang-Ping, Shan Wan-Shui, and Lou Ming-Wu

7.1 Introduction

Hand-foot-and-mouth disease (HFMD) is an acute infectious disease caused by a variety of enteroviruses which commonly affects infants and preschoolers. It is characterized by fever, skin rashes, and/or herpes at hand, foot, and oral cavity as well as herpetic angina. The condition is rarely complicated by aseptic meningitis, brainstem encephalitis, neurogenic pulmonary edema, acute flaccid paralysis, and myocarditis. The pathogens inducing HFMD mainly include echovirus, Coxsackie virus group A (serotype 4, 5, 9, 10, and 16) and group B (serotype 2 and 5), and enterovirus 71 (EV71). Among these pathogens, EV71 and Cox A16 are the most common.

In 1958, Robinson, a Canadian physician, isolated Cox A16 in stool specimen and throat swab from patient with HFMD. Meanwhile, he detected four times increase of the serum antibody. It was preliminarily defined Cox A16 as the pathogen, which is the first enterovirus ever found by a scientist that can cause HFMD disease.

In the year of 1959, HFMD prevailed in Birmingham, UK. Alsop et al. isolated Cox A16 in herpetic fluid from patient and further proved the etiological relationship between Cox A16 and the disease. Thereafter, the disease was officially nominated as hand-foot-and-mouth disease. In 1974, Schmidt et al. performed pathogenic detection in 20 cases of meningitis or encephalitis in California, USA, during the period from 1969 to 1974. They firstly isolated the virus, identified as EV71, in the stool specimen from one pediatric patient with encephalitis (1969). During the 1970s and 1980s, EV71 infection and Cox A16 infection prevailed alternatively, which constituted the major pathogens of HFMD. Since 1990s, EV71 has been the most common pathogen causing hand-foot-and-mouth disease across the world. It has strong infectivity, and its infection has a high incidence rate. EV71 infection can cause serious complications and even death.

7.2 Etiology

Hand-foot-and-mouth disease is caused by enterovirus, which has many pathogenic types. All of these pathogenic types are categorized into the genus of enterovirus and the family of *Picornaviridae*. Based on the pathogenicity, infectivity, and antigenicity of enteroviruses, it can be divided into polio virus (PV), Coxsackie virus (Cox), ECHO virus, and new enterovirus (type 68–71).

7.2.1 Coxsackie Virus

In the early epidemics of HFMD, Coxsackie virus was the pathogen, which caused mild clinical symptoms with favorable prognosis. Death and serious complications were rarely reported. However, during the epidemics of HFMD in Malaysia in 1997, Chinese Taiwan in 1998, and mainland

Yuan Jing (✉)
Department of Infection, Shenzhen Third People's Hospital Guangdong, Shenzhen, China
e-mail: 13500054798@139.com

Huang Wen-Xian
Shenzhen Children's Hospital, Futian, Shenzhen, Guangdong, China

Zeng Hong-Wu
Department of Radiology, Shenzhen Children's Hospital Guangdong, Shenzhen, China
e-mail: homerzeng@126.com

Li Jian-Ming • Gou Ji-zhou • Yang Guang
Zheng Guang-Ping • Shan Wan-Shui
The Shenzhen No.3 People's Hospital, Guangdong College, Shenzhen, China

Ou Shan-Xing
General Hospital of Guangzhou Military Command of PLA, Yuexiu, Guangzhou, Guangdong, China

Lou Ming-Wu
Longgang Central Hospital of Shenzhen, Longgang, Shenzhen, Guangdong, China

P.-X. Lu, B.-P. Zhou (eds.), *Diagnostic Imaging of Emerging Infectious Diseases*, DOI 10.1007/978-94-017-7363-8_7

China from 1999 to 2004, Cox A16 and EV71 concurrently prevailed. Therefore, the two viruses needed to be etiologically differentiated to provide basic data for the studies of their pathomechanisms.

7.2.2 EV71

Since EV71 was firstly isolated in 1969, it has been occupying an increasingly important position in the etiology of HFMD. EV71 virus is a symmetrically spherical icosahedral structure without envelope and spikes, whose diameter is about 24–30 nm. The viral nucleic acid is single-stranded positive RNA and its capsid is formed by 60 subunits. And the capsid is a pentamer-like structure assembled by four types of capsid proteins (VP1–VP4). VP4 is embedded inside the capsid of viral particles and is closely attached to the viral core, while the other three capsid proteins are exposed on the surface of the viral particle. Therefore, the antigenic determinant is basically located on VPl–VP3.

Due to the morphological structure and physiochemical properties of EV71, it survives and can be transmitted in hot and humid environment. EV71 can survive for 1 year at a temperature of 4 °C and can be preserved for a long period of time at a temperature of −20 °C. The organic substances can protect the virus for the virus can survive for several months in feces and sewage. The enterovirus is tolerant to the positive ion, and a divalent cation environment can improve its resistance virus to heat. EV71 is stable at an environment with a pH value of 3–9 and cannot be inactivated by stomach acid and bile. Its infectivity remains to be unaffected in an environment of 25 °C and pH 3.0 for 4 h. However, the virus is intolerant to strong alkali and is resistant to diethyl ether, deoxycholate, detergents, and weak acid as well as common disinfectants such as 75 % alcohol and 5 % soda water. EV71 is also sensitive to various oxidants such as 1 % potassium permanganate, 1 % hydrogen peroxide, and chlorine-containing disinfectants, and the virus can be inactivated by formaldehyde and iodine. In addition, EV71 virus is sensitive to high temperature, dryness, and ultraviolet, and can be inactivated at 56 °C for 30 minutes. Its tolerance to acid means that it can be transmitted via fecal-oral route, and its tolerance to heat indicates its self-replication at a high temperature.

7.3 Epidemiology

7.3.1 Introduction

Hand-foot-and-mouth disease is an infectious disease occurring worldwide. Local or large-scale epidemics of HFMD occur in many countries and regions. The disease was firstly described by Seddon from New Zealand in 1957. In 1958, Robinson from Canada isolated CVA16 in stool specimen and throat swabs from patient and detected a four times increase of serum antibody, indicating Cox A16 to be the pathogen.

In 1997, an outbreak of HFMD occurred in Malaysia, and the main pathogen was defined to be EV71. During that epidemic of HFMD, a total of 5999 cases was reported, including 41 cases of death. In 1998, the ever largest-scale EV71-induced epidemic occurred in Chinese Taiwan, with a total of 129,106 cases reported, including 405 severe cases and 78 deaths. In 782 outpatients and inpatients, the detection rate of EV71 was 59.6 %, and the detection rate of CVA16 was 28.9 %. During the years of 2000–2001, EV71-induced epidemic occurred in Singapore, with 7 deaths of children patients. By virus culture, 71 cases showed positive, including 59 cases of EV71 (83 %). In 2005, a total of 764 cases of pediatric patients was reported from the Children's Hospital in Ho Chi Minh City, Vietnam, with 411 cases (53.8 %) detected to be enteroviral infection. Among these 411 cases, 173 were detected EV71 positive, including 51 severe cases and 3 deaths.

In 2008, laboratory-detected HFMD was firstly reported in China, with a total of 8639 cases. The positive rate of viral nucleic acid of EV71, CVA16, and other enteroviruses was 54.01 %, 14.77 %, and 31.22 %, respectively. In severe and death cases, the positive rate of EV71 nucleic acid was 81.59 % and 91.29 %, respectively.

In 2010, large-scale epidemic of HFMD occurred again in China, with a total of 987,779 cases reported, including 15,501 severe cases and 537 deaths. The death toll was four times as high as that reported in 2008. Some scholars compared the epidemics in 2008 and 2010, indicating that the mortality rate in males was higher than that in females. In addition, the scholars found that the death occurred at a median of day 3 from onset to death, commonly in children aged 0–2 years, and the peak death rate was in children aged 4–7 months.

7.3.2 Source of Infection

Person is the infection source of HFMD, including the infected patients, asymptomatic virus carriers, and persons with latent infection.

The patient excretes the viruses via throat 1–2 weeks after the onset and excretes the viruses in feces about 3–5 weeks after onset. The herpetic fluid contains a large quantity of viruses, which overflow when the herpes ruptures.

The blood, nasopharyngeal secretions, and feces of patient contain viruses several days before the onset of symptoms. Therefore, the patient is highly contagious during the incubation period. The ratio of symptomatic to asymptomatic patients is 4:1 in children aged 0–4 years, 1:2 in children aged 5–12 years, and 1:8 in children aged above 12 years. In healthy individuals, the virus-carrying rate is 13 % in children aged under 5 years and 25 % in adults aged above 20 years. Several days prior to the onset in symptomatic patients, the pathogenic virus can be detected in the throat and feces. In general, the infectivity is the strongest within 1 week after the onset.

7.3.3 Route of Transmission

The transmission route of EV71-induced HFMD is diversified, and the main transmission routes include fecal-oral route and/or respiratory droplets as well as close contact to infected individual. The contaminated hand is the key medium for its transmission.

7.3.4 Susceptible Population

Populations are generally susceptible to EV71 infection, but predominantly latent infection. Specific immunity can be acquired after both symptomatic and latent infections. However, the duration of specific immunity remains to be defined. No cross-immunity exists between different types of pathogenic viruses. And all age groups can be infected, but infants and young children are the most susceptible. The incidence rate is the highest in group aged ≤3 years, and the cases aged under 4 years account for 85–95 % of all reported cases. During the outbreaks, children under 5 years commonly account for above 90 % of the total reported cases.

7.3.5 Immunity After Infection

EV71 infection can induce the production of neutralizing antibodies, indicating a long-lasting immunity to the same type of pathogenic virus. Therefore, the infected person can be protected against infection of the same type of virus again. However, due to the pathogenicity of various types of enterovirus, the antibodies produced after infection fail to protect against other types of pathogenic enterovirus. Therefore, HFMD can repeatedly occur.

7.4 Pathogenesis and Pathological Change

7.4.1 Pathogenesis

Hand-foot-and-mouth disease is an acute infectious disease caused by enteroviruses. More than 20 types of enterovirus are pathogenic to induce the disease, the most commonly Cox A16 and EV71.

Intracellular oxidation-reduction reaction accelerates cytopathic effect and virus replication, and scavenger receptor SCARB2 mediates viruses into target cells. In addition to effects of pro-inflammatory factors, HFMD occurs. Currently, it is generally accepted that retrograde viral infection of EV71 causes central nervous system lesions. EV71-induced pulmonary edema is neurogenic, namely, neurogenic pulmonary edema, whose underlying mechanism still remains elusive. Authority theories about the pathogenesis of pulmonary edema include the blast theory and the permeability defect theory. In addition, abnormal secretion of inflammatory mediator, abnormal clotting mechanism, and increased pulmonary vascular permeability may also play important roles in the pathogenesis of pulmonary edema.

Hyperglycemia, increased WBC count, and acute flaccid paralysis constitute high-risk factors of neurogenic pulmonary edema. After the central nervous system is impaired, the level of endothelin-1 (ET-1) significantly increases. ET-1 is capable of inducing chemotaxis, adhesion, and activation of neutrophils to vascular endothelial cells and promoting the release of inflammatory mediators to impair the gas-blood barrier. Its increase may contribute to occurrence of pulmonary edema.

7.4.2 Pathological Change

The clinical symptoms of HFMD induced by Cox A16 are mild and typical, generally including ulceration in oral cavity as well as maculopapules and herpes on the skin of palms and/or soles. Pathohistologically, light microscopy demonstrates intraepidermal blisters and debris of neutrophils and eosinophils within the blister, intercellular and intracellular edema at the surrounding epidermal of blister, as well as infiltration of scattering chronic inflammatory cells in the superficial dermis under the blister. Under an electron microscope, epithelial cell is demonstrated with acidophilic inclusion. In mild cases of HFMD, only the skin of distal limbs and oral mucosa is affected. Most patients can be cured with therapies, with good prognosis.

EV71 is a serotype of enterovirus and is one of important types including severe HFMD. In addition to the abovementioned pathological manifestations, EV71-induced HFMD often involves the central nervous system, heart, lungs, and other major organs, with following pathological changes.

1. Central Nervous System

   EV71 is highly neurotropic, causing lesions commonly at the thalamus, midbrain, pons, medulla oblongata, cerebellar dentate nuclei, and spinal cord. The neuron at the lesion is degenerative and necrotic, with poorly defined or even absent neuronal nissl body, formation encephalomalacia focus, and satellites of neurotropic cells (Fig. 7.1). In addition, there are hyperplastic neurogliocyte and formation of gliocyte nodules. Clinically, the patients experience corresponding neurological symptoms, such as myoclonus, myasthenia, acute flaccid paralysis, eclampsia, and convulsions. In severe and critical cases, the patients may even experience coma and cerebral edema. The cerebral and spinal meninges are demonstrated with infiltration of lymphocytes and mononuclear

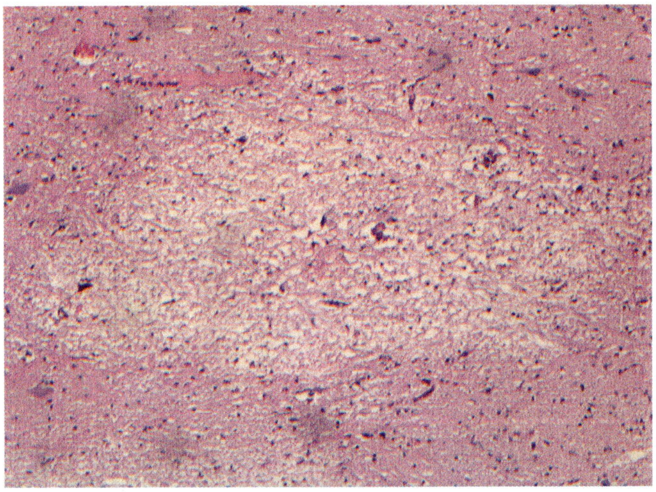

Fig. 7.1 Lesion of cerebral infarction, with degenerative and necrotic neuron as well as poorly defined or absent neuronal nissl body, H&E ×100

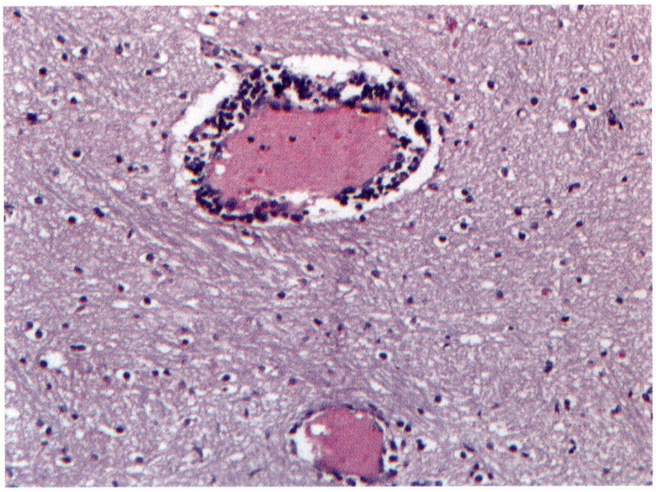

Fig. 7.2 Perivascular lymphocytic sleeve in the brain tissue, H&E ×200

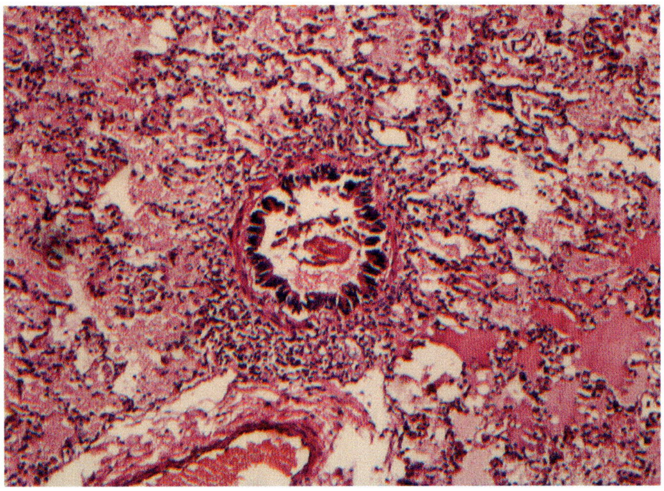

Fig. 7.3 Edema fluid in alveolar cavity and infiltration of peribronchiolar inflammatory cells, H&E ×200

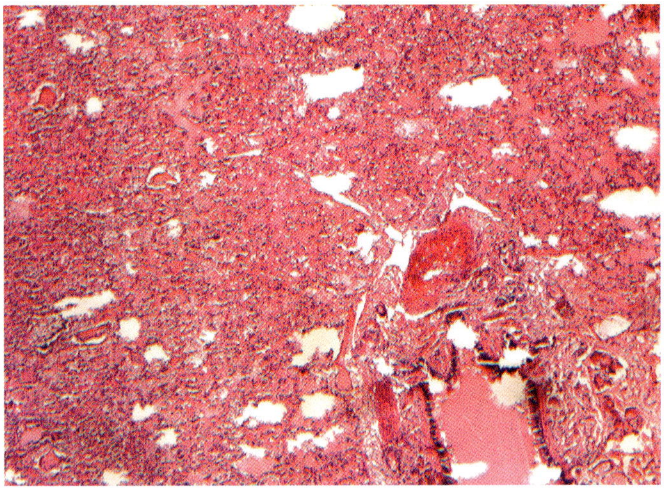

Fig. 7.4 Hemorrhage of alveolar cavity and pulmonary septum, H&E ×100

macrophages. Lesions at the cerebrum and cerebellum are relatively mild, with mild lymphoblastic leptomeningitis. In the cortex and white matter, the perivascular space is obviously widened, with light-pink-stained flocky substances and occasionally perivascular lymphocytic sleeve inside (Fig. 7.2).

2. Lungs

Different from lung lesions of other infectious diseases such as human-infected highly pathogenic avian influenza, EV71 is most likely to damage the ventral, dorsal, and intermediate sections of the medulla oblongata. Nerve centers related to respiration and vasomotion are located at these parts. Therefore, in addition to direct invasion of virus to lung tissue, neurogenic pulmonary edema is the main reason for acute pulmonary edema. The occurrence of acute pulmonary edema is related to the impaired respiratory center at the brain stem caused by brain lesions and increased intracranial pressure caused by encephaledema. The respiratory disease in patients with EV71-induced HFMD is mainly severe viral pneumonia. Its main pathological changes include dilated and congestive vascular capillaries in the alveolar septum, a large quantity of infiltrated mononuclear cells, a large quantity of fluid from edematous lungs in the alveolar space, monocyte effusion, and formation of pulmonary hyaline membrane. These pathological changes cause pulmonary edema, local lung consolidation, and hemorrhagic infarction, constituting the main reason for respiratory distress in pediatric patients (Figs. 7.3 and 7.4).

3. Heart

EV71-induced brain stem encephalitis may cause dysfunctional autonomic nervous system. The sympathetic nerves innervating the heart, by releasing adrenaline, activate β-adrenergic receptors and then stimulate adenosine cyclase to produce cAMP. The production of cAMP leads to stronger myocardial contraction, tachycardia, and high blood pressure. Based on autopsy of death cases, it has been confirmed that the heart is slightly involved, with mild hypertrophy. The epicardium was demonstrated with patchy lymphocytic infiltration, and the myocardium was always shown with no inflammation. Occasionally, focal myocardial cells were demonstrated with degeneration and necrosis, with interstitial edema as well as infiltration of lymphocytes and plasmocytes.

In addition, other organs also show different degrees of pathological changes. For instances, hepatic sinusoid dilation, congestion, and hepatocyte edema were shown in tissues of hepatic lobule. The kidneys may be demonstrated with renal interstitial congestion, epithelial cell edema, and adrenal medulla congestion. The small intestinal mucosa is congestive and thinner, with accompanying multifocal epithelial cell necrosis, shedding of cell membrane and hyperplasia of submucosal lymphoid tissue, expanded germinal center, splenic sinus congestion, and reactive hyperplasia.

7.5 Clinical Typing and Laboratory Test

7.5.1 Incubation Period

The incubation period of EV71 infection generally lasts for 2–7 days and occasionally lasts for up to 12 days. The patients in incubation period are asymptomatic, with EV71 detectable in throat swabs or stool specimen. Most patients do not experience onset of symptoms immediately after infection, namely, latent infection or asymptomatic infection. Pediatric patients, especially infants and young children, have a high incidence rate after being infected, with various symptoms. In both symptomatic and asymptomatic patients, respiratory excretion of virus persists for 1–3 weeks, and fecal excretion of the virus persists for 7–11 weeks.

7.5.2 Clinical Typing

Based on severity and prognosis, EV71 infection can be clinically classified into four types: common type, severe type, critical type, and atypical type.

7.5.2.1 Common Type

The onset is acute onset, with mild fever and a body temperature of about 38 °C. Simultaneously or within 1–2 days after the onset, scattered ulcerative herpes occur at the mucosa of oral cavity; maculopapules and herpes occur at the skin of hands, feet, and buttocks. Red inflammatory halo surrounds the skin rashes. And the prognosis is good.

7.5.2.2 Severe Type

The severe type refers to patients with mild encephalitis, encephalomyelitis, aseptic meningitis, or acute flaccid paralysis. The patients experience neurological symptoms of low spiritual stage, drowsiness, headache, vomiting, tendency to be frightened, shaking limbs, or paralysis. By physical examination, the patients show meningeal irritation sign and weakened or absent tendon reflex. Most of the patients have no sequelae, with good prognosis.

7.5.2.3 Critical Type

Critically ill patients, especially those aged under 3 years, may experience neurogenic pulmonary edema, pulmonary hemorrhage, circulatory failure (shock) brain stem encephalitis, cerebral edema and herniation, respiratory failure, severe pneumonia, sepsis, and multiple organ failure. Most of the patients sustain relevant sequelae and the mortality rate is high.

7.5.2.4 Atypical Type

In rare patients, the patients experience no typical rashes or oral herpes and/or ulceration but only fever and some other atypical symptoms. The atypical type of patients may only experience meningitis and encephalitis but no skin rashes.

7.5.3 Laboratory Test

7.5.3.1 Peripheral WBC Count

For common type of patients, the WBC count is generally within normal range. For severe type of patients, the WBC count may significantly increase.

7.5.3.2 Blood Biochemistry

In some cases, slight increases of ALT, AST, and CK-MB may be demonstrated. In severe type of patients, blood glucose level may be increased.

7.5.3.3 Cerebrospinal Fluid Examination

For the patients with the nervous system involved, cerebrospinal fluid examination demonstrates clear fluid, increased pressure, increased WBC count (with more multinucleated cells than monocytes in the critical type of cases), normal or slightly increased protein, and normal levels of sugar and chloride.

7.5.3.4 Etiological Examination

Virus isolation is the basis to define the diagnosis:

1. Throat swab

   At the beginning of enterovirus infection, within about 1–2 weeks, the virus may be isolated from pharyngeal secretions.
2. Fecal examination

At the early stage after enterovirus infection, the virus can be excreted in feces for 3–8 weeks or longer. Therefore, the virus can be isolated in the feces.

3. Other examination for virus isolation

   The virus can also be isolated from cerebrospinal fluid, blood, or other potentially infected tissues.

   Viral nucleic acid detection can be performed by using RT-PCR. Positive finding of EV71 nucleic acid constitutes the basis to define the diagnosis.

7.5.3.5 Serological Test

Comparing to viral antibody titers in the acute and convalescent stages, an at least four times increase or IgM antibody positive is the basis to define the diagnosis.

7.6 Clinical Diagnosis

EV71 infection commonly occurs in preschoolers; especially young children aged under 3 years have been demonstrated with the highest incidence rate. The source of infection includes symptomatic patients and individuals with latent infection. The virus spreads mainly via digestive tract, respiratory tract, and close contact to secretions. The patients commonly experience maculopapules and herpes on hands, feet, oral cavity, and other body parts. Occasionally, the patients may experience encephalitis, encephalomyelitis, meningitis, pulmonary edema, and circulatory failure. Based on epidemiological data and clinical manifestations, the clinical diagnosis can be made.

7.6.1 Basis for Diagnosis

7.6.1.1 Epidemiological Data

The disease occurs during epidemic seasons and the patients are commonly aged under 3 years.

7.6.1.2 Clinical Manifestations

The patients mainly experience symptoms of fever, maculopapules, and herpes on hands, feet, oral cavity, and buttocks. Some patients may also experience symptoms of upper respiratory tract infection.

7.6.1.3 Physical Signs

Some patients only experience rashes/herpes on hands, feet, and buttocks and herpetic angina.

7.6.1.4 Nervous System Involvement as well as Respiratory and Circulatory Failure

The severe type of patients may experience neurological symptoms due to involvement of the nervous system, as well as respiratory and circulatory failure. In some rare cases, especially those aged under 3 years, the patients may experience encephalitis, encephalomyelitis, meningitis, pulmonary edema, circulatory failure, and other symptoms.

7.6.1.5 Laboratory Test

1. Peripheral WBC count

   In common type of patients, the WBC count is within normal range. In severe type of patients, the WBC count may obviously increase.

2. Blood biochemistry

   In some cases, slight increases of ALT, AST, and CK-MB can be detected. In severe cases, the blood glucose level may be increased.

3. Cerebrospinal fluid examination

   In the patients with the nervous system involved, cerebrospinal fluid is shown to be clear, with increased pressure, increased WBC count (with more multinucleated cells than monocytes in critical cases), normal or slightly increased protein, as well as normal levels of sugar and chloride.

7.6.1.6 Etiological Examination

1. Virus isolation

   The virus isolation is the basis for definitive diagnosis. Throat swab, stool specimen, cerebrospinal fluid, blood, or other potentially infected tissues can be sampled for virus isolation.

2. Viral nucleic acid detection

   EV71 nucleic acid positive by RT-PCR is also the basis for definitive diagnosis.

7.6.1.7 Serological Test

Comparing the serum viral antibody titers in the acute stage and the convalescent stage, an at least four times increase of antibody titer or IgM antibody positive also constitutes basis for the diagnosis.

7.6.1.8 Diagnostic Imaging

1. Chest CT

   Chest CT may demonstrate changes of bronchitis, pneumonia, pulmonary edema, and pulmonary hemorrhage.

2. MRI

   By MRI, the lesions are mainly located in the brain stem and the gray matter of the spinal cord.

7.6.2 Basis for Definitive Diagnosis

The diagnosis should be based on comprehensive analysis of epidemiological data, clinical manifestations, and laboratory findings. And the diagnosis can be defined based on evidence from serological test and etiological examination.

1. After the onset, EV71 nucleic acid is detected positive or EV71 virus is isolated from stool specimen or mouth-rinsed fluid.
2. EV71 nucleic acid is detected positive or EV71 virus is isolated from cerebrospinal fluid or herpetic fluid.
3. EV71 IgM antibody is serologically detected in the early stage.
4. Serum neutralizing antibody in the convalescent stage shows an at least four times increase as high as that in the acute stage.

Clinically typical cases, with any *one* of the above four conditions, can be defined with HFMD.

7.7 Radiological Demonstrations

7.7.1 Radiology of the Neurological Complications

Compared to CT scan, MRI is definitively superior in examining the central nervous system due to its favorable soft tissue contrast and multiparameter imaging. Therefore, MRI is the radiological modality of choice to detect and assess the neurological complications of HFMD.

7.7.1.1 Aseptic Meningitis

Aseptic meningitis, also known as viral meningitis, is a common complication occurring at the central nervous system induced by EV71. Its diagnosis is mainly based on clinical symptoms, biochemistry of cerebrospinal fluid, and virus isolation. Plain MR imaging always shows no abnormalities, and contrast MR imaging demonstrates no meningeal enhancement, indicating its difference from bacterial meningitis. In the case with HFMD complicated by viral encephalitis, necrosis and edema can be displayed at the bilateral temporal lobes and frontal lobes, with long T1 and long T2 signal from the diseased lobes. The ependyma of lateral ventricle is demonstrated thickened, with slightly hyperintense T2WI signal. And some indirect signs, including meningeal enhancement and subdural effusion, can also be shown.

7.7.1.2 Brain Stem Encephalitis

The complications of brain stem encephalitis are commonly induced by EV71 infection, with diversified radiological demonstrations.

Location of Lesion

The main lesion is located at the dorsal interface between pons and medulla oblongata, which are longitudinal lesions. The lesion may extend upward and downward to involve medulla oblongata, midbrain, thalamus, cerebellar dentate nucleus, and even into the cervical spinal cord. MRI shows abnormal patchy signals.

Signal Change

The main lesion (at the dorsal interface between pons and medulla oblongata) is demonstrated with long T1 and long T2 signals. We analyzed the cases of brain stem encephalitis by large sampling and found that the signal changes are diversified, which is related to the duration of the illness course.

1. Signal of the main lesion at the acute stage can be classified into three types based on plain and contrast imaging: (1) negative by plain MR imaging but slight enhancement by contrast imaging (Fig. 7.5); (2) positive by plain MR imaging but no enhancement by contrast imaging (Fig. 7.6) (3) as well as isointense or slightly hypointense T1WI signal, slightly hyperintense T2WI signal, hyperintense FLAIR, and DWI signals by plain imaging but no enhancement by contrast imaging; and (4) positive by plain MR imaging and slight to moderate enhancement by contrast imaging (Fig. 7.7) as well as isointense or slightly hypointense T1WI signal, slightly hyperintense T2WI signal, hyperintense FLAIR, and DWI signals by plain imaging.
2. Signal of the main lesion at the convalescent stage varies according to the patient's condition. In the cases with improved condition, no abnormal signal can be demonstrated by MRI. In the cases with deteriorated condition, the main lesion may progress into malacia lesion with long T1 and long T2 signals (Fig. 7.7). Meanwhile, they may show circulatory and respiratory dysfunctions.
3. Signal of other lesions at the medulla oblongata, midbrain, thalamus, and cerebellum dentate nucleus (Fig. 7.8) is demonstrated as long T1 and long T2 signal at the acute stage. FLAIR and DWI demonstrate hyperintense signal and no enhancement by contrast imaging. The radiological demonstrations resemble to those of common enterogenous viral encephalitis. The lesions apart of the main lesion show no progression into malacia. The quantity of lesions demonstrated by MRI is significantly related to the clinical symptoms. That is, to say, the cases with more brain parts involved show more severe clinical symptoms (Fig. 7.9).

7.7.1.3 Encephalitis

In clinically diagnosed cases of encephalitis, the positive rate by MRI is low. Lu et al. analyzed data of 25 cases with clinical diagnosis of encephalitis in the year of 2010. The analysis demonstrated that seven cases showed positive by MRI,

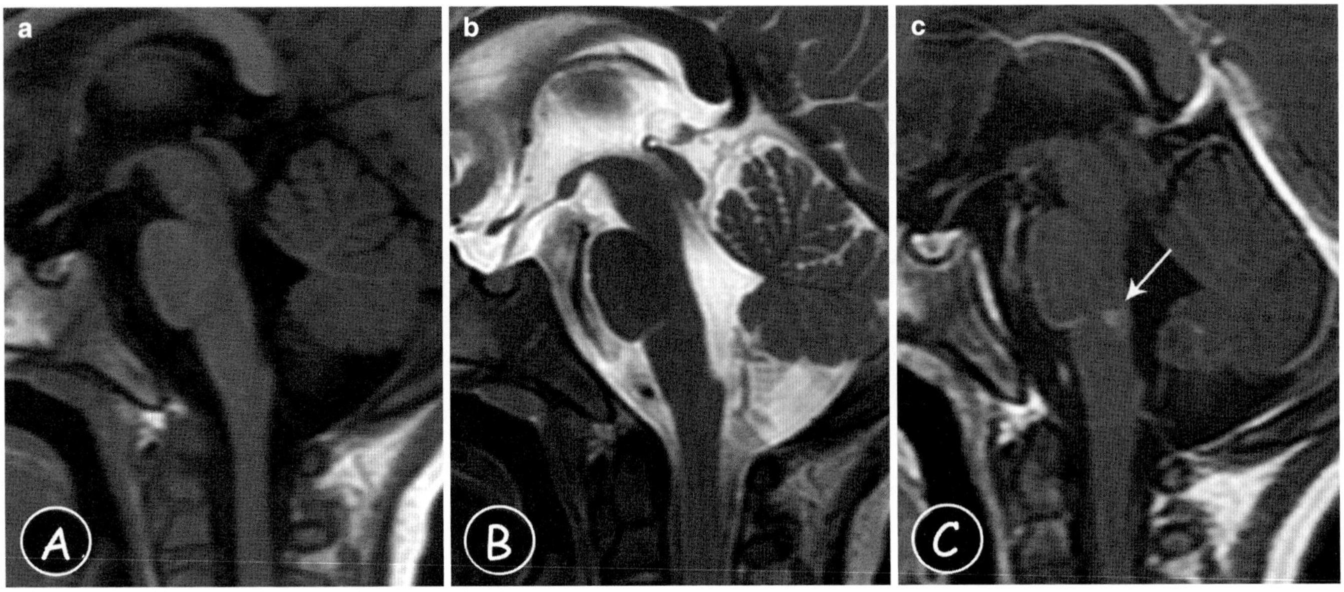

Fig. 7.5 (**a–c**) A girl aged 27 months with EV71-induced HFMD complicated by brain stem encephalitis at day 7 after onset. Sagittal view T1WI (**a**) and T2WI (**b**) showed no abnormal signal in the brain stem. Contrast sagittal view (**c**) imaging showed small patchy highly enhanced lesion at the dorsal interface between pons and medulla oblongata

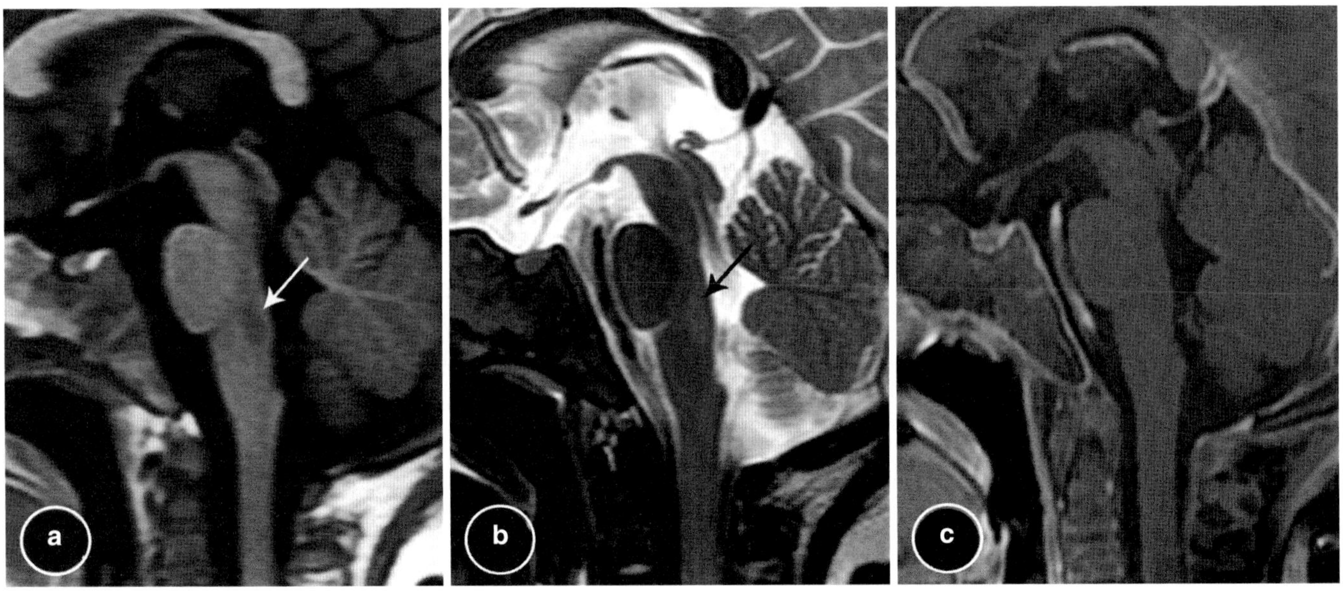

Fig. 7.6 (**a–c**) A boy aged 17 months with EV71-induced HFMD complicated by brain stem encephalitis at day 11 after onset. Sagittal view T1WI (**a**) showed longitudinal slightly hypointense signal at the dorsal interface between pons and medulla oblongata. Sagittal view T2WI (**b**) showed hyperintense signal of the lesion, and contrast imaging (**c**) displayed no enhancement of the lesion

with long T1 and long T2 signal at the right parietal lobe that was slightly enhanced by contrast imaging (Fig. 7.10). The signal changes were demonstrated to be not characteristic.

7.7.1.4 Myelitis

Myelitis mainly involves the central gray matter of the spinal cord, predominantly the anterior horn. The lesion may be either unilateral or bilateral, demonstrated as slightly long T1 and long T2 signals and slight to moderate enhancement. The cervical spinal cord is more commonly involved [16] (Fig. 7.11). In critical and severe cases, cervical myelitis may manifest as acute transverse myelitis. By MRI, it is demonstrated as diffuse swelling of the cervical spinal cord with slightly long T1 and long T2 signals. The gray and white matters are concurrently involved with poorly defined boundary. The signal from the cervical spinal cord commonly extends into the abnormal

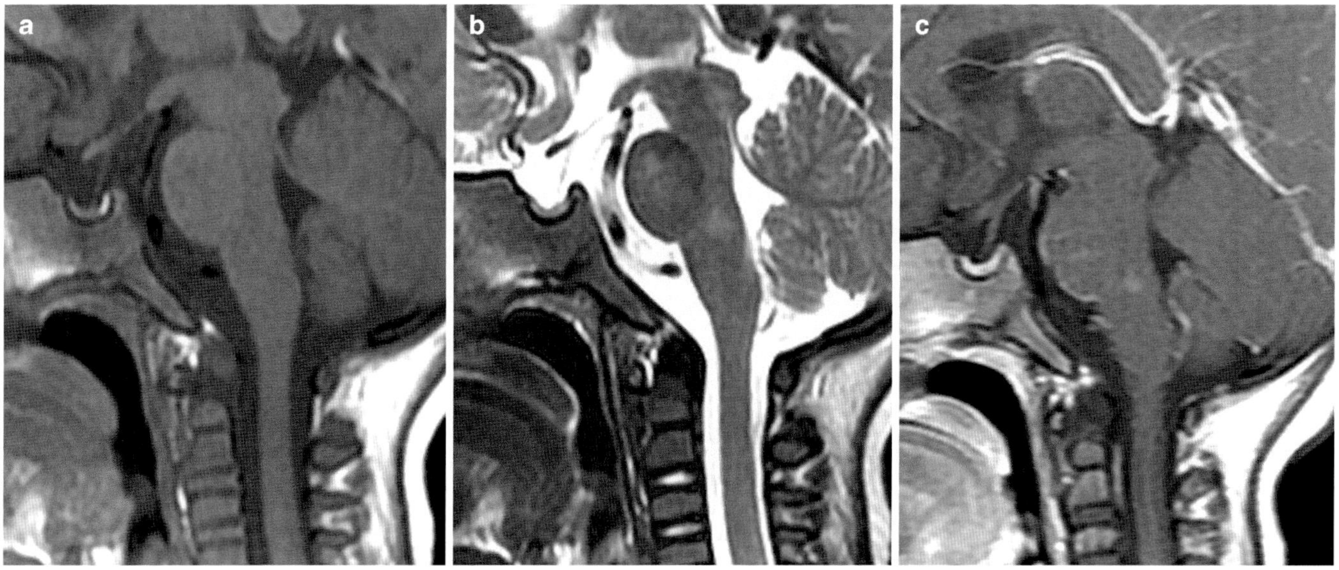

Fig. 7.7 A boy aged 28 months was diagnosed with EV71-induced HFMD complicated by brain stem encephalitis at day 11 after onset. Sagittal view T1WI (**a**) showed no apparently abnormal signal at the dorsal interface between pons and medulla oblongata. Sagittal view T2WI (**b**) showed hyperintense signal of the lesion. Contrast imaging (**c**) displayed slight enhancement of the lesion

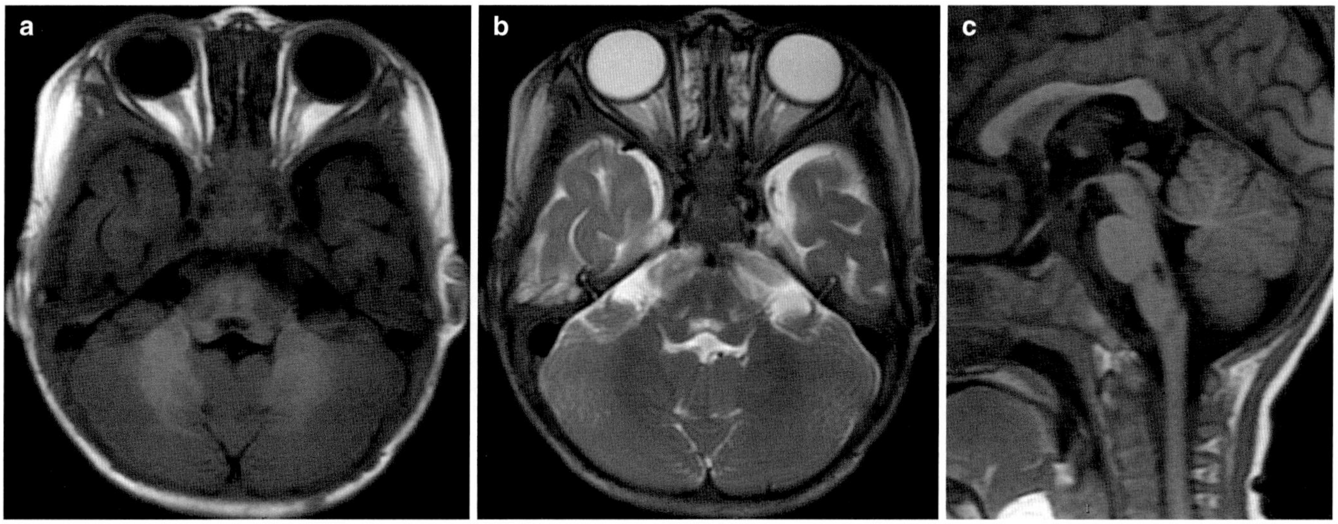

Fig. 7.8 A boy aged 4 months with EV71-induced HFMD complicated by brain stem encephalitis. By reexamination after 1 month, transverse T1WI (**a**) showed patchy malacia lesion at the dorsal medulla oblongata. Transverse T2WI (**b**) showed hyperintense signal and sagittal view T1WI (**c**) displayed longitudinal malacia lesion at the interface between pons and medulla oblongata

signal from the medulla oblongata (Fig. 7.12), which is a sign of critical condition in the cases with brain stem encephalitis accompanied by transverse myelitis of the cervical spine. In pediatric patients with enlarged lumbar spinal cord and involved central gray matter, temporary neurogenic bladder may occur (Fig. 7.13). It is caused by impaired low-level nerve center of micturition reflex due to enlarged lumbar spinal cord, which further leads to neurogenic voiding dysfunction of the bladder and urinary retention. During the convalescent stage, MRI commonly demonstrates no abnormalities. The lesion rarely progresses into malacia lesion.

Generally, EV71-induced HFMD can be complicated by disorders of the central nervous system, with brain stem encephalitis as the most common. The lesions are mainly located at the interface between pons and medulla oblongata. By contrast MRI, the lesions that are demonstrated to be negative by plain imaging can be enhanced. Sagittal thin-layer imaging is recommended. Myelitis commonly

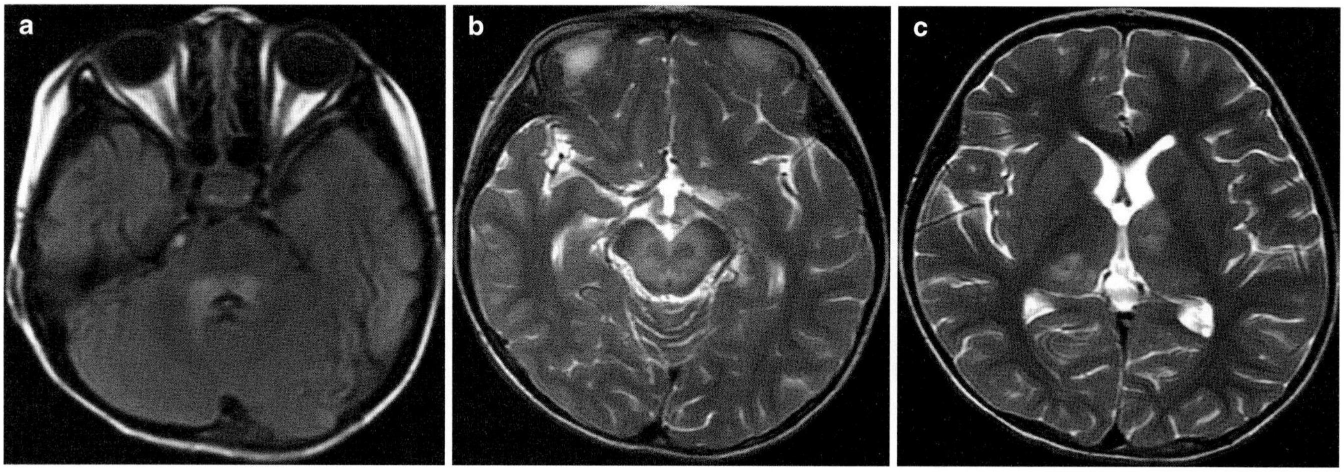

Fig. 7.9 A boy aged 28 months with EV71-induced HFMD complicated by brain stem encephalitis at day 11 after onset. Transverse FLAIR (**a**) showed patchy hyperintense signal at the dorsal pons. Transverse T2WI (**b**, **c**), respectively, displayed patchy hyperintense signal at the midbrain and bilateral dorsal thalamus

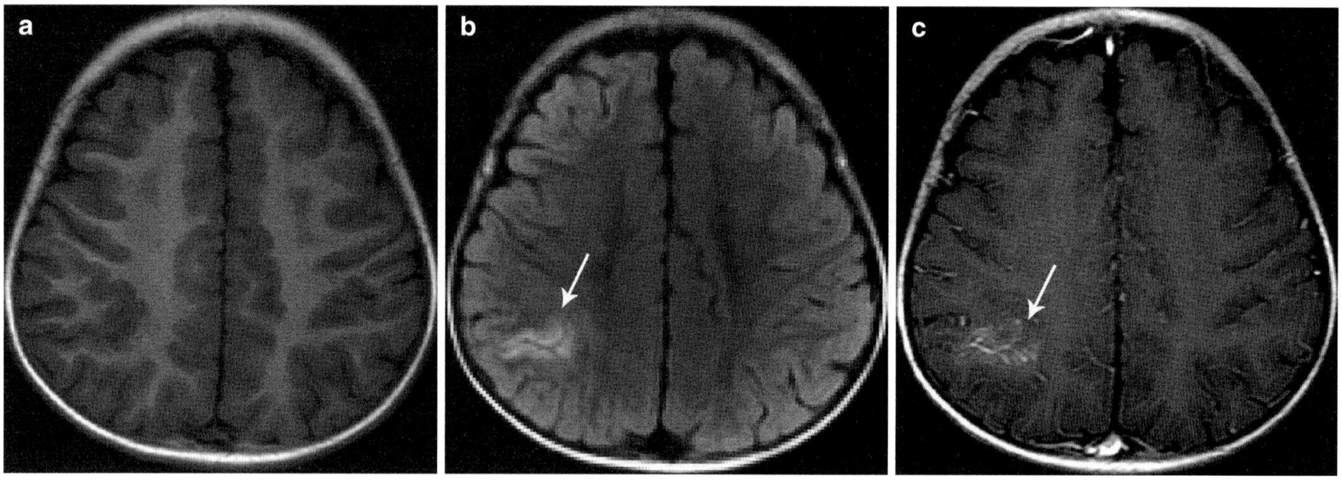

Fig. 7.10 (**a**–**c**) A boy aged 2 years with EV71-induced HFMD complicated by encephalitis at day 7 after onset. Transverse T1WI (**a**) showed flaky slightly long T1 signal at and under the cortex of right parietal lobe. FLAIR (**b**) showed hyperintense signal. Contrast imaging (**c**) displayed moderate enhancement of the lesion

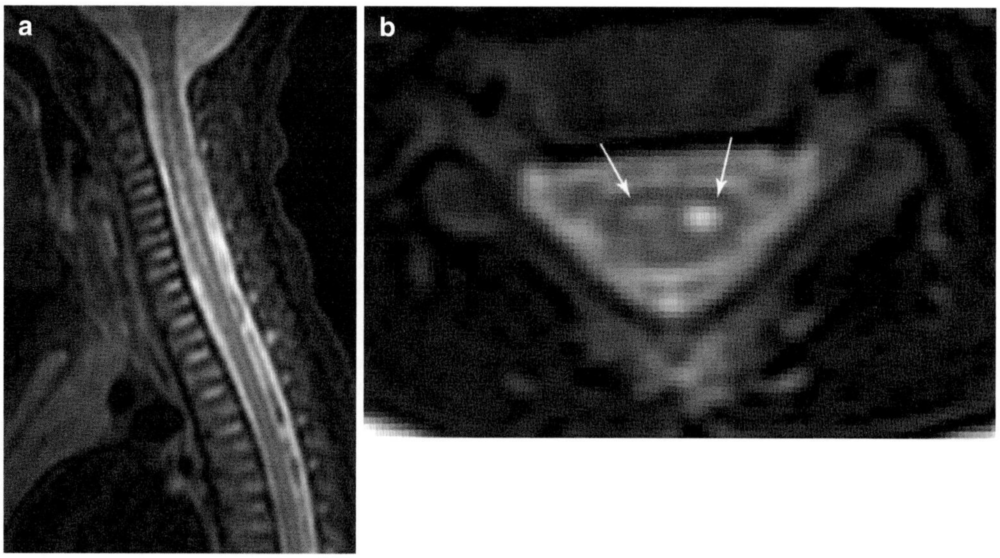

Fig. 7.11 A boy aged 2 years and 3 months with EV71-induced HFMD. At day 5 after onset, his upper limbs were asthenic, especially the left upper limb. Sagittal view T2WI (**a**) showed linear hyperintense signals at the center of cervical spinal cord. Transverse T2WI after fat suppression (**b**) showed small oval hyperintense signal at the central gray matter of cervical spinal cord, which was more obvious at the left side

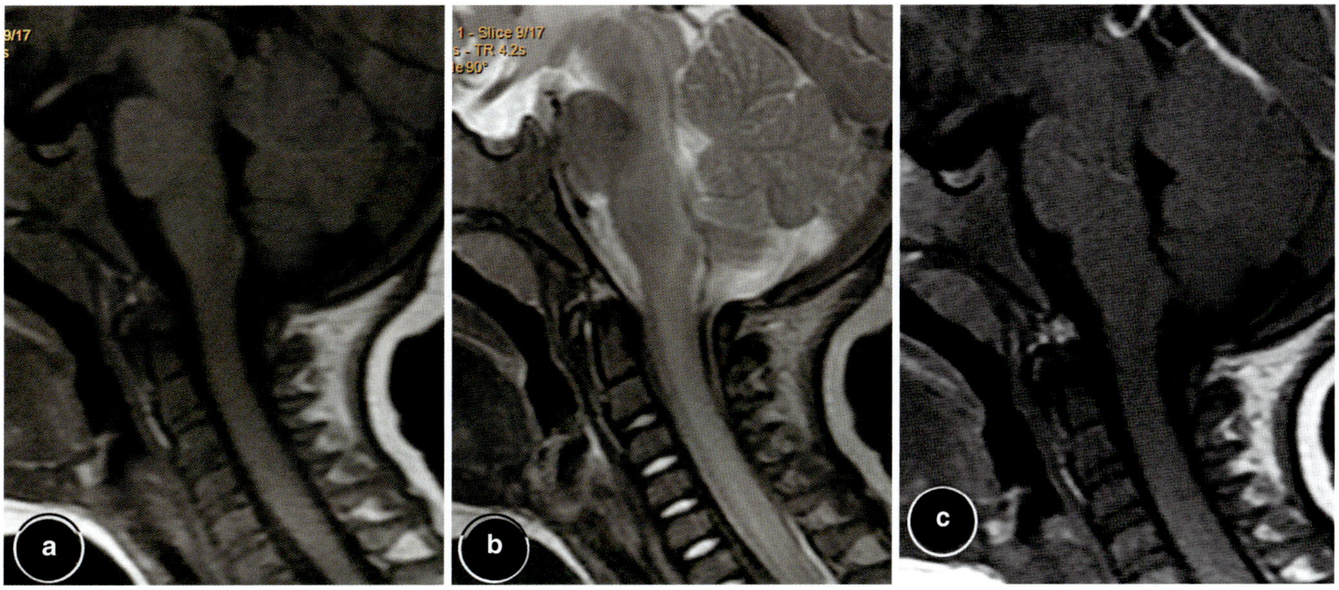

Fig. 7.12 A boy aged 27 months with EV71-induced HFMD complicated by brain stem encephalitis and myelitis at day 6 after onset. Sagittal view T1WI (**a**) showed obviously swollen cervical spinal cord and slightly hypointense flaky signal in the brain stem and cervical spinal cord. Sagittal view T2WI (**b**) showed slightly hyperintense large flaky. Contrast imaging (**c**) displayed no obvious enhancement of lesion

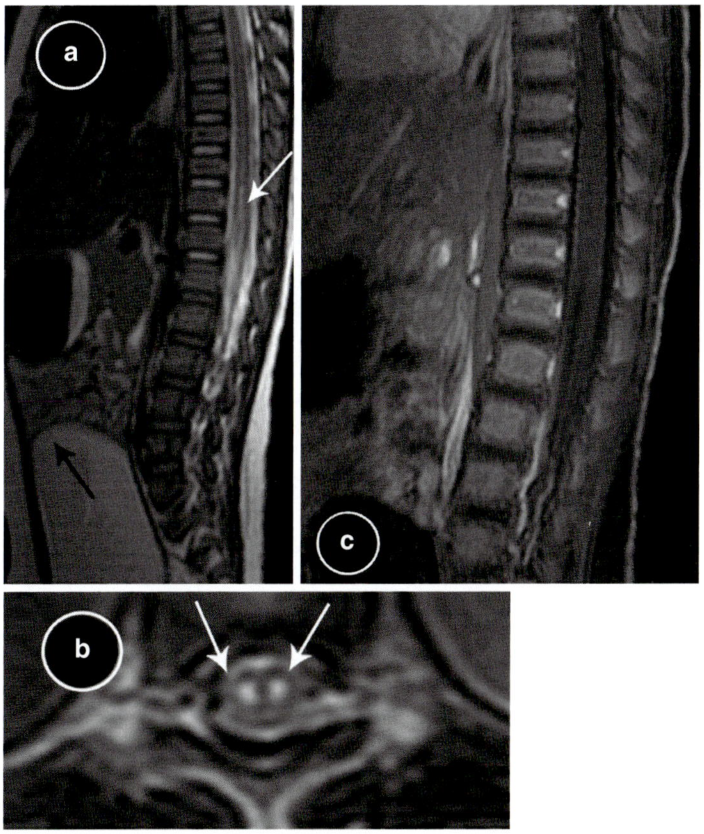

Fig. 7.13 A boy aged 5 months with EV71-induced HFMD complicated by flaccid paralysis of both lower limbs and dysuresia. Sagittal view T2WI (**a**) showed enlarged lumbar spinal cord with longitudinal flaky hyperintense signal (*white arrow*), enlarged bladder with its superior border reaching the level of fourth lumbar vertebra (*black arrows*). Transverse T2WI (**b**) at the first lumbar vertebra showed round-like hyperintense signals from bilateral central gray matters (*white arrows*). Contrast imaging (**c**) showed no enhancement of the lesions

involves the central gray matter, especially the central gray matter of the cervical spinal cord. And myelitis is commonly accompanied by brain stem encephalitis. Therefore, for clinically suspected cases of myelitis, brain plain and contrast MRI are recommended. In addition, brain stem encephalitis accompanied by cervical transverse myelitis is a sign of critical condition. In the cases with myelitis and enlarged lumbar spinal cord, temporary neurogenic bladder may occur.

7.7.2 Radiological Demonstrations of Respiratory Complications

Chest radiological demonstrations for HFMD are diversified, which are closely related to the severity and staging of the disease. Based on the radiological findings, the complications can be classified into four types: bronchitis, pneumonia, pulmonary edema, and pulmonary hemorrhage.

7.7.2.1 Bronchitis Type

Its pathological basis is pulmonary interstitial inflammation. The lesions are always extensive, possibly involving each lobe of both lungs and commonly distributing bilaterally. The lesions are more commonly located at the middle and inner zone of both lower lung fields.

1. Bronchial wall and surrounding tissue inflammation

   Chest X-rays demonstrate thickened lung markings with poorly defined boundaries, which are fine blurry linear shadow. The blurry linear shadow distributes along airways and runs anatomically along the bronchi (Fig. 7.14).
2. Interstitial inflammation of alveolar wall and interlobular septum

   Chest X-ray demonstrates short linear shadow interweaving into network-like appearance or diffusely decreased transparency of lung fields with slightly ground-glass density (Fig. 7.15).
3. Inflammation of lobular acinus or inflammation around bronchiole

   Chest X-ray demonstrates small nodular density shadows with poorly defined boundaries, which scatter within the abovementioned interstitial lesions.

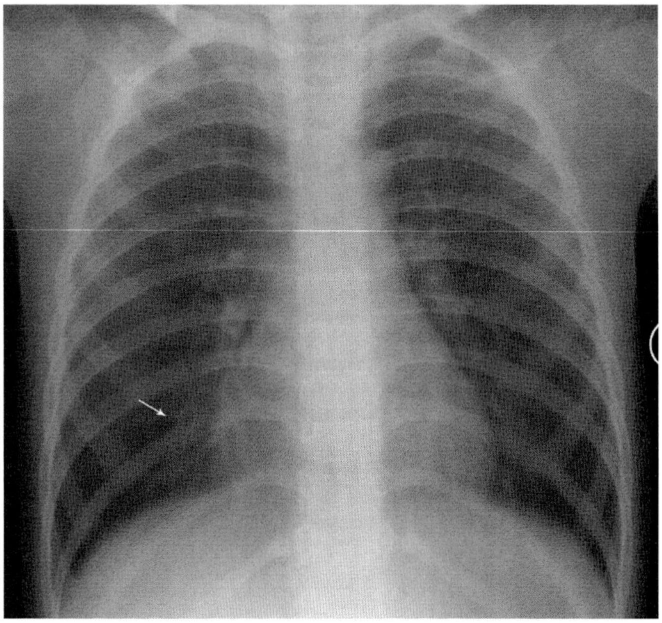

Fig. 7.14 A girl aged 3 years with EV71-induced HFMD complicated by peribronchitis at day 4 after onset. Chest X-ray showed thickened pulmonary markings of both lungs and poorly defined lung markings at the right lower lung field (*white arrow*)

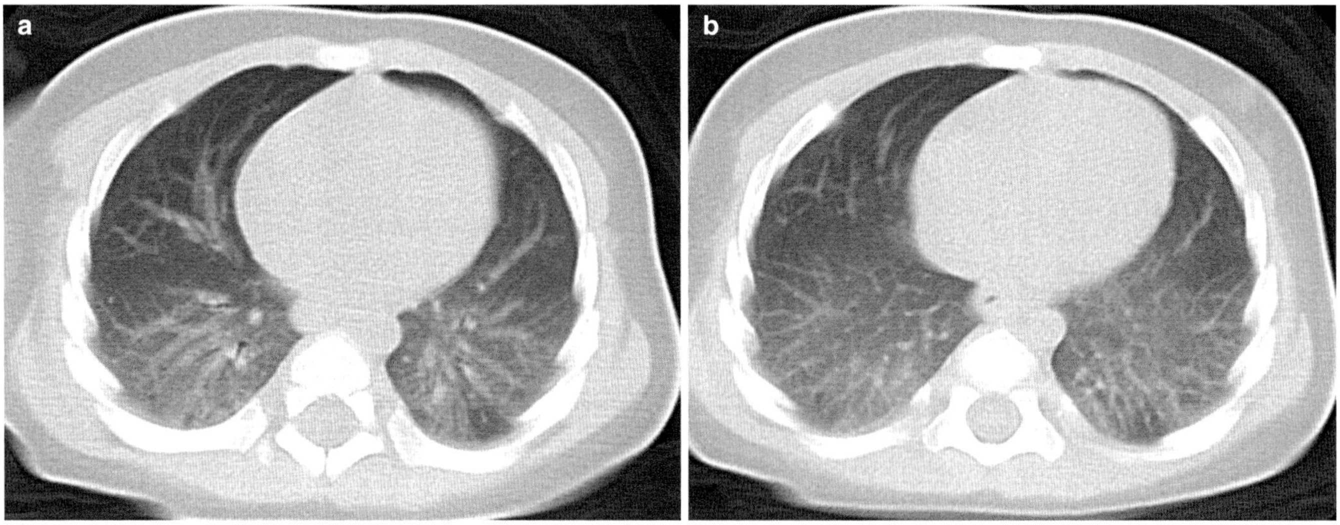

Fig. 7.15 (**a**, **b**) A boy aged 4 months with HFMD complicated by pulmonary interstitial inflammation. He was radiologically demonstrated with decreased transparency of both lower lung lobes in slightly ground-glass density and poorly defined thickened lung markings. The findings indicated lesions at both lower lung lobes, predominantly interstitial change

7.7.2.2 Pneumonia Type

The inflammation invades alveolar ducts, alveolar sacs, and alveoli to cause inflammatory exudative consolidation of pulmonary lobule and further bronchopneumonia.

In addition to increased and thickened lung markings with poorly defined boundaries, chest X-ray/CT demonstrates multiple small patchy high-density opacities or ground-glass density opacities with poorly defined boundaries and different sizes, which distribute along the lung markings. The lesions may integrate into flakes (Figs. 7.16 and 7.17) and even lobar change with uneven density (Fig. 7.18).

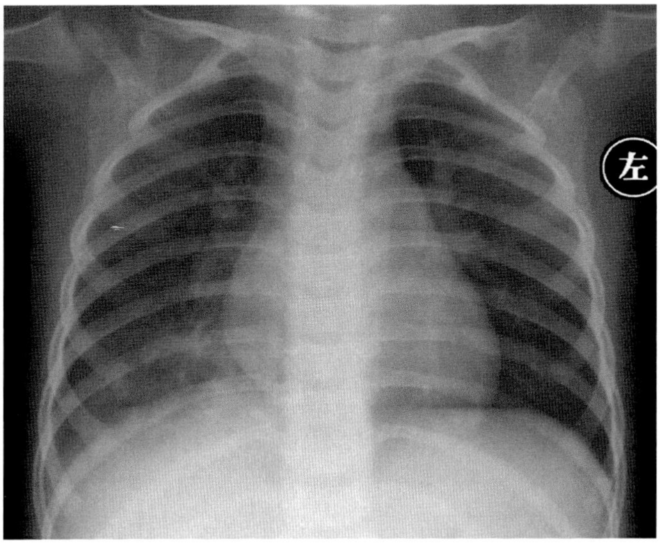

Fig. 7.16 A girl aged 2 years with EV71-induced HFMD complicated by pneumonia of the right lower lung at day 7 after onset. Chest X-ray showed flaky light blurry opacity above diaphragm in the right lower lung field and poorly defined right diaphragmatic surface

Chest radiological signs of severe HFMD are diversified, which are predominantly flaky and flocculent opacity, as well as ground-glass density opacity. The condition may be complicated by pulmonary interstitial infiltration, with rapid dynamic changes, which are radiologically characteristic.

7.7.2.3 Pulmonary Edema Type

Pulmonary edema complicating HFMD is commonly neurogenic, which occurs in pediatric patients with EV71-induced HFMD complicated by brain stem encephalitis. It is caused by impairment of the circulatory and respiratory nerve center. Based on the occurring phase and location, it can be classified into interstitial pulmonary edema and alveolar pulmonary edema.

Interstitial Pulmonary Edema

1. Changes of lung marking and hilum

   The fluid fills into the pulmonary interstitium to cause decreased transparency of lungs and ground-glass density change. Due to increased pulmonary venous pressure, the blood in lungs is redistributed, with more blood distributed in the upper lungs. Therefore, the blood vessels in the upper lungs are thicker than those in the lower lungs, showing thickened, increased, and poorly defined lung markings in the upper lungs but thinner lung markings in the lower lungs (Fig. 7.19).
2. Septal linear opacity

   It is also known as Kerley line that can be classified into Kerley A line, Kerley B line, and Kerley C line, with the Kerley B line as the most common. Kerley A line is located in the upper and middle fields of both lungs and is shown as a linear high-density opacity (5–6 cm in length and 0.5–1.0 mm in width) coursing diagonally from the periphery to the hilum. It is caused by accumulated fluid around the

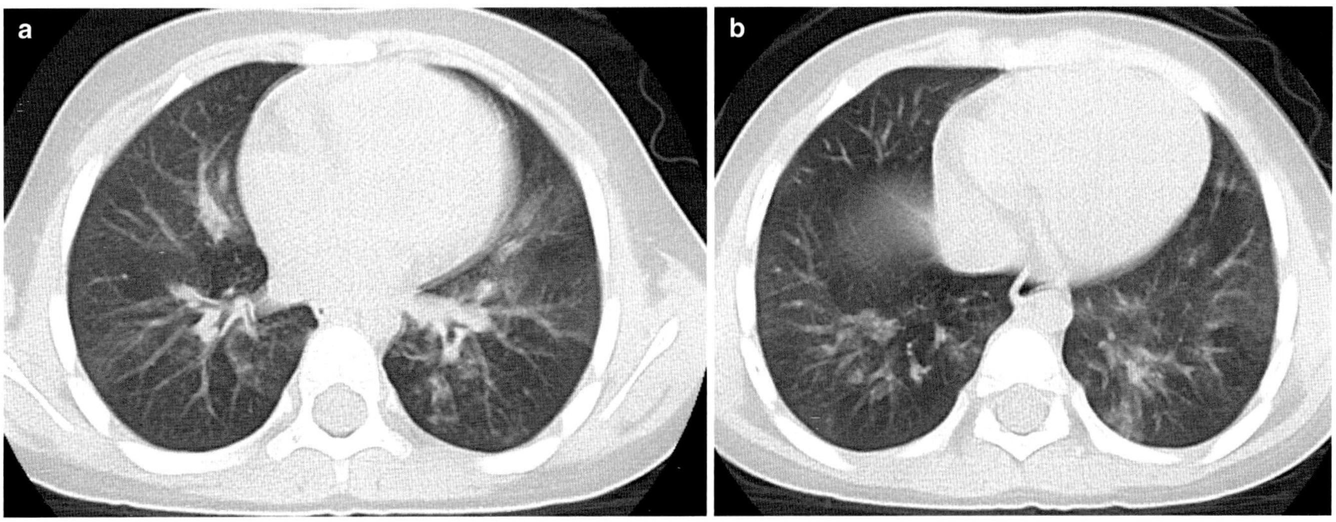

Fig. 7.17 (**a**, **b**) A girl aged 3 years with EV71-induced HFMD complicated by pneumonia of both lungs. She was radiologically demonstrated with multiple patchy blurry opacities at the lingular segment of left upper lung lobe and both lower lung lobes. Some of the patchy blurry opacities were shown with ground-glass density

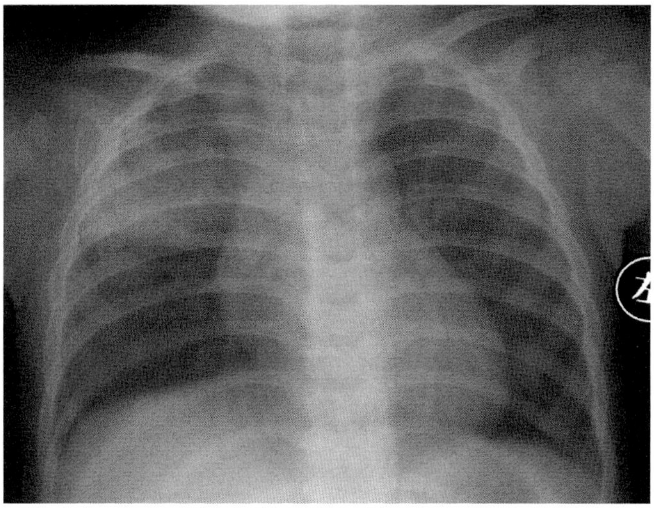

Fig. 7.18 A girl aged 13 months with HFMD complicated by pneumonia at day 3 after onset and high fever for 1 day. Chest X-ray showed large flaky triangular high-density opacity at the right upper and middle lung fields. The opacity was shown with uneven density as well as straight clear inferior margin, which was horizontal fissure

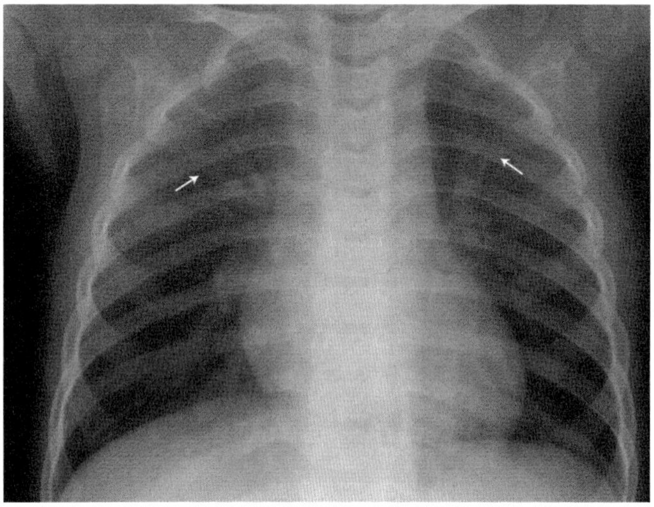

Fig. 7.19 A 2-year-old patient with HFMD complicated by interstitial pulmonary edema. Chest X-ray showed obviously thickened vascular markings in both upper lungs and thicker lung markings in both upper lungs than in both lower lungs, with poorly defined boundaries (*arrows*). The vascular markings at the right lower lung field was shown to be thinner

pulmonary deep veins and lymphatic vessels. Kerley B line is the most important X-ray sign for diagnosis of interstitial pulmonary edema. It is located in the lower lung fields adjacent to the costophrenic angle and is shown as a short straight linear high-density opacity (2–3 cm in length). It is perpendicular to the pleura and is caused by thickened edema of interlobular septum. Kerley C line is located in the lower lung fields and is shown as reticular high-density opacity. It overlaps with Kerley B line.

3. Subpleural effusion

   When fluid passes through pulmonary interstitium into thin connective tissue under the visceral pleura to cause subpleural interstitial edema and lymphangiectasis, interlobar subpleural edema line is radiologically displayed. The interlobar fissure is widened and shows no change along with posture change.

Alveolar Pulmonary Edema (Fig. 7.20)
The lesions are symmetrically distributed with the hilus as the center. A large flake of cloudy high-density opacity is demonstrated within the lung fields, mostly in the middle and inner zone. In the typical cases, butterfly-wing-like change is displayed, which may also be unilateral. Generally speaking, pulmonary edema is distributed more in the lower lung than in the upper lung and more in the medial lung than in the lateral lung. Lesion is rarely found at the apex of lung, and its density gradually decreases from the medial lung to the lateral lung. Alveolar pulmonary edema may be accompanied by a small quantity of pleural effusion, which is commonly bilateral. After clinical symptomatic treatment, the intrapulmonary lesions can be obviously absorbed within a short period of time.

7.7.2.4 Pulmonary Hemorrhage Type

HFMD is rarely complicated by pulmonary hemorrhage, which is commonly caused by EV71. Hemorrhage may occur in alveolus or interstitium, and alveolar hemorrhage is more common (Fig. 7.21).

1. Reduced transparency of lung fields and small spots of high-density opacities

   Due to pulmonary edema and mild hemorrhage, the reduced alveolar air inflation causes decreased transparency of lungs. During this stage, the diagnosis of pulmonary hemorrhage can hardly be diagnosed based only on radiological findings.
2. Small patchy opacities

   Along with increased volume of bleeding, bloody edema fluid fills in the alveoli and interstitium of the diseased area, which may be shown with integration into small flakes. The changes are radiologically demonstrated as flaky and flocculent dense opacity with even density but no fixed structure.
3. Large flaky opacities

   Along with further increased volume of bleeding, the pathological sections display mass or large mass like bleeding, which indicates the advanced stage of hemorrhage. It is radiologically demonstrated as even and dense opacity in one or both lungs, namely, the white lung.
4. Abnormal heart shadow

   The hear shadow is demonstrated to be enlarged or progressively enlarged. Cardiac dysfunction may accelerate the occurrence and progression of pulmonary edema and pulmonary hemorrhage.

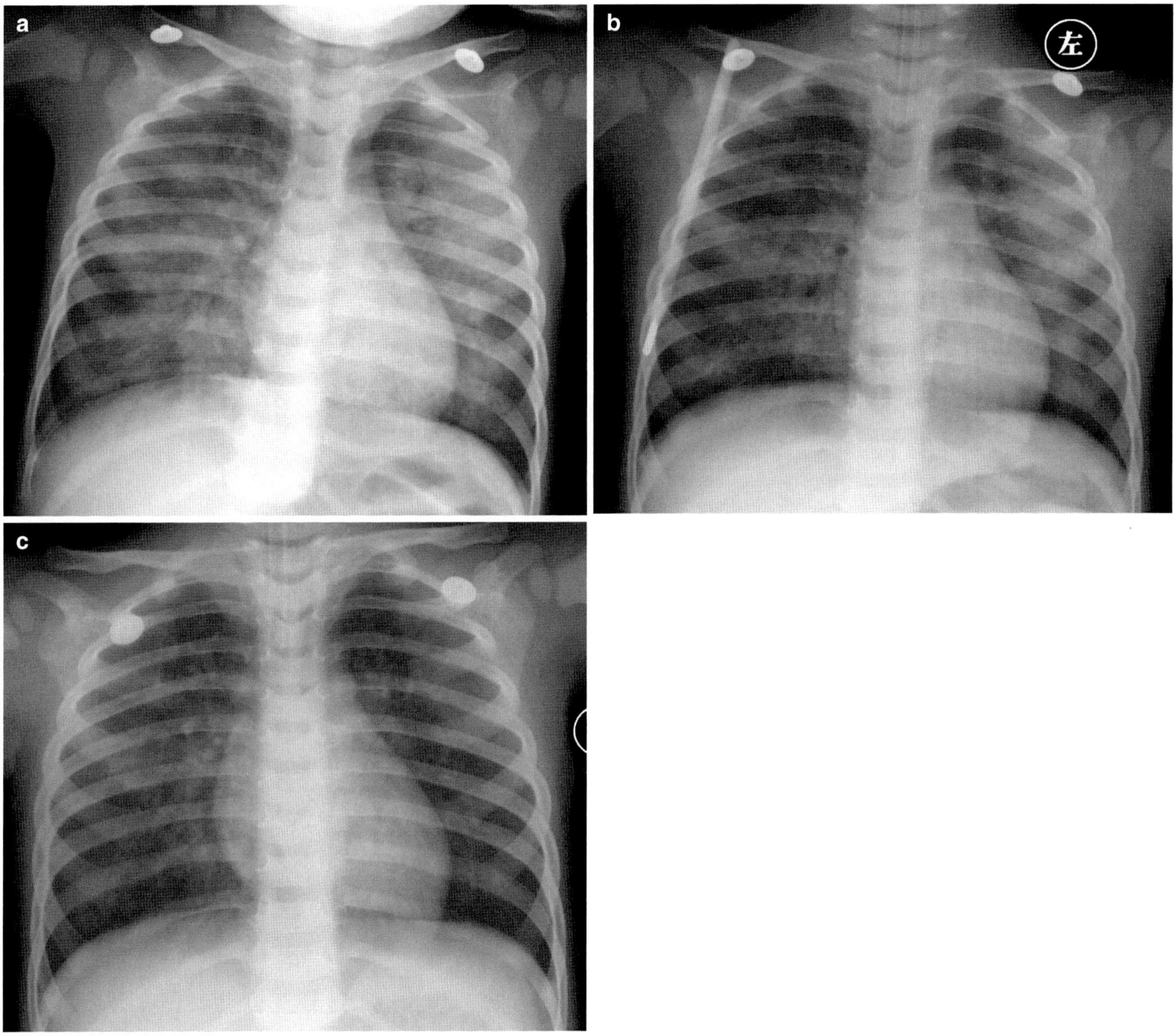

Fig. 7.20 A girl aged 2 years with EV71-induced HFMD complicated by alveolar pulmonary edema and brain stem encephalitis. (**a**) Chest X-ray showed patchy and cloudy opacities in both lung fields. The opacities were dense around both lung hili and were distributed like butterfly wings. The heart shadow was not enlarged. (**b**) The follow-up chest X-ray after 1 h showed obviously decreased patchy and cloudy opacities in both lungs, with decreased density. (**c**) The follow-up chest X-ray after 26 h showed that most of the patchy and cloudy opacities were absorbed

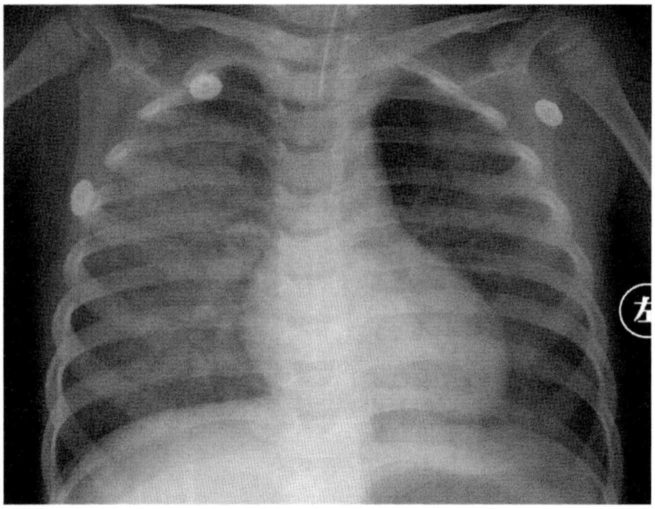

Fig. 7.21 A girl aged 20 months with HFMD complicated by pulmonary hemorrhage. By endotracheal cannulation, dark red blood was aspirated. Radiologically, the both lung fields were demonstrated with patchy and cloudy opacity, especially around hili. The right lung field was displayed with large flake of high-density opacity, showing white lung. The heart shadow was shown to be slightly enlarged. Death occurred 24 h after the radiological examination

Further Reading

1. Lu CY, Lee CY, Kao CL, et al. Incidence and case-fatality rates resulting from the 1998 enterovirus 71 outbreak in Taiwan. J Med Virol. 2002;67(2):217–23.
2. Robinson CR, Doane FW, Rhodes AJ. Report of an outbreak of febrile illness with pharyngeal lesions and exanthem: Toronto, summer 1957; isolation of group A Coxsackie virus. Can Med Assoc J. 1958;79(8):615–21.
3. Schmidt NJ, Lennette EH, Ho HH. An apparently new enterovirus isolated from patients with disease of the central nervous system. J Infect Dis. 1974;129(3):304–9.
4. Zeng H, Wen F, Gan Y, et al. MRI and associated clinical characteristics of EV71-induced brainstem encephalitis in children with hand-foot-mouth disease. Neuroradiology. 2012;54(6):623–30.
5. Huang CC, Liu CC, Chang YC, et al. Neurologic complications in children with enterovirus 71 infection. N Engl J Med. 1999; 341(13):936–42.
6. Zhou BP, Li CR. EV71 induced hand-foot-and-mouth disease. Beijing: People's Health Publishing House; 2009. p. 159–83.
7. Li J, Chen F, Liu T, et al. MRI findings of neurological complications in hand-foot-mouth disease by enterovirus 71 infection. Int J Neurosci. 2012;122(7):338–44.
8. Huang CC. Neurologic complications of enterovirus 71 infection in children: lessons from this Taiwan epidemic. Acta Paediatr Taiwan. 2001;42(1):5–7.
9. Chen Y, Cai QL, Chen F, et al. Pediatric severe hand-foot-and-mouth disease complicated by encephalitis or brainstem encephalitis: MRI analysis. J Pract Radiol. 2010;26(9):1341–3, 9.
10. Zeng HW, Sun J, Huang WX, et al. EV71 induced hand-foot-mouth disease complicated by disorders of the central nervous system: clinical and radiological analysis. J Pract Radiol. 2010;26(11):1653–56,74.
11. Li ZY, Gan YG, Lin FF, et al. Pediatric hand-foot-mouth disease complicated by brainstem encephalitis: MRI findings. J Clin Radiol. 2011;30(2):243–6.
12. Shen WC, Tsai C, Chiu H, et al. MRI of Enterovirus 71 myelitis with monoplegia. Neuroradiology. 2000;42(2):124–7.
13. McMinn P, Stratov I, Nagarajan L, et al. Neurological manifestations of enterovirus 71 infection in children during an outbreak of hand, foot, and mouth disease in Western Australia. Clin Infect Dis. 2001;32(2):236–42.
14. Fu HN, Zou YX. EV71 induced hand-foot-mouth disease complicated by acute flaccid paralysis: clinical data analysis. J Clin Pediatr. 2012;30(4):347–50.
15. Chen CY, Chang YC, Huang CC, et al. Acute flaccid paralysis in infants and young children with enterovirus 71 infection: MR imaging findings and clinical correlates. AJNR Am J Neuroradiol. 2001;22(1):200–5.
16. Lu M, Meng G, He YX, et al. Pathology of enterovirus 71 infection: an autopsy study of 5 cases. Zhonghua Bing Li Xue Za Zhi. 2009;38(2):81–5.
17. Parratte B, Bonniaud V, Tatu L, et al. Anatomy and physiology of the lower urinary tract. Prog Urol. 2007;17(3):331–5.
18. Chang LY, Lin TY, Hsu KH, et al. Clinical features and risk factors of pulmonary oedema after enterovirus-71-related hand, foot, and mouth disease. Lancet. 1999;354(9191):1682–6.
19. Cheng JL, Liu K, Wang H, et al. Pediatric severe hand-foot-mouth disease complicated by pulmonary edema: chest X-ray analysis. J Clin Radiol. 2012;04:553–5.
20. Hao TR, Xu ZQ, Zhang XH, et al. Chest X-ray diagnosis of neurogenic pulmonary edema as complication of critical and severe hand-foot-mouth disease: analysis of 6 cases. Radiol Pract. 2011;26(05):543–5.
21. Han XZ, Li HB. Neurogenic pulmonary edema caused by severe hand-foot-mouth disease. J Pract Clin Pediatr. 2009;10:732–3.
22. Mu HG, Chen PY, Sang L, et al. Clinical and chest X-ray analysis of hand-foot-mouth disease. Radiol Pract. 2009;07:781–3.
23. Ho M, Chen ER, Hsu KH, et al. An epidemic of enterovirus 71 infection in Taiwan. Taiwan Enterovirus Epidemic Working Group. N Engl J Med. 1999;341(13):929–35.
24. Prager P, Nolan M, Andrews IP, et al. Neurogenic pulmonary edema in enterovirus 71 encephalitis is not uniformly fatal but causes severe morbidity in survivors. Pediatr Crit Care Med. 2003;4(3):377–81.
25. Shekhar K, Lye MS, Norlijah O, et al. Deaths in children during an outbreak of hand, foot and mouth disease in Peninsular Malaysia--clinical and pathological characteristics. Med J Malaysia. 2005; 60(3):297–304.
26. Yan XF, Ge YL, Xie XB, et al. Clinical analysis of children with severe hand-foot-and-mouth disease in Shanghai. Zhonghua Er Ke Za Zhi. 2012;50(4):271–5.
27. Huang RW, Wu XL, Yang RY. Analysis of death cases from hand-foot-and-mouth disease. Chin J Clin Obstetr Gynecol Pediatr (Electronic Edition). 2011;7(04):318–20.
28. Chang LY, Lin TY, Huang YC, et al. Comparison of enterovirus 71 and coxsackie-virus A16 clinical illnesses during the Taiwan enterovirus epidemic, 1998. Pediatr Infect Dis J. 1999;18(12):1092–6.
29. He YX, Fu D, Cao DZ, et al. Critical care and therapy based different illness state of 80 patients with severe hand-foot-and-mouth disease seen in Shenzhen. Zhonghua Er Ke Za Zhi. 2009;47(5):338–43.
30. Wei D, Li KX, Chen E. Autopsy report of two cases with enterovirus type 71 infection brainstem encephalitis and literature review. Zhonghua Er Ke Za Zhi. 2010;48(3):220–3.
31. Chen KT, Chang HL, Wang ST, et al. Epidemiologic features of hand-foot-mouth disease and herpangina caused by enterovirus 71 in Taiwan, 1998–2005. Pediatrics. 2007;120(2):e244–52.

8 Pulmonary Tuberculosis

Deng Qun-Yi, Pu-Xuan Lu, Yu Wei-Ye, Li Guo-Bo, Liu Guo-Hui, Zhang Wei-Ren, He Yu-Lin, Liu Zhi, Chen Jian-Bo, Fang Mu-Tong, Liu De-Cun, Zeng Jian-Feng, Ma Wei, Peng Xiao-Hui, Gong Hong-Han, Xu Ren-Gen, and Zhang Hong-Mei

8.1 Introduction

8.1.1 Definition of Pulmonary Tuberculosis

Pulmonary tuberculosis (PTB) is an infectious disease in the lungs that is caused by *Mycobacterium tuberculosis*. The bacteria spread primarily via the respiratory tract directly from the patients excreting the bacteria. The onset of symptoms does not necessarily occur in healthy individuals infected by the bacteria but does occur in infected individuals with compromised immunity.

8.1.2 History of PTB

PTB was one of the major infectious diseases threatening human health, and it has plagued human society for thousands of years. As early as before the third century, scholars of ancient Chinese medicine recognized that the disease is a serious chronic infectious disease. Since the seventeen century, PTB has been prevailing in European countries and remains to be more common in America.

On March 24, 1882, a famous German scientist, Robert Koch, announced in Berlin to the scientific community that *Mycobacterium tuberculosis* had been detected in sputum from patients with PTB. Since then, the pathogen of PTB was defined, which is the first and the most important milestone in the history of TB control. In 1921, A. Calmette and Guerin successfully cultivated attenuated *Mycobacterium tuberculosis*, bacillus Calmette-Guerin (BCG) vaccine, which has been used to prevent against tuberculosis in children. In 1944, S. A. Waksman discovered streptomycin, whose anti-TB effects opened up a new gate for TB treatment. In 1966, scholars from Italy and Switzerland jointly developed a highly effective anti-TB drug, rifampicin, which provided a new way for effective treatment against TB within a short period of time. On the previous achievements, in 1971, W. Fox et al. developed a combined chemotherapy with isoniazid and rifampicin for treatment against TB within a short period of time.

8.1.3 Impact of TB Prevalence on Human Health

Since Koch discovered *Mycobacterium tuberculosis* in 1882, about 200 million cases of death had occurred worldwide from TB. Currently about two billion cases of infection have been reported worldwide, and some eight million new cases of active TB are reported each year. Factors including population growth, HIV/AIDS infection and transmission, population flows, and inappropriate treatment in the public health system and hospitals (especially hospitals specializing in tuberculosis) result in the slow development of TB control. In the 1990s, outbreaks of multidrug-resistant tuberculosis (MDR-TB), especially extensive drug-resistant tuberculosis (XDR-TB), occurred in many regions and countries worldwide, which presented new challenges to TB control. The newly emerging types of TB have constituted major public health problems as well as obstacles to effective TB control across the world. The WHO announced the Global

Deng Qun-Yi (✉) • Pu-Xuan Lu
Department of Radiology, Shenzhen Third People's Hospital Guangdong, Shenzhen, China
e-mail: dengqunyi@hotmail.com; lupuxuan@126.com

Yu Wei-Ye • Li Guo-Bo • Liu Guo-Hui • Liu Zhi
Chen Jian-Bo • Fang Mu-Tong • Liu De-Cun • Zeng Jian-Feng
Ma Wei • Zhang Hong-Mei
The Shenzhen No.3 People's Hospital, Guangdong College, Shenzhen, China

Zhang Wei-Ren
Tuberculosis Prevention and Control of Hospital, Heilongjiang Province, Heilongjiang, China

He Yu-Lin • Gong Hong-Han
The First Affiliated Hospital of Nanchang University, Donghu, Nanchang, Jiangxi, China

Peng Xiao-Hui • Xu Ren-Gen
The Second People's Hospital of Jiangxi Province, Jiangxi Province, Nanchang, China

P.-X. Lu, B.-P. Zhou (eds.), *Diagnostic Imaging of Emerging Infectious Diseases*, DOI 10.1007/978-94-017-7363-8_8

Tuberculosis Emergency in 1993 to call for global initiatives and national commitments to TB control. Meanwhile, March 24 was designated as the World Tuberculosis Day to raise people's awareness of TB prevention and control.

8.2 Etiology

As early as in 1882, a German bacteriologist, Robert Koch (1843–1910), discovered and proved that *Mycobacterium tuberculosis* is the pathogenic bacteria of TB. In 1886, Lehmann and Neumann officially nominated the bacteria as *Mycobacterium tuberculosis* (*M. tuberculosis*). *M. tuberculosis* is categorized into the genus of Mycobacterium, the family of Mycobacteriaceae, and the order of Actinomycetales. *Mycobacterium tuberculosis* complex includes four types: human, bovine, African, and murine. The pathogenic type to human is the most commonly human *M. tuberculosis*, followed by bovine *M. tuberculosis*.

8.2.1 Biological Properties of *M. tuberculosis*

M. tuberculosis is slender and slightly curved, sometimes with branches. Its diameter is about 0.4 μm, and its length 1–4.0 μm, with its both ends slightly blunt. The bacterium cannot move, with no capsule, no flagella, and no spores. *M. tuberculosis* grows slowly and requires high nutrition. *M. tuberculosis* colonies takes at least 2–4 weeks' culture to form. *M. tuberculosis* can be hardly stained. After heated in 5 % carbolfuchsin, it can resist acidic ethanol destaining and thus stained red. Therefore, it is also known as acid-fast bacillus. *M. tuberculosis* has a strong resistance to adverse environment and some physical and chemical factors but is intolerant to heat. It is sensitive to ultraviolet ray. Hence, it is normally disinfected by heat or ultraviolet ray. And its exposure to high-pressure steam (121 °C) for 20 min is the optimal way for sterilization.

8.2.2 Transmission of *M. tuberculosis* and Susceptible Population

As for the spread of *M. tuberculosis*, the main source of infection includes patients with secondary pulmonary tuberculosis whose sputum smear or culture shows positive and untreated TB patients who excrete the bacteria. Droplets of 1–5 μm in diameter are most likely to deposit in the alveoli and droplets from their passionate speaking, coughing, and sneezing can spread the bacteria. More excreted bacteria and longer period for contacts indicate higher likelihood of infection. After sputum of TB patients dries, the bacteria can be carried in dusts, which are likely to be inhaled to cause infection. The susceptible population is mainly individuals with compromised immunity, such as infants, young children, the elderly, patients with HIV infection, users of immunosuppressive agents, patients with chronic disease, and diabetic patients with poor blood glucose control. In addition, individuals living in underdeveloped regions or overworking and malnutrition population are more likely to be infected.

8.2.3 Virulence of *M. tuberculosis*

M. tuberculosis does not contain endotoxin and does not produce exotoxin and invasive enzymes. Its bacterial pathogenicity is mainly related to bacteria composition, toxic metabolites, and immunopathological damage induced by the bacteria. The bacterial components include lipids, proteins, and polysaccharide. In the cell wall of *M. tuberculosis*, there is a large amount of lipid whose content is closely related to its virulence. Cord factor, phospholipid, wax D, and cerebroside-sulfuric acid cerebroside all play an important role in pathomechanism of TB. A variety of proteins contained in *M. tuberculosis* can cause delayed hypersensitivity, which further leads to tissue necrosis and systemic poisoning symptoms. Meanwhile, they participate in the formation of tubercles. Protein and polysaccharide possess antigenicity, which can stimulate the body to produce antibodies, and then immune responses are triggered.

8.2.4 Introduction of Laboratory Tests for the Diagnosis of TB

The etiological examinations for the diagnosis of TB include smear acid-fast staining for microscopy and mycobacterium culture. Mycobacterium culture is referred to as the gold standard for the diagnosis of TB. Due to the slow growth of mycobacterium that splits averagely every 18 h, the traditional way of mycobacterium culture needs a comparatively longer period of time, roughly 1.5 months. The automatic liquid culture system speeds up the cultivation of mycobacterium and renders automatic detection possible. Most of the positive results can be detected in 5–20 days.

Molecular tests for the diagnosis of TB include real-time fluorescence PCR, DNA probe hybridization, and gene chip technology. Cepheid, a company in the USA, recently developed a rapid automatic molecular diagnostic system (GeneXpert). With GeneXpert, it is possible to simultaneously detect *M. tuberculosis* and rifampin-resistant gene mutations within 2 h. The WHO recommended GeneXpert System for the rapid diagnosis of TB.

8.3 Epidemiology

8.3.1 Procedures of Its Prevalence

8.3.1.1 Source of Infection

The main source of infection includes TB patients who excrete bacteria, namely, TB patients with sputum smear or culture positive. TB patients with sputum smear positive are more highly infectious. It has been estimated that a TB patient with sputum smear positive can infect 10–20 individuals per year, while a TB patient with bacteria culture positive can infect 2–4 individuals per year.

8.3.1.2 Route of Transmission

M. tuberculosis spreads mainly via the respiratory tract. When bacteria-positive TB patients cough, sneeze, or talk loudly, droplet with singular *M. tuberculosis* as the core can suspend in the air and then is inhaled by other persons to cause new infection. Its infectivity is different, which is closely related to the amount of excreted bacteria and respiratory symptoms of coughing and sneezing that produce a large quantity of droplets. *M. tuber*culosis excreted by TB patients dries and is attached to dust to form bacteria carrying dust, which can also be inhaled into the human body to cause infection.

8.3.1.3 Susceptible Population

Individuals who have not been infected by *M. tuberculosis* or have not received BCG vaccines are susceptible population of TB. Since the newborns have not been infected by *M. tuberculosis*, they are also categorized into the susceptible population. Individuals with HIV/AIDS, diabetes, silicosis, neoplasm, and transplanted organ or those in long-term use of immunosuppression or corticosteroids are also vulnerable to tuberculosis. Poverty, poor living conditions, and malnutrition are high-risk factors TB in underdeveloped regions. Genetic factor of host plays an important role in the occurrence and development of TB, and individual differences in susceptibility or resistance to TB are associated with certain genes of host.

8.3.2 Prevalence of TB

According to estimates from the WHO, about one-third of the world's population have latent infection of tuberculosis. In 2012 alone, about 8.6 million individuals suffered from tuberculosis, with 1.3 million deaths from TB and 0.53 million pediatric cases. Among the diseases caused by single infectious pathogen, PTB is the second top killer in the world after HIV/AIDS. Asia has witnessed the most new cases of tuberculosis, accounting for 60 % of global new cases. However, in terms of population, the proportion of new cases in sub-Saharan Africa is the largest, with more than 255 new cases of TB per 100,000 individuals. According to data released by the WHO, the global incidence rate of TB declines slowly, which may be related to the increase of flowing population, the increase of HIV/AIDS patients, and the prevalence of MDR-TB. It has been estimated by the WHO that patients with multidrug-resistant TB account for 3.4 % of the total number of TB patients. In individual countries, patients with MDR-TB account for about 20 % of the total TB patients. China, following India, ranks the second in the world in terms of the total number of active tuberculosis patients. China is one of the 22 countries with high TB burden, and China is also one of the 27 countries with high prevalence of MDR-TB.

8.4 Pathogenesis and Pathological Changes

8.4.1 Pathogenesis and Basic Pathological Changes of TB

The pathogenic bacterium of TB is *M. tuberculosis*, and its main pathogenic types include the human type and the bovine type. The human-type *M. tuberculosis* is the most likely to cause TB, and the respiratory tract is the most common and most important way for its transmission. *M. tuberculosis* does not produce toxins, and its pathogenicity is related to bacteria composition, mainly including lipids, proteins, and polysaccharides.

Lipid: Cord factor of glycolipid derivatives can lead to granuloma formation. Wax D can enhance the antigenicity of bacterial protein to trigger strong allergic reactions and result in caseous necrosis and systemic poisoning symptoms. Phospholipids can transform macrophages in inflammatory lesion into epithelial cells, which is the main component of tubercles. In addition, lipids can protect the bacteria from being digested by macrophages and prolong the surviving time of bacteria in the macrophages.

Protein: Protein is antigenic, whose binding to wax D can cause allergic reactions, thus resulting in tissue necrosis and systemic poisoning symptoms. In addition, it contributes to the formation of tubercles.

Polysaccharide: Polysaccharides can cause local neutrophilic infiltration and participate in the immune response as a hapten.

The immune responses of tuberculosis are primarily cellular immune responses. Macrophages in alveolar constitute the first line of defense to inhibit *M. tuberculosis* and the main effector cells responsible for immune clearance. On the one hand, macrophages can resist infection by directly killing the bacteria, secreting cytokines, and

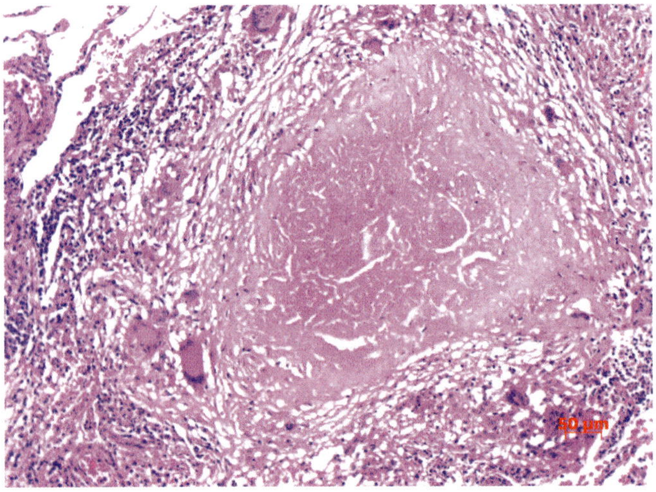

Fig. 8.1 Pulmonary tuberculosis. The lung tissues were demonstrated with observable tubercles, containing caseous necrosis. Necrosis was shown to be surrounded by epithelioid cells, inflammatory exudates, and lung tissue. H&E staining

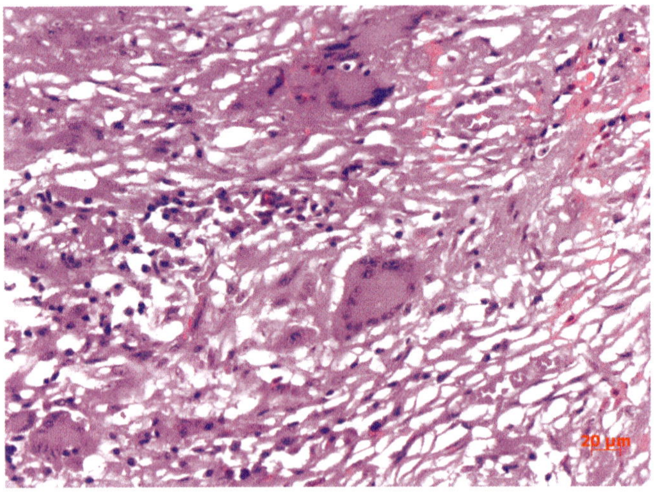

Fig. 8.2 Epithelioid cells and Langerhans giant cells in tubercle, H&E staining

presenting antigen to T cells. On the other hand, the bacteria can also affect the macrophages through a series of mechanism to avoid being killed by the macrophages. The bacteria can survive in macrophages for a long time after infecting human body.

The basic pathological changes of TB include:

1. *Exudate-based lesion*

   The lesion occurs at early stage of tuberculous inflammation or in patients with compromised immunity, large amount of infected bacteria with strong virulence, or strong allergic reactions. The lesion is mainly characterized by serous inflammation or serous fibrinous inflammation. Early local lesion is infiltrated with neutrophils, which are soon replaced by macrophages. *M. tuberculosis* can be

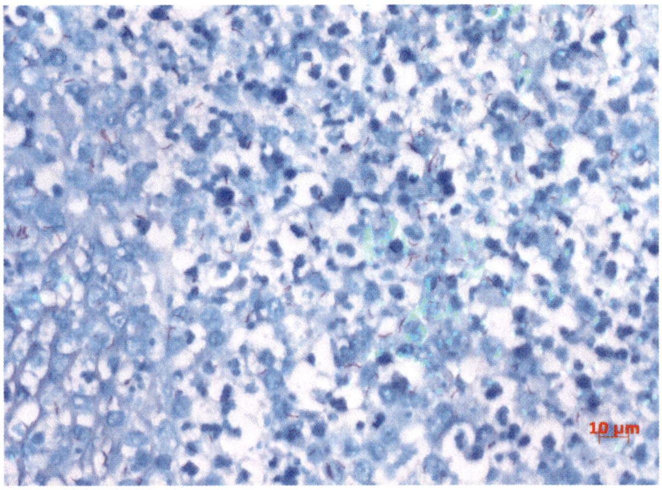

Fig. 8.3 Acid-fast bacilli. The bacilli were shown as red short rods, Acid-fast staining

   detected in exudates and macrophages in the local lesion. The exudates can be completely absorbed or transformed into hyperplasia- or necrosis-based lesion.

2. *Hyperplasia-based lesion*

   In cases with small amount of infected bacteria and weak virulence or strong immune responses, the lesion is mainly hyperplasia based, which develops into diagnostically significant tubercle. Tubercle is composed of epithelioid cells, Langerhans giant cells, peripheral lymphocytes, and reactively hyperplasic fibroblasts (Figs. 8.1, 8.2, and 8.3). Typical tubercle has central caseous necrosis as well as peripheral epithelioid cells and Langerhans giant cells.

3. *Necrosis-based lesion*

   In cases with large amount of infected bacteria, strong virulence, and compromised immunity or strong allergic reactions, the abovementioned exudate- or hyperplasia-based lesion may develop into caseous necrosis. Microscopy demonstrates unstructured and red-stained particles, which are of certain significance for the diagnosis of TB. In most cases, caseous necrotic tissues contain a certain amount of *M. tuberculosis*, constituting the source of bacterial dissemination in the body. The caseous necrosis can also be dissolved and spread, leading to deterioration and progression of TB.

The above three types of lesions commonly coexist or with one type as the main lesion. Under certain conditions, the three types of lesions are interchangeable.

8.4.2 Pathological Features of Tuberculosis

Tuberculosis is a chronic granulomatous disease caused by *M. tuberculosis*. It can affect all body organs, but pulmonary tuberculosis is the most common. Due to different responses in the human body between primary infection and reinfection of *M. tuberculosis* cause, the pulmonary lesions are different. And pulmonary TB can be categorized into primary and secondary pulmonary TB.

8.4.2.1 Primary Pulmonary Tuberculosis

Primary tuberculosis is characterized by the occurrence of primary complex. After *M. tuberculosis* is inhaled into the lungs, grayish white inflammatory solid lesion about 1 cm in diameter firstly forms in the vicinity of the pleura of the lower part of the upper lung lobe or the upper part of the lower lung lobe with good ventilation. Caseous necrosis can be found at the center of most primary lesions, surrounded by exudates, which is more common in the right lung. The bacteria then rapidly invade lymphatic vessels to be disseminated to the hilar lymph nodes along with lymph flow. Consequently, tuberculous lymphangitis and lymphadenitis occur, manifested as enlarged hilar lymph nodes and caseous necrosis. Primary lung lesions, tuberculous lymphangitis, and hilar lymph node tuberculosis are collectively known as the primary complex, which is the most common in pediatric cases of pulmonary TB. Under the condition of malnutrition or compromised immunity, the lesions expand, with caseous necrosis and cavity. In some cases, the lesions even disseminate in the lungs to cause miliary TB. Otherwise, the lesions may even disseminate in the whole body to cause systemic miliary TB.

8.4.2.2 Secondary Pulmonary Tuberculosis

Secondary pulmonary tuberculosis is caused by reactivated *M. tuberculosis* after primary infection. It is rarely exogenous reinfection. Various morphologies of TB lesions coexist in patients with secondary pulmonary tuberculosis. According to pathological feature and clinical course, the lesions of secondary pulmonary TB can be classified into the following five types:

1. *Focal tuberculosis*

   The lesion is about 0.2–1.0 cm in diameter, which is hyperplasia based with a small quantity of central caseous necrosis.
2. *Infiltrative tuberculosis*

   Infiltrative lesions are mostly developed from focal lesions. The common early lesions are demonstrated with mixed pathological changes of different degrees of inflammatory infiltration and fibrous nodules. The lesion is exudate based, with central caseous necrosis that is surrounded by inflammatory tissue.
3. *Chronic fibrocavitary tuberculosis*

   Chronic fibrotic cavity type is pathologically characterized by singular or multiple chronic cavities with relatively thick fibrous capsules in the lungs. The cavities are surrounded by significant fiber changes and scattered new and old lesions. The cavity wall can be divided into three layers. The inner layer is caseous necrosis, containing a large quantity of *M. tuberculosis*. The middle layer is tuberculous granulation tissue, and the outer layer is fibrous connective tissue.
4. *Caseous pneumonia*

   The caseous lesion-based infiltrative TB is known as caseous pneumonia. Microscopy mainly demonstrates large flakes of caseous necrosis. The alveolar cavity is demonstrated with serous fluid and fibrinous exudates with macrophage-based inflammatory cells.
5. *Tuberculoma*

   When large flake of caseous necrosis is surrounded by fibrous tissue or blocked by cavity, it is subjected to shrinkage. Those with a diameter of less than 2 cm are fibrous caseous lesions, and those with a diameter of above 2 cm are known as tuberculoma (Fig. 8.4).

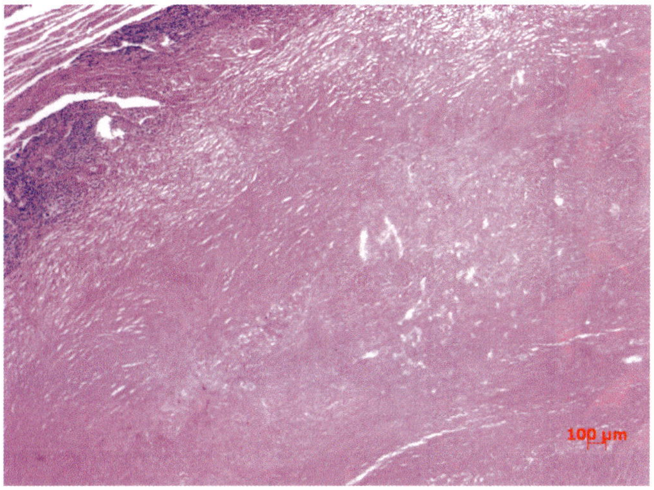

Fig. 8.4 Tuberculoma. Large flake of caseous necrosis was shown to be surrounded by fibrous tissue, H&E staining

8.5 Classification of TB and Their Clinical Diagnosis

According to the new classifying criteria of tuberculosis implemented in China in 2004, tuberculosis can be classified as follows:

1. *Primary pulmonary tuberculosis* including primary complex and intrathoracic lymphoid tuberculosis

   Primary pulmonary TB is common in children and young adults. Clinical manifestations include irregular low-grade fever, anorexia, night sweats, and other tuberculosis poisoning symptoms. In some cases, the patients may experience acute onset and high fever. And some patients may show symptoms of cervical lymphadenectasis. Chest X-ray rarely displays typical dumbbell-like and bipolar shape signs. But CT is superior to chest X-ray in the diagnosis of pulmonary TB.

2. *Hematogenous disseminated pulmonary tuberculosis* including acute, subacute, and chronic hematogenous disseminated pulmonary TB

   M. tuberculosis spreads along with the blood flow to the lungs. The clinical manifestations include obvious tuberculosis poisoning symptoms such as chills, high fever, night sweats, and accompanying respiratory symptoms such as cough, expectoration, and shortness of breath. By physical examination, pulmonary rales are relatively less and hepatosplenomegaly is common. By chest X-ray, acute hematogenous disseminated pulmonary TB is displayed as typical miliary opacities, with even density, size, and distribution. Some patients can be detected with tubercles on the choroid of ocular fundus.

3. *Secondary pulmonary tuberculosis* including infiltrative pulmonary tuberculosis, cavitary pulmonary tuberculosis, tuberculoma, caseous pneumonia, and *fibrocavitary* tuberculosis

   The clinical manifestations of secondary pulmonary TB are diversified. The patients commonly experience no obvious symptoms at the early stage. Along with progress of the condition, the patients gradually show symptoms of fatigue, weariness, poor appetite, weight loss, low-grade fever, night sweats, and other tuberculosis poisoning symptoms as well as uncurable cough. In some cases, sudden hemoptysis is the first symptom, rarely with signs of pulmonary TB. The patients may experience low breath sounds or local rales and dullness to percussion. Chest X-ray demonstrates multiple patches, nodules, and cord-like opacities, cavity opacity, tuberculoma, and calcification in both lungs. Coexistence of old and new lesions is characteristically pulmonary TB, predominantly at the upper lung lobes. Based on positive result by sputum smear for acid-fast staining or Mycobacterium culture, the diagnosis can be defined.

4. *Tuberculous pleurisy* including dry tuberculous pleurisy, exudative tuberculous pleurisy, and tuberculous empyema

   Many patients experience pleural pain and sometimes accompanying fever, cough, fatigue, and anorexia. Shortness of breath after activities is associated with the quantity of pleural effusion. By physical examination, signs of pleural effusion can be found, and sometimes pleural fricatives can be heard at the early stage. Chest X-rays show typical signs of pleural effusion and accompanying radiological changes of pulmonary TB.

5. *Extrapulmonary tuberculosis* including tracheobronchial tuberculosis, renal tuberculosis, tuberculous meningitis, and tuberculous pericarditis

   Extrapulmonary TB can be classified into various types and thus is nonspecific. Extrapulmonary TB is commonly concurrent to intrapulmonary TB. Tuberculosis at different body parts has its own features whose definitive diagnosis should be based on bacteriologic and pathologic evidence.

8.6 Diagnostic Imaging

8.6.1 Radiological Demonstrations of Pulmonary Tuberculosis

8.6.1.1 Primary Pulmonary Tuberculosis

Primary Pulmonary Tuberculosis including primary complex and intrathoracic lymphoid tuberculosis

Primary Complex by Radiology

1. Primary lesion

   After invasion of *M. tuberculosis* into the lungs, acute exudative inflammation occurs in the bronchioles and alveoli. The lesion is commonly located at the lung margin of posterior segment of upper lung lobe and dorsal segment of lower lung lobe. The primary lesion is mostly singular in size of 0.5–2.0 cm. It may be spot-, nodule-, or patch-like in shape with poorly defined boundary. And its density is centrally high and peripherally low.

2. Lymphangitis

   The pathogenic bacteria in the primary lesion can be disseminated to the lung hilum along with lymph flow. During its course to the lung hilum, it can cause lymphangitis. Radiologically, cord-like and strip-like opacity is demonstrated between the primary lesion and the lung hilum, which is poorly defined.

3. Hilar and mediastinal lymphadenectasis

   Along with lymph flow, the pathogenic bacteria gain their access into the lung hilum and mediastinal lymph nodes to cause inflammation, with manifestation of enlarged lymph nodes at the hilum and mediastinum. Radiologically, pulmonary primary lesion, lymphangitis, hilar, and mediastinal lymphadenectasis are demonstrated, namely, typical dumbbell-shaped lesion of primary complex (Fig. 8.5).

Intrathoracic Lymphoid Tuberculosis by Radiology

Pulmonary TB mainly manifested as enlarged lymph nodes at the hilum and mediastinum is known as intrathoracic lymphoid TB. Hilar lymphadenectasis can be classified into mass type and inflammation type.

Radiological demonstrations of mass-type hilar lymphadenectasis:

1. Location: Mass type of right hilar lymphadenectasis is commonly located at the superior margin of the right hilum in the right hilar angle area around the course of the right inferior pulmonary artery. The mass type of left hilar lymphadenectasis is often located at the superior

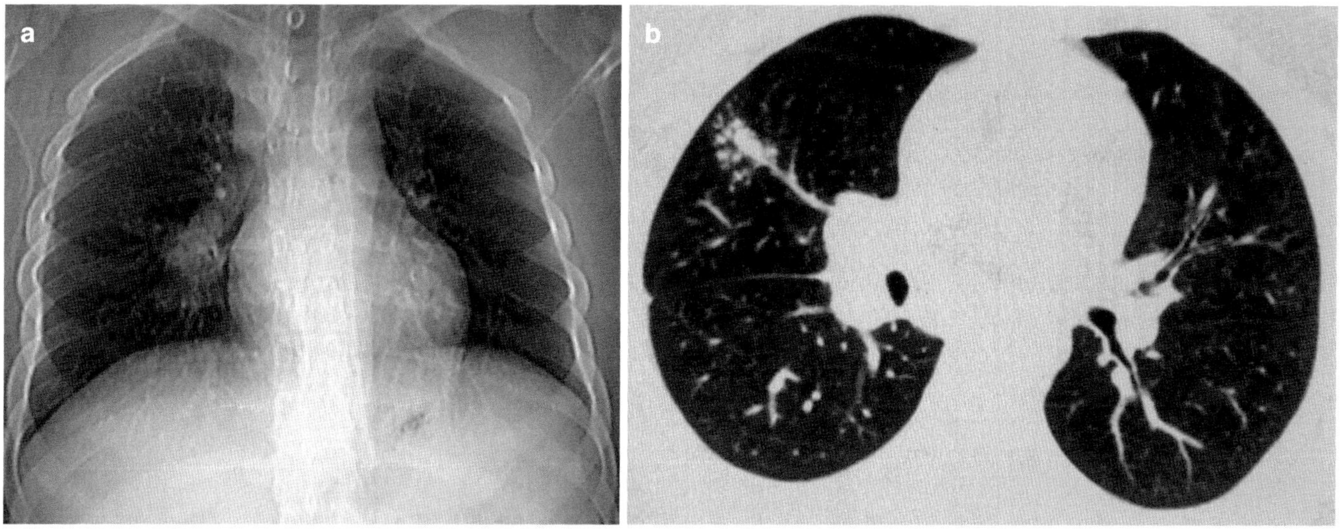

Fig. 8.5 (**a**, **b**) A male patient aged 16 years with primary tuberculosis. (**a**) Plain chest X-ray demonstrated spots of opacity at the margin of lateral zone in the middle right lung field, overlapping with ribs, and nodular opacity at the lower end of the middle bronchial segment adjacent to the right inferior pulmonary artery. (**b**) The lung window by CT scan demonstrated rare spots of opacity at the lateral segment of the middle right lung lobe and fusion of some spots. A cord-like opacity was displayed between the cluster of spots and the right lung hilum. The right lung hilum was shown to be enlarged due to right hilar lymphadenectasis

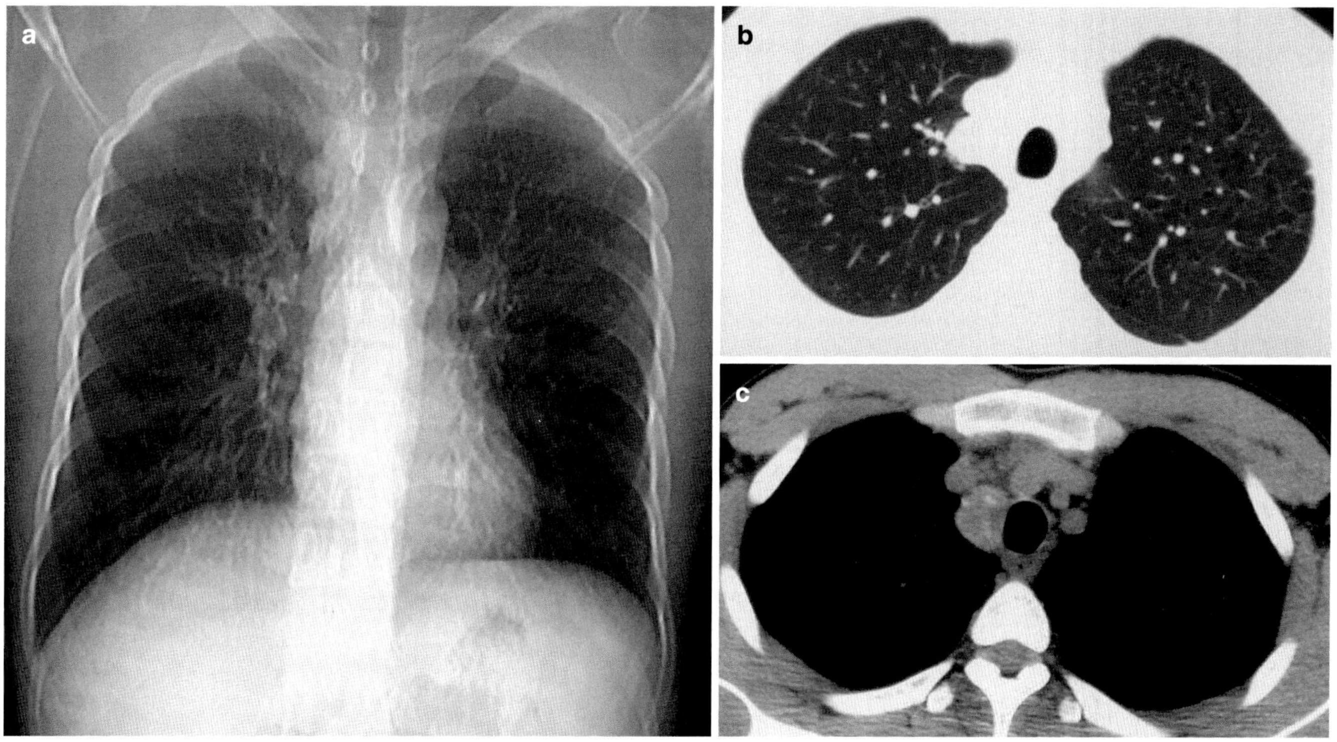

Fig. 8.6 (**a**–**c**) A male patient aged 21 years with intrathoracic lymphoid TB. (**a**) Plain chest X-ray demonstrated nodular opacity at the margin of right upper mediastinum. And the nodular opacity was semiarch in shape protruding to the lung field. (**b**) The lung window by CT scan displayed a nodular opacity beside the bronchus of the right upper mediastinum. The nodular opacity was arch shaped, protruding to the lung field. (**c**) The mediastinal window showed nodular opacity beside the right trachea, with spots of calcifications within and at the margin of the nodular opacity

and lateral margin of left pulmonary artery arch around the course of the left inferior pulmonary artery. The mass type of right hilar lymphadenectasis is more common.

2. Morphology: The totally exposed lymph nodes are nodular, round, or oval in shape, with intact and well-defined boundary. The partially exposed lymph nodes, due to overlapping partly with the vascular vessels in the hilar area, are semiarch-like protruding to the lung field (Fig. 8.6).
3. Density: The density may be either even or uneven. When caseous necrosis or liquefaction occurs in the lymph

nodes, the density of the lesion is uneven. And sometimes calcification can be demonstrated. Enhanced scans show circular enhancement. When several lymph nodes are integrated into a lager mass, it shows separated enhancement. Obvious contrast can be demonstrated between enlarged lymph nodes and adjacent vascular vessels in the hilar area.

Radiological Demonstrations of Inflammation-Type Hilar Lymphadenectasis

1. Due to caseous necrosis and capsular rupture of some lymph nodes, some lymph nodes are demonstrated with coarse unsmooth margin that is poorly defined. Otherwise, exudative inflammation around the lymph nodes causes the lymph nodes to be radiologically poorly defined.
2. The major bronchial lumens in the hilar area are normally unobstructed, with well-defined and smooth inner wall. Occasionally, enlarged lymph nodes invade adjacent bronchi or tuberculosis of adjacent bronchi occurs to cause thickened bronchial wall and narrowed bronchial lumen.

Radiological Demonstrations of Mediastinal Lymphadenectasis

Mediastinal lymphadenectasis induced by tuberculosis is often located beside the trachea and in the tracheobronchial area, which is more common in the right lung. In most cases, several or several groups of lymph nodes are enlarged, with various sizes. The enlarged lymph nodes in the same group may be integrated, showing radiological sign of large mass opacity (Fig. 8.7).

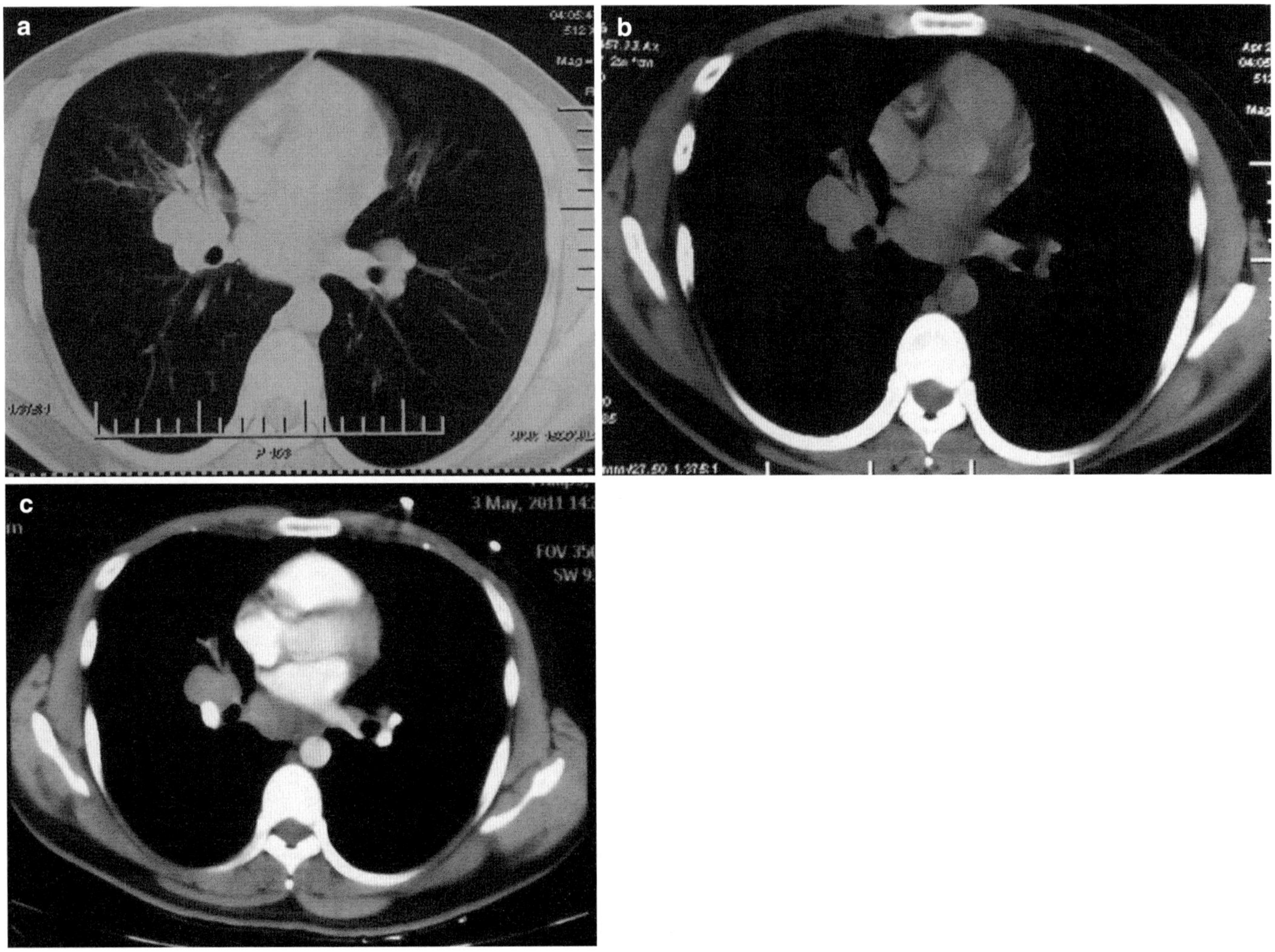

Fig. 8.7 (**a**–**c**) A male patient aged 16 years with intrathoracic lymphoid TB. (**a**, **b**) The lung and mediastinum windows by CT scan demonstrated nodular lesions of enlarged lymph nodes at the right lower hilum and posterior mediastinum and obstructive pneumonia in the right middle lung lobe. (**c**) Contrast CT scans demonstrated consistently homogeneous enhancement of hilar major vascular vessels and thoracic aorta, which had obvious contrast to the adjacent nodular lymph nodes

8.6.1.2 Hematogenous Disseminated Pulmonary Tuberculosis

Acute Hematogenous Disseminated TB by Radiology

1. Pulmonary interstitial miliary nodule

   It is manifested as diffusively distributed miliary nodules in the interstitium of both lungs, which are about 1–3 mm in diameter. Their density, size, and distribution are even, mostly are well defined.
2. Ground-glass opacity

   It is manifested as focalized ground-glass opacity formed by integrated miliary nodules. The opacity has low density and is poorly defined.
3. Interlobular septal thickening and intralobular reticular opacity

   They are radiological signs induced by alveolar septal congestion and edema at the acute stage, commonly coexisting with ground-glass opacity. For most patients, they can subside after treatment.
4. Clustered thin-walled cystic cavity opacity

   In rare patients, it appears at the progressive stage and is reversible.
5. Lobular central branch opacity and tree-bud sign

   After delayed or inappropriate treatment, acute hematogenous disseminated TB progresses. The caseous substances formed in TB lesions involve alveolar cavities and spread through the bronchi. Therefore, randomly distributed nodules in both lungs and focally distributed lobular central branch opacity and tree-bud sign are radiologically displayed, which can be well or poorly defined (Fig. 8.8).

Subacute and Chronic Hematogenous Disseminated Tuberculosis by Radiology

1. The lesions are commonly located at the upper and middle parts of unilateral or bilateral lung fields.
2. Exudative, hyperplastic, and even caseous lesions can coexist in upper lung field, manifesting as small nodular,

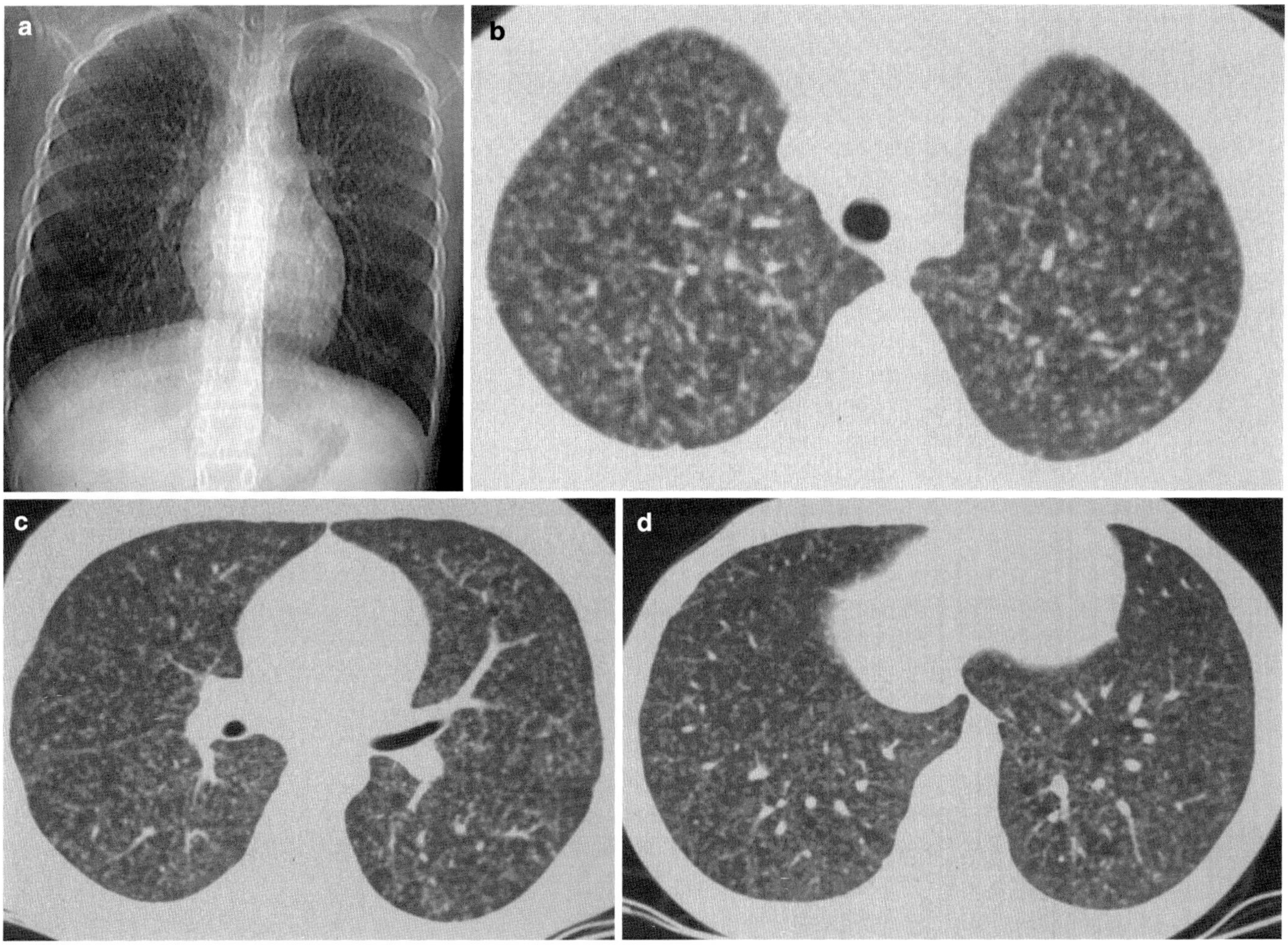

Fig. 8.8 (**a–d**) A female patient aged 14 years with acute hematogenous disseminated TB. (**a**) Plain chest X-ray demonstrated diffusively distributed miliary opacities in the upper, middle, and lower fields of both lungs. The miliary opacities were shown with the same size, even density, and even distribution. (**b–d**) The lung window by CT scan displayed diffusively distributed miliary opacities in the upper, middle, and lower fields of both lungs. The miliary opacities were shown with the same size, even density, and even distribution

patchy and mass opacities. In the middle lung field, the lesions are predominantly demonstrated as small nodular and miliary opacities. Therefore, the condition is manifested as long illness course of the lesions in the upper lung field and comparatively new lesions in the middle lung field (Fig. 8.9).

3. Compensatory emphysema can be displayed between the lesions or in the lower part of the affected lung.

8.6.1.3 Secondary Pulmonary Tuberculosis

Secondary pulmonary TB refers to pulmonary TB occurring at any time after primary pulmonary TB, mainly including infiltrative pulmonary TB, tuberculous lobar pneumonia and caseous pneumonia, tuberculoma, and chronic *fibrocavitary* TB. Secondary pulmonary TB is one of the main types of pulmonary TB and is the most common type of pulmonary TB.

Infiltrative Pulmonary TB by Radiology

In cases of secondary pulmonary TB, the signs of primary pulmonary TB can sometimes be observed. The calcifications within the intrapulmonary primary lesions are demonstrated to be spotlike or nodular, with high density. Old peripheral inflammation around the lesions is common, with high central density and blurry boundary in shapes of patches and small flakes (Fig. 8.10).

Secondary pulmonary TB:

1. The lesions of secondary pulmonary TB are commonly located at the apical posterior segment of the upper lung lobe and the dorsal segment of the lower lung lobe.
2. In overwhelming majority of the cases, the lesions are multiple. The lesions may be demonstrated within one lung lobe or one lung segment or within unilateral or bilateral lung fields.

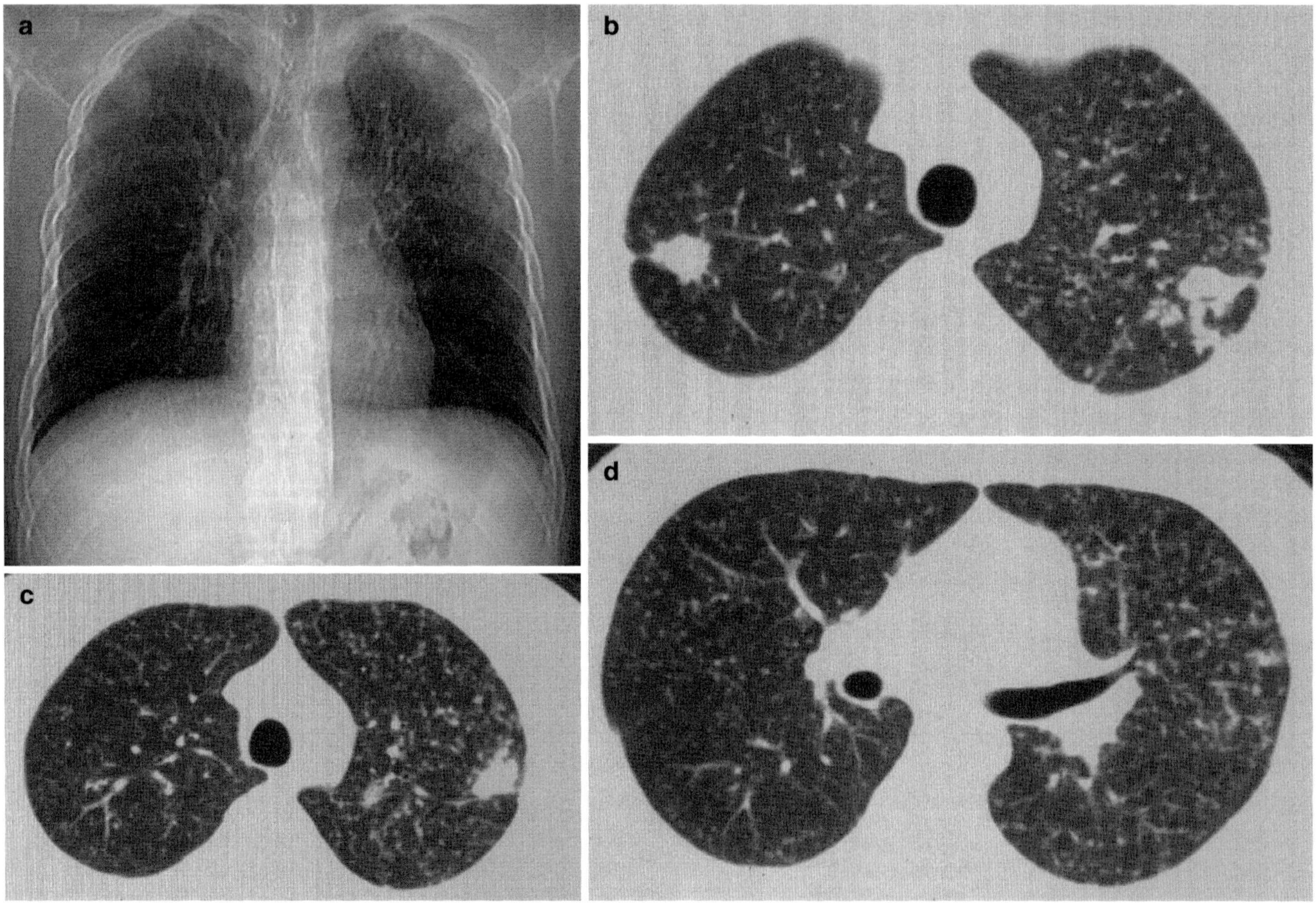

Fig. 8.9 (**a–d**) A male patient aged 24 years with subacute hematogenous disseminated TB. (**a**) Plain chest X-ray demonstrated patches of opacity with poorly defined boundary in the right upper lung field and lateral zone of left upper and middle lung fields. Small spots of and miliary opacities were displayed to be diffusively distributed in the upper and middle fields of both lungs, with poorly defined boundaries. (**b–d**) The lung window by CT scan demonstrated patches of opacity in the apical segment of the right upper lung lobe and lateral zone of apical posterior segment of the left upper lung lobe. The patches of opacity were accompanied by diffuse miliary opacities in both lungs, with uneven distribution

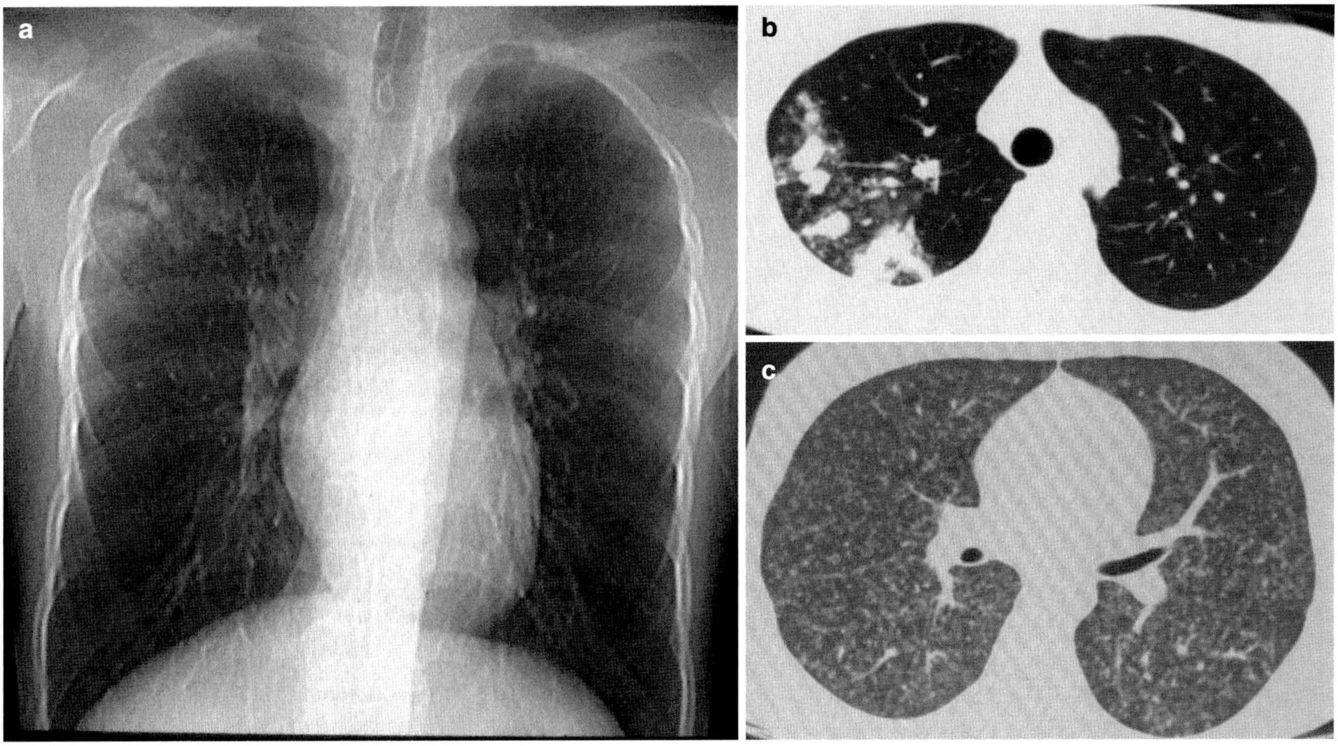

Fig. 8.10 (**a–c**) A male patient aged 20 years with secondary pulmonary TB (specifically infiltrative pulmonary TB). (**a**) Plain chest X-ray demonstrated spots and small nodular and patches of opacity at the right upper lung field and interface of right upper and middle lung fields. Most of the opacities were poorly defined. (**b**, **c**) The lung and mediastinum windows by CT scan displayed spots and small nodular and patches of opacity at the right upper lung lobe. Most of the small nodular opacities were well defined. Calcifications were observable at the apical segment of right upper lung lobe

3. Exudative lesions are radiologically demonstrated as cloud-like opacity with spots, small flakes, or flakes of homogeneous or heterogeneous high-density shadows.
4. Hyperplastic lesions are radiologically demonstrated as spots and small nodular or patchy mass-like opacity with relatively high density.
5. Caseous dissolution occurs within the lesions to cause formation of semitransparent areas with low density or cavities. Radiologically, they are light-transparent areas with different sizes and shapes. Around the cavities, spots and small nodular opacity are demonstrated, which are known as satellite lesions (Fig. 8.11).
6. Calcified lesions are radiologically demonstrated as spots and small nodular or linear opacity with high density.
7. Fibrous lesions are radiologically demonstrated as cord-like or stellate-shaped opacity, with relatively high density and rough margins.
8. Within a short period of time, progression and absorption of the lesions are slower than the lesion of lobar pneumonia and lobular pneumonia.
9. The lesions of secondary pulmonary TB may be accompanied by pleural effusion.
10. Secondary pulmonary TB may be complicated by hematogenous disseminated pulmonary TB. In addition to the infiltrative lesions in lung fields, the lesions of acute or chronic hematogenous disseminated pulmonary TB can be detected.

In cases of infiltrative pulmonary TB, two or more types of basic lesions such as exudation, proliferation, caseation, cavity, calcification, and fibrosis may be detected within the lungs of one patient. Radiologically, it is demonstrated with multiple lesions of different densities and various shapes. Especially, the apical posterior segment of both upper lung lobes is radiologically demonstrated with multiple lesions of various shapes and different densities. These signs are typical radiological signs of infiltrative pulmonary TB.

Tuberculous Lobar and Caseous Pneumonia by Radiology

Tuberculous Lobar Pneumonia by Radiology

Tuberculous lobar pneumonia is one of the uncommon types of secondary pulmonary TB. It is also known as bronchopneumonic TB:

1. The lesions are commonly located at the apical posterior segment of the upper lung lobe.

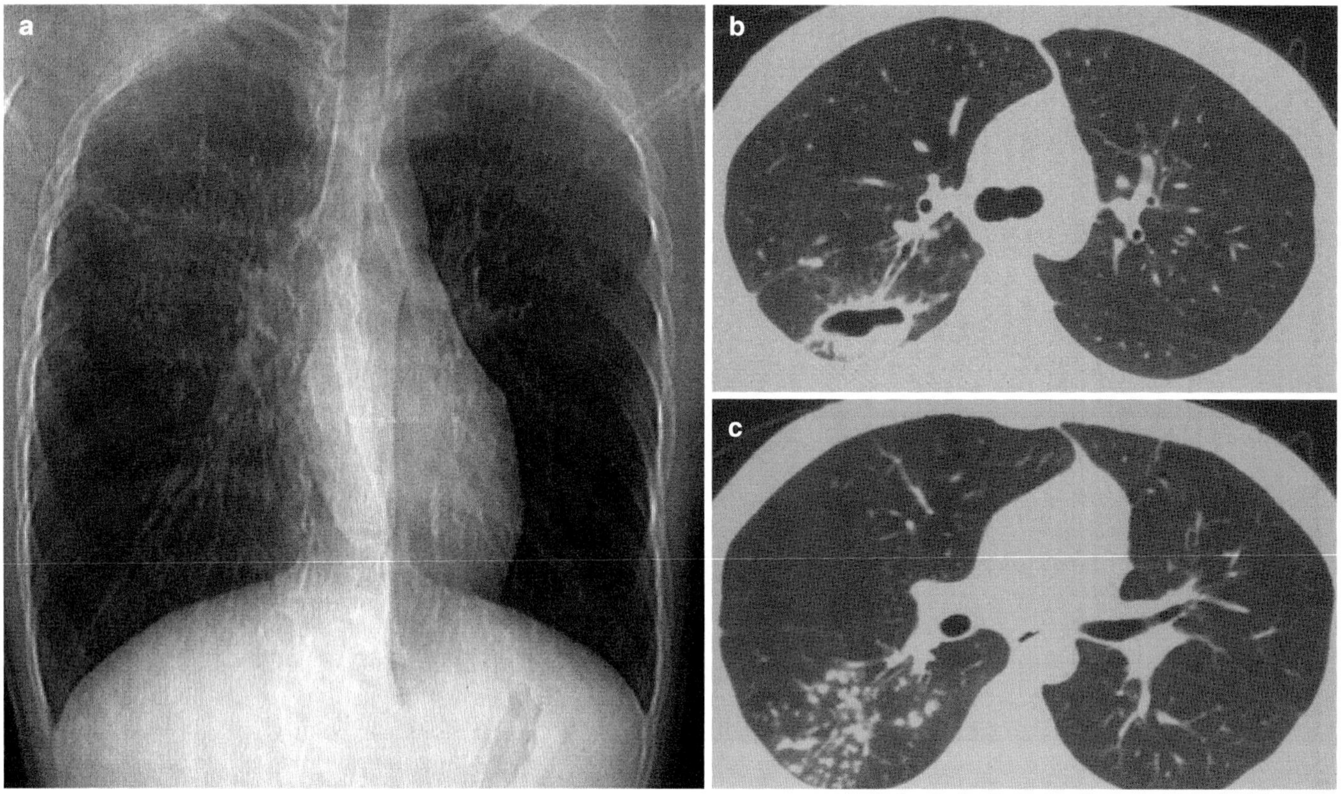

Fig. 8.11 (**a–c**) A male patient aged 25 years with secondary pulmonary TB (specifically cavitary pulmonary TB). (**a**) Plain chest X-ray demonstrated a thin-walled transparent area at the middle zone of right upper lung field, and its inferior wall overlapped with spots and small patches of opacities at the right middle lung field. (**b**, **c**) The lung window by CT displayed a transparent area at the posterior segment of right upper lung lobe. Between the transparent area and the lung hilum, there were dual tracks of draining bronchi. Around the transparent area, spots of satellite lesions were shown. Spots of bronchial disseminated lesions were detected at the right lower lung lobe

2. The lesion is radiologically shown as large flake of opacity, occupying one lung segment, one lung lobe, or even unilateral lung field. At its central area, a large area of consolidation can be found, with poorly defined boundary. Air bronchogram sign is displayed in the large flake of consolidation.
3. In the cloudy opacity, spots and small nodular lesions with high density are displayed. Radiologically, it is displayed as a large flake of lesion surrounded by small lesions. These small lesions scatter with uneven distribution. These radiological signs facilitate the differential diagnosis from lobar pneumonia. Its mechanism involves exudative and proliferative pathological changes of the lesions in the lungs induced by *M. tuberculosis* infection.
4. Within the large flake of consolidation opacity or at its margin, small low-density semitransparent areas or small transparent areas can be detected. These small areas indicate small caseous necrosis or small dissolution and liquefaction of the lesions.
5. Scattering polymorphic spots and small nodular or patches of TB lesions in isolateral or contralateral lung field of the lesions facilitate the diagnosis (Fig. 8.12).

Caseous Pneumonia by Radiology

Caseous pneumonia is one of the most serious types of secondary pulmonary TB. Its pathogenesis involves invasion of the lungs by large quantities of *M. tuberculosis* via the bronchi within a short period of time. Due to compromised immunity, the hosts who are hypersensitive to the antigen of *M. tuberculosis* show rapidly deterioration and progression of the condition into lobar or lobular caseous pneumonia. In some cases, caseous pneumonia is resulted from caseous necrosis of exudative lesions of tuberculous lobar pneumonia (Fig. 8.13):

1. Lobar caseous pneumonia is radiologically shown as large flakes of cloud-like opacities that gradually develop into large flake of consolidation with intermediate density. The consolidation is more common at the upper lung lobes and occupies one lung segment, one lung lobe, or even unilateral lung, with poorly defined boundary.
2. The density of lesion is heterogeneous. And the lesion is radiologically demonstrated as large flake of consolidation with extensive multiple semitransparent or transparent

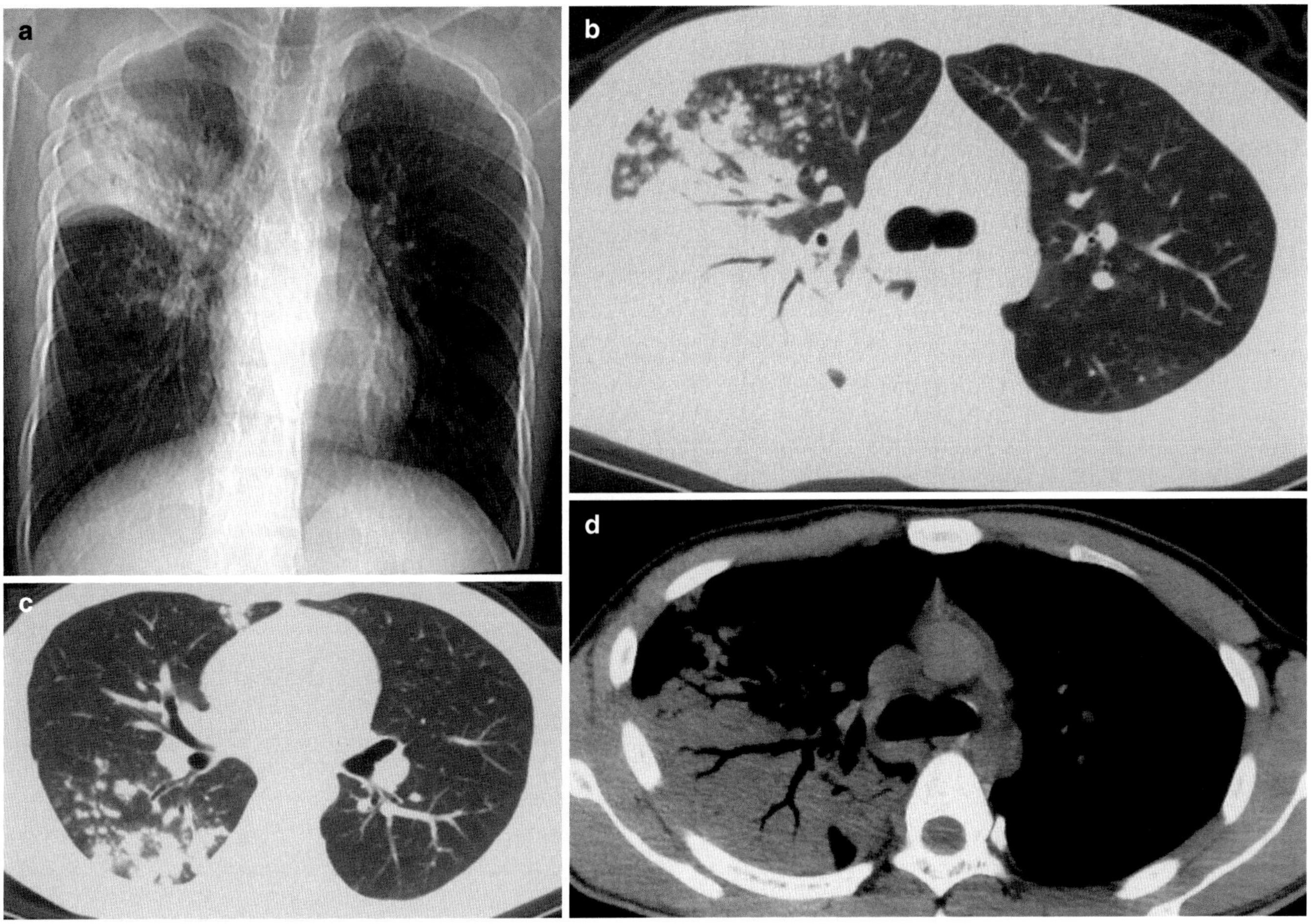

Fig. 8.12 (**a–c**) A male patient aged 36 years with secondary pulmonary TB (specifically tuberculous lobar pneumonia). (**a**) Plain chest X-ray demonstrated large flaky opacity at the right upper lung field, with poorly defined boundary, and spot of opacity at the right middle lung field. (**b**, **c**) The lung window by CT scan displayed large flaky opacity at the right upper lung lobe, with air bronchogram sign inside. The lesion had poorly defined boundary, which was accompanied by small flakes and spots of opacities. Small flakes and spots of opacities were also shown at the middle and lower lobes of the affected lung

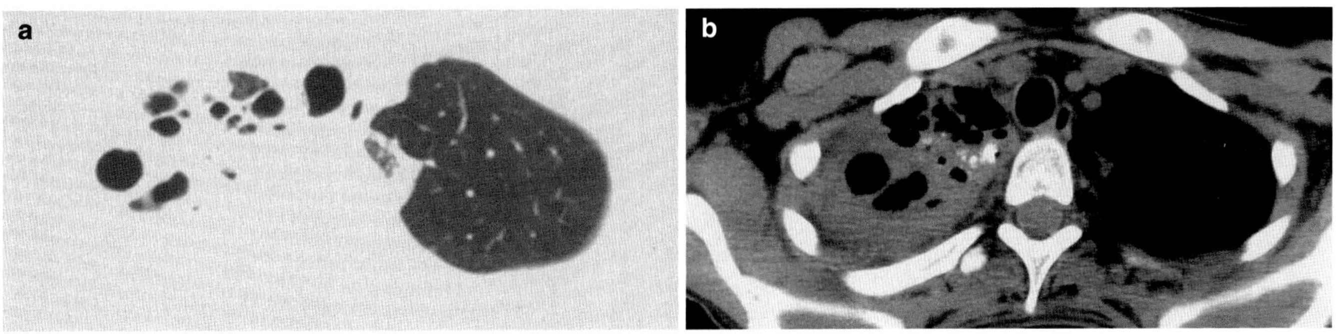

Fig. 8.13 (**a**, **b**) A female patients aged 30 years with secondary pulmonary TB (specifically caseous pneumonia). The lung and mediastinum windows by CT scan displayed large flaky opacity at the right upper lung lobe. Within the lesion, multiple transparent areas were shown with different sizes and irregular shape. The mediastinum window by CT scan demonstrated spots of calcification in the lesion. The left upper lung lobe was demonstrated with cord-like opacity

areas inside. The semitransparent or transparent areas are worm-bitten-like in shape with low density. The shape of cavities is also diversified and irregular, with poorly defined and unsmooth cavity wall.
3. Bronchial disseminated lesions can be detected in isolateral or contralateral lung field.
4. For lobular caseous pneumonia, multiple scattering small flakes and small nodular and spots of opacities are detected in the upper and middle parts of one or both lungs. Within these opacities, caseous necrotic lesions can be detected with different sizes and irregular shape, which are semitransparent or transparent areas with low density.
5. In the middle and advanced stages, extensive or serious damages to lung tissues cause shrinkage of the lung lobe. Meanwhile, the adjacent pleura is thickened.

Pulmonary Tuberculoma by Radiology

Tuberculoma refers to spherical lesion that derives from encapsulated caseous lesion by fibrous tissue (Fig. 8.14):

1. Tuberculoma commonly occurs in the apical posterior segment of the upper lung lobe and the dorsal segment of the lower lung lobe. Its common location is consistent with the lesion of secondary pulmonary TB.
2. The lesion is mostly singular but rarely multiple.
3. The lesion is round or oval in shape. The lesion with a diameter of less than 2 cm is known as fibrous caseous lesion, and the lesion with a diameter of above 2 cm is known as tuberculoma.
4. The lesion of tuberculoma has well-defined and intact boundary.
5. The density of the lesion can be even, possibly with inner dissolved area that is semitransparent. The dissolved area is commonly close to the hilum. Cavity can also be detected.
6. In the lung field near the spherical lesion, scattering proliferative or fibrous lesions are common. The lesions are radiologically demonstrated as spots and small nodular and cord-like opacities, namely, the satellite lesions.
7. Cord-like opacity is detected between the spherical lesion and the hilum, which is actually residual draining bronchus after cavity-derived tuberculoma.
8. Calcification can be detected in or at the margin of the spherical lesion. The typical radiological sign is stratified ring shape calcification opacity or scattering spots of calcifications.
9. By contrast CT, the spherical lesion shows no enhancement or only slight enhancement. Its capsule may be demonstrated with ring-shaped enhancement.

Chronic Fibrocavitary Pulmonary TB by Radiology

Chronic *fibrocavitary* pulmonary TB occurs at the advanced stage of pulmonary TB. During the long-term development of pulmonary TB, deterioration and improvement occur alternatively, which causes serious damage to local or most of the lung tissue. Meanwhile, extensive hyperplasia and repair of fibrous tissues occur around the lesions of pulmonary TB to cause fibrous cavity.

1. The apical posterior segment of the upper lung lobe or the dorsal segment of the lower lung lobe is displayed with fibrous cavities of irregular shape, which are surrounded by extensive cord-like opacity. The lesions often cause

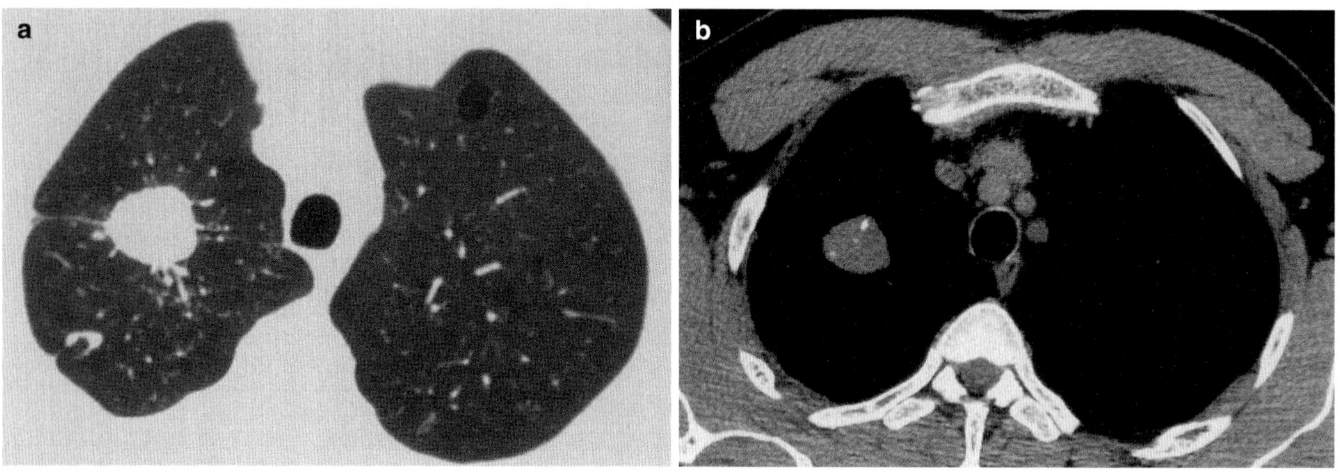

Fig. 8.14 (**a**, **b**) A male patient aged 39 years with secondary pulmonary TB (specifically pulmonary tuberculoma). The lung and mediastinum windows by CT scan demonstrated round-like nodular opacity at the apical segment of the right upper lung lobe, with well-defined and smooth boundary. Meanwhile, several linear opacities in different lengths radiated from the nodular opacity. Around the nodular opacity, there were spots of satellite lesions. And spots of calcifications were displayed in the nodular opacity

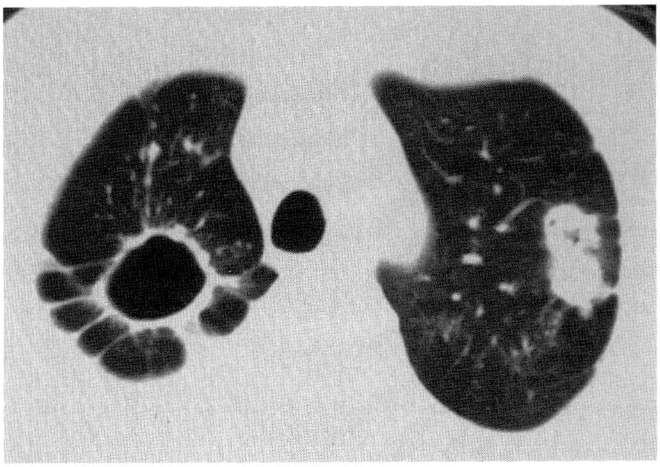

Fig. 8.15 A male patient aged 44 years with secondary pulmonary TB (specifically chronic fibrocavitary TB). The posterior segment of the right upper lung lobe was demonstrated with a transparent area, with smooth and intact inner margin. Its outer margin was displayed with several cord-like opacities that radiated from the outer margin and most of them connected with the adjacent pleura. Around the transparent area, scattering spots of opacities are displayed. The apical posterior segment of the left upper lung lobe was shown with spots and patches of opacities

elevated hilum of the affected lung and willowlike lung markings. Bronchial mediastinum is demonstrated to shift toward the affected lung.

2. The upper and middle lung fields of the isolateral or contralateral lung are demonstrated with old and new TB lesions of different types, including exudative, proliferative, caseous, cavities, fibrous, or calcified lesions with the lungs of one patient. The cavity may be singular with several transparent areas of different sizes and different shapes. The cavity wall is shown with spots or linear calcification.
3. The middle and lower parts of the affected lung and the lung field of the contralateral lung are commonly demonstrated with bronchial disseminated lesions.
4. The unaffected lung fields are displayed with compensatory emphysema. CT scans can detect pulmonary bullae.
5. Due to the shrinkage of the upper lung as well as adhesion and traction of thickened pleura, the upper mediastinum and trachea are obviously displayed with shift toward the affected lung.
6. Secondary bronchiectasis is demonstrated with multiple thin-walled small bubbles, bead-like or honeycomb-like in appearance. Bronchial dual-track sign may also be shown (Fig. 8.15).

8.6.1.4 Tuberculous Pleurisy

Tuberculous Dry Pleurisy

Dry tuberculous pleurisy refers to the type of tuberculous pleurisy with no obvious exudates or with only a small quantity of cellulose exudates. In most cases, it develops into pleural effusion. At the early stage, radiological examination may show no abnormalities due to the small quantity of cellulose exudates on the surface of pleura. When the cellulose exudates accumulate into a certain amount in the pleural cavity and the thickness of pleura reaches 2–3 mm, alternative lung and mediastinum windows by CT scans can more sensitively show pleural thickening or slight pleural protrusion to the lung field due to a small quantity of liquid density area with poorly defined boundary (Fig. 8.16).

Tuberculous Exudative Pleurisy

The fluid of exudative tuberculous pleurisy is commonly serous, mostly in unilateral thoracic cavity. At the early stage, pleural effusion is free, indicating its change along with posture. Therefore, the fluid flows to the lowest part of the pleural cavity. Along with the development of the condition, some patients experience absorption of the fluid after active and appropriate treatment. However, some patients experience delayed or inappropriate treatment or compromised immunity and thus sustain pleural thickening and adhesion due to a large amount of deposited cellulose in the pleural effusion. Pleural thickening and adhesion further cause separated or encapsulated pleural effusion. In some cases, the patients may even experience pleural thickening and calcification in the advanced stage (Fig. 8.17).

8.6.1.5 Tracheal and Bronchial TB

Tracheal and bronchial TB is mainly caused by direct invasion of *M. tuberculosis* in the sputum. Otherwise, it can also be caused by its direct invasion of the lining of airway after the lesion of tuberculous lymphadenitis ruptures or by its dissemination along with lymph flow around the bronchus.

1. Endobronchial TB is demonstrated with thickened bronchial wall and small nodular protrusions from the bronchial inner walls. Otherwise, the wall of segmental bronchus may be displayed to be thickened (Fig. 8.18).
2. In some cases of bronchial stenosis, enlarged lymph nodes in the hilum or the mediastinum directly invade the adjacent bronchus or trachea, causing narrowing, distortion, deformation, or displacement of the lumen (Fig. 8.19).
3. The middle and lower lung fields of unilateral or bilateral lungs may be demonstrated with spots and small patches of bronchial disseminated lesions.
4. In cases of bronchial dilation, the bronchus in the diseased area is displayed with bead-like or honeycomb-like changes. The bronchus is displayed with luminal dilation, thickened wall, and unsmooth inner wall.
5. In cases of focalized pulmonary emphysema, proliferative and caseous lesions in the bronchial wall cause bronchial stenosis. At its distal lung field, segmental or focalized lobar increased transparency is displayed.

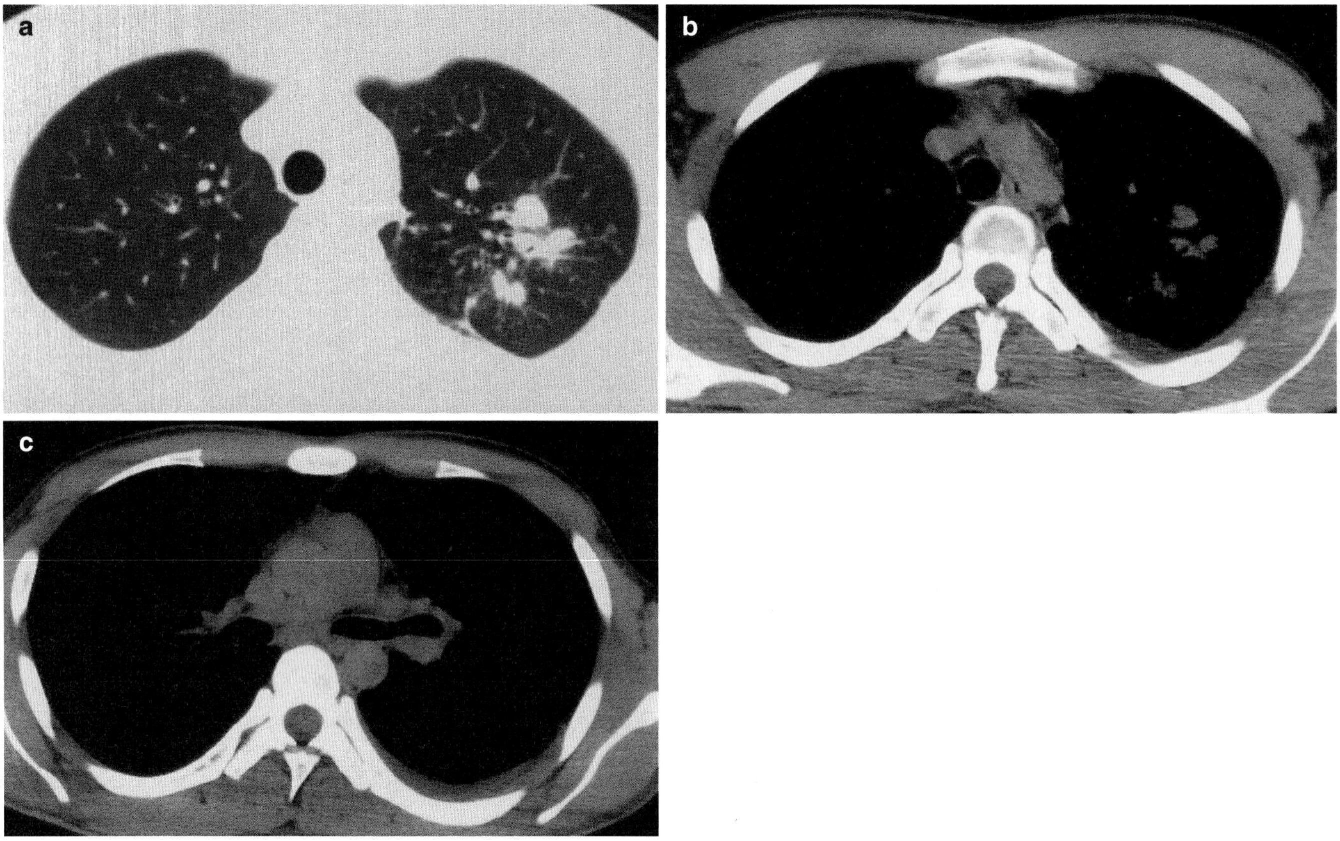

Fig. 8.16 (**a**–**c**) A male patient aged 22 years with tuberculous pleural effusion. The lung and mediastinum windows by CT scan demonstrated spots and patches of opacities at the apical posterior segment of the left upper lung lobe and arch- and crescent-shaped fluid opacity at the dorsal part of left thoracic cavity

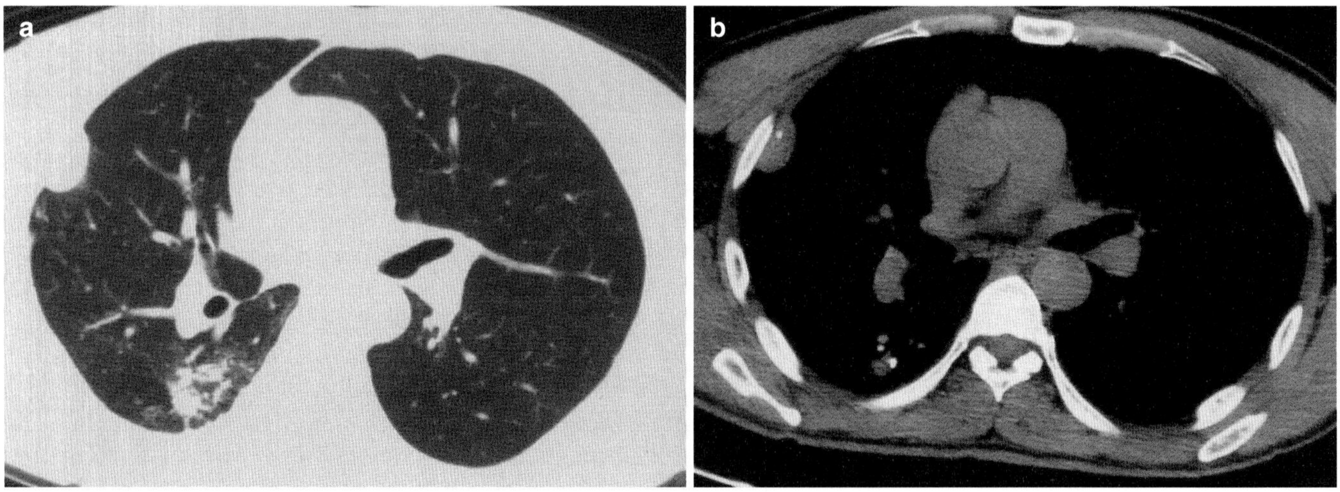

Fig. 8.17 (**a**, **b**) A male patient aged 43 years with pleural TB (specifically tuberculous focal encapsulated pleural thickening and calcification). The lung and mediastinum windows by CT showed patches of opacity at the dorsal segment of the left lower lung lobe and calcification in the lesion. Exteriorly and anteriorly adjacent to the right pleura, a D-shaped soft tissue density opacity was displayed. The pleura was shown with smooth and clearly defined surface, with calcification inside

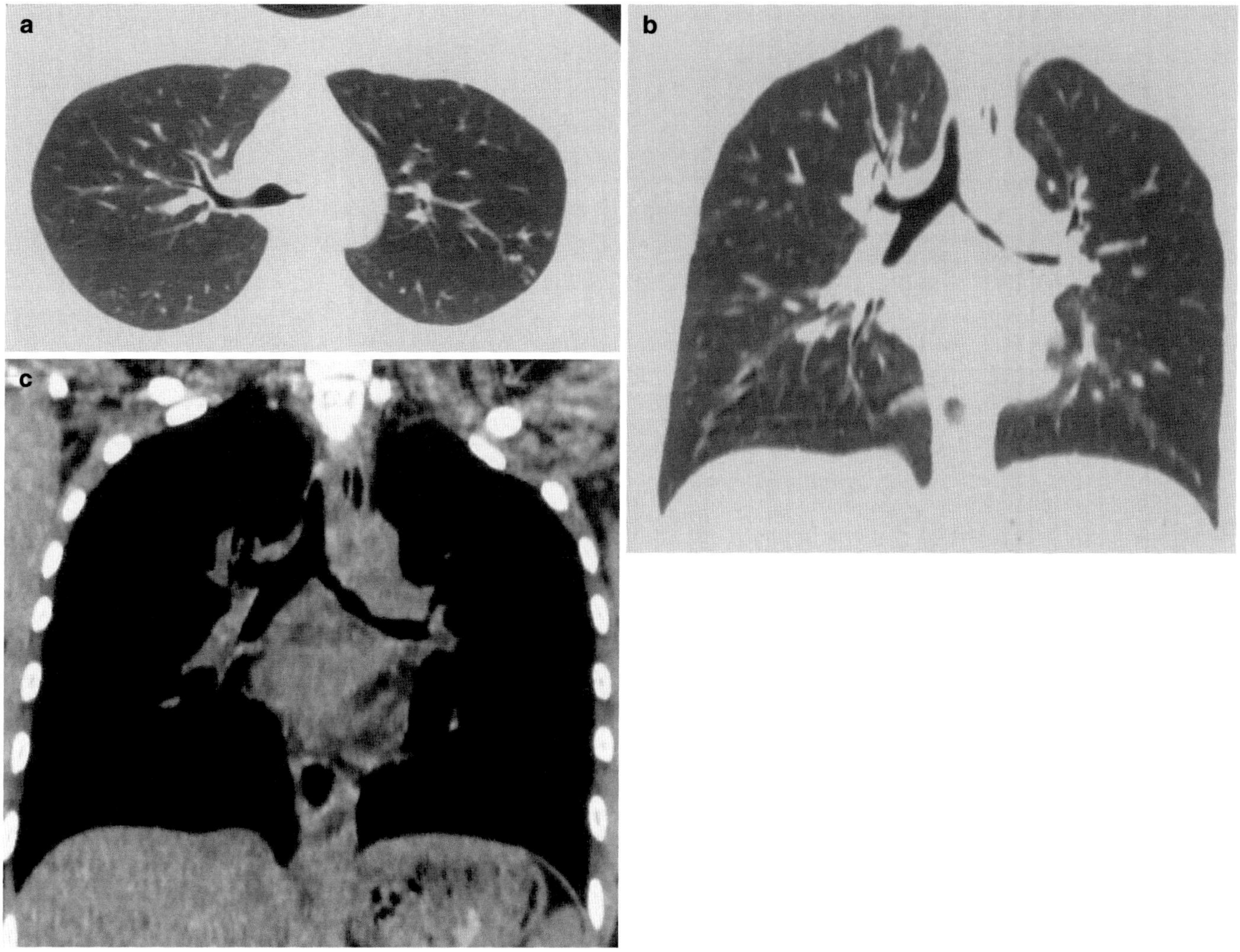

Fig. 8.18 (a–c) A female patient aged 24 years with bronchial TB. The lung and mediastinum windows by CT displayed coronally reconstructed images of the chest. The lateral zone of the apical posterior segment of the left upper lung lobe was shown with scattering spots of opacity. The left major bronchi were commonly narrowed, with thickened bronchial wall

6. Pulmonary segmental or lobar atelectasis causes bronchial stenosis and occlusion, which further develop into decreased segmental or lobar volume but increased density (Fig. 8.20).
7. Calcification of the bronchial wall is radiologically demonstrated as spots and linear calcification.

8.6.1.6 Tuberculous Meningoencephalitis

M. tuberculosis invade the subarachnoid space directly or along with blood flow to cause lesions at the pia mater and arachnoid membrane and further lesions at the brain nerves, parenchyma, blood vessels, and spinal cord. The condition is known as tuberculous meningoencephalitis. MRI is superior to CT in detecting the TB lesions. However, CT is superior to MRI in detecting calcification of intracerebral tuberculous granuloma:

1. Increased density of meninx is radiologically demonstrated as extensively thickened outlines of the cistern and sulcus as well as meninx with increased density. By contrast CT scans, obvious enhancement is displayed (Fig. 8.21).
2. Parenchymal miliary lesions are displayed as fine and uniform density miliary nodular opacities extensively distributing in the cerebral cortex or brain tissue. Contrast CT scans demonstrate enhancement.
3. Ring-shaped, disk-like, mass-like, and spots of opacities are characteristic radiological signs of brain tuberculomas. Contrast scans display ring-shaped enhancement with central low density and peripheral high density.

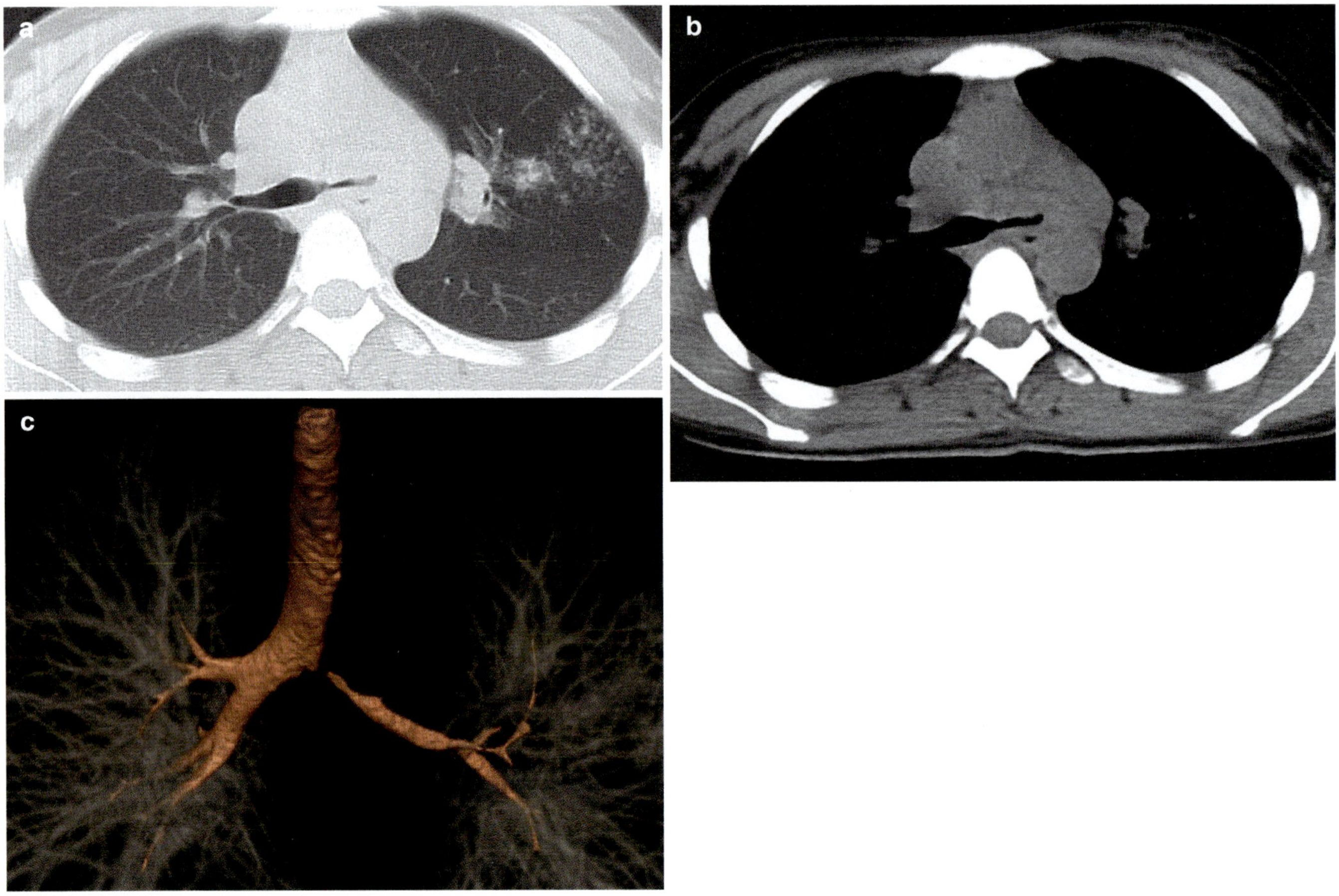

Fig. 8.19 (**a–c**) A female patient aged 25 years with left bronchial TB. (**a**) The left lung was displayed with acinar nodular disseminated lesions. (**b**) The left major bronchi were shown with obviously thickened and rough wall as well as stenosis. (**c**) Three-dimensional reconstruction demonstrated stenosis of the left major bronchi

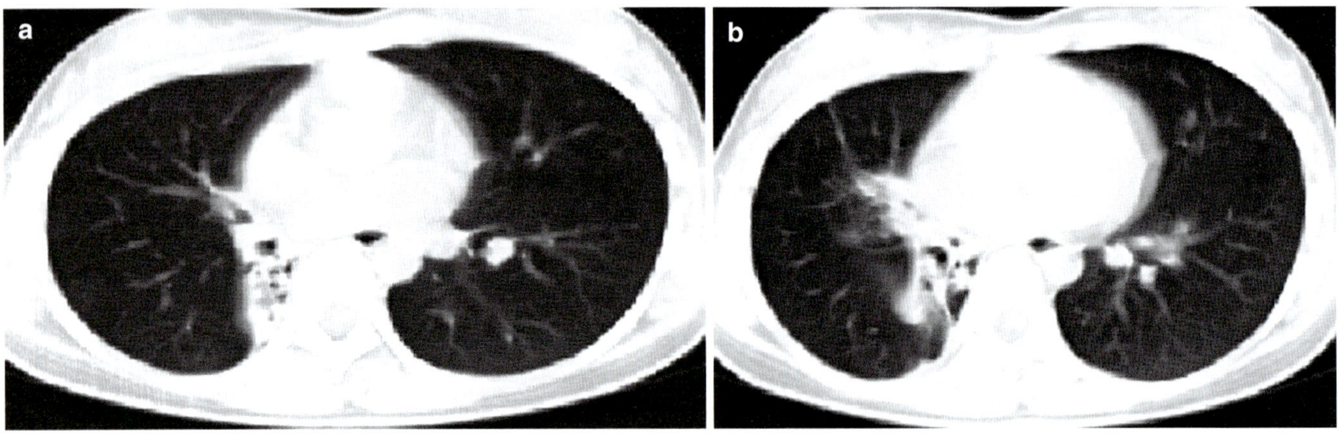

Fig. 8.20 (**a–e**) A female patient aged 35 years with bronchial TB in the right lower and middle lung lobes. (**a–d**) Chest CT showed obvious narrowing of the right major bronchi and patchy and grid-like opacity in the dorsal segment of the right lower lung lobe. (**e**) Three-dimensional reconstruction demonstrated stenosis of the right major bronchi and the bronchi in the right middle lung lobe

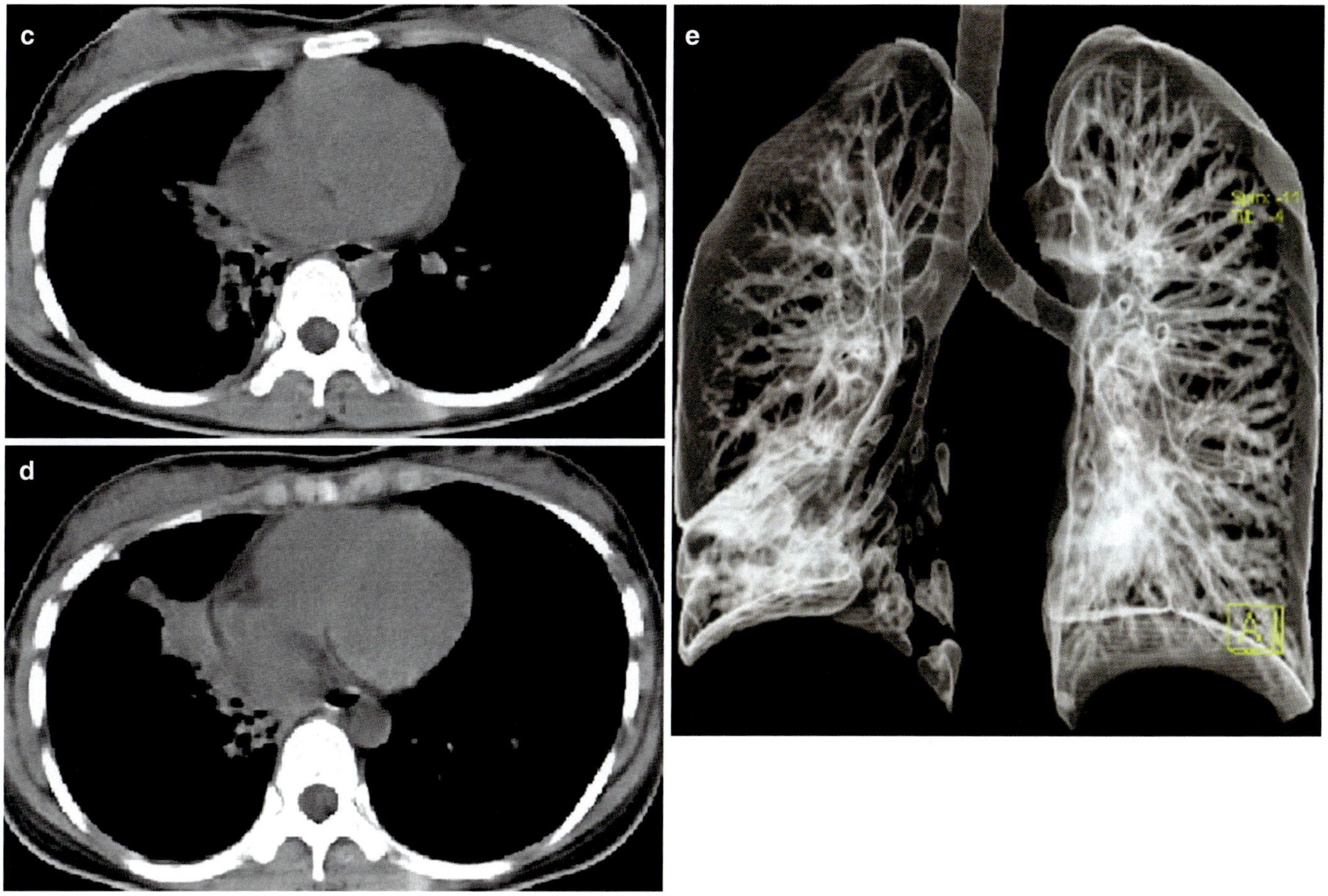

Fig. 8.20 (continued)

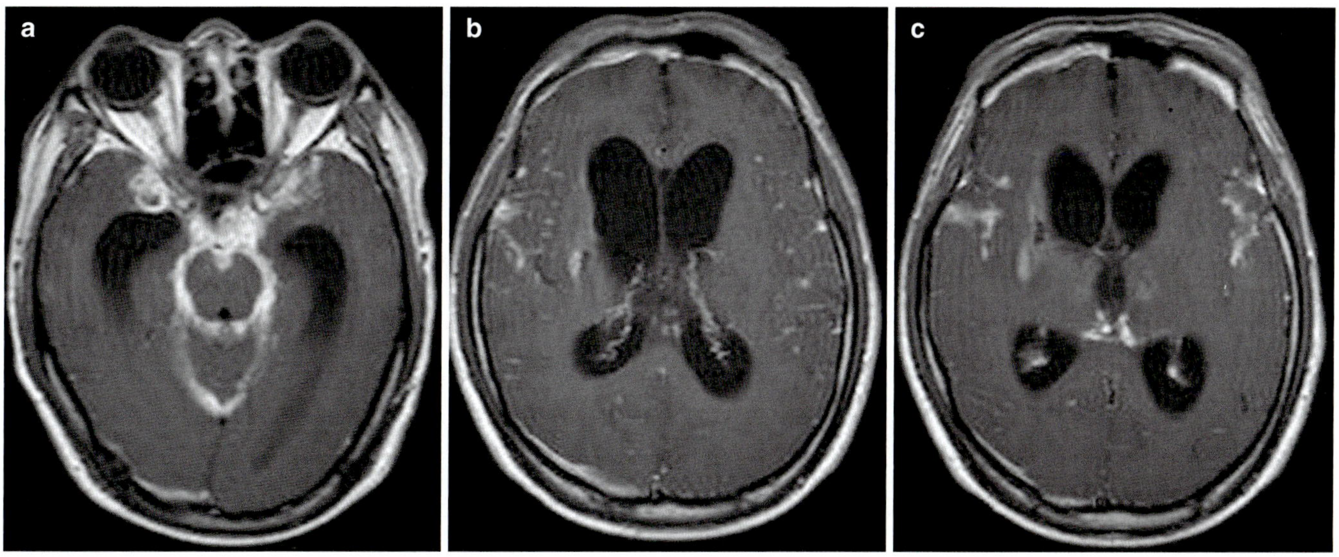

Fig. 8.21 (**a**–**c**) A male patient aged 46 years with tuberculous meningoencephalitis. Contrast MRI demonstrated obvious enhancements of basal cisterns including lateral fissure cistern, ambient cistern, interpeduncular cistern, and meninges

Surrounding edema and space-occupying effect are relatively slight.

4. Brain ventricular dilation and effusion

   The passages for cerebrospinal fluid are obstructed at different positions with different severities. Therefore, cerebral ventricle is subject to dilation. In mild cases, the anterior horn of lateral ventricle turns into obtuse. In moderate cases, the lateral ventricle is subject to slight dilation. In severe cases, the lateral ventricle is subject to obvious dilation and accompanying compressed adjacent brain parenchyma.
5. Brain edema is demonstrated as flaky decreased density area with poorly defined boundary. It commonly surrounds the cerebral TB lesions. By contrast CT scans, the brain edema is displayed with no enhancement.
6. Cerebral infarction can be demonstrated with singular or multiple hypodense lesions. They are different in size and shape and are commonly found in the area supplied by the middle cerebral artery. By contrast scans, the lesion of cerebral infarction shows no enhancement.
7. Cord-like or nodular-like opacity with increased density is a radiological sign of tuberculous arteritis. Contrast scans show bead-like enhancement.
8. Calcifications can occur in brain tuberculomas and in the meninges.
9. (1) MRI findings of tuberculous meningoencephalitis include abnormal signal shadow at the basal cistern, brain convex meninges, and lateral fissure in the early stage with slightly hyperintense T1WI signal and hyperintense T2WI signal. After injection of Gd-DTAP, T1WI shows enhancement of the basal cistern and diffuse enhancement of the meninges. (2) MRI is superior in demonstrating the lesions at optic chiasma, brain stem, and temporal lobe. (3) MRI can accurately demonstrate the shape and size of the lesions as well as the range of edema. Brain tuberculoma is displayed as isointense signal with the brain gray matter by T1WI but mostly heterogeneous signal by T2WI. The T2WI signals are mostly hypointense and rarely slightly hyperintense. After injection of Gd-DTAP, brain tuberculomas is demonstrated with nodular or ring-shaped enhancement (Fig. 8.22).

8.6.1.7 Hepatic and Splenic Tuberculosis

Hepatic TB by Radiology

1. Miliary hepatic TB is radiologically demonstrated with enlarged liver and multiple miliary low-density lesions in the liver.
2. Nodular hepatic TB is displayed with nodular low-density lesions. In some cases, the nodular opacity has uneven density, with fine spots and spots of calcifications. Contrast scans display marginal enhancement (Fig. 8.23).

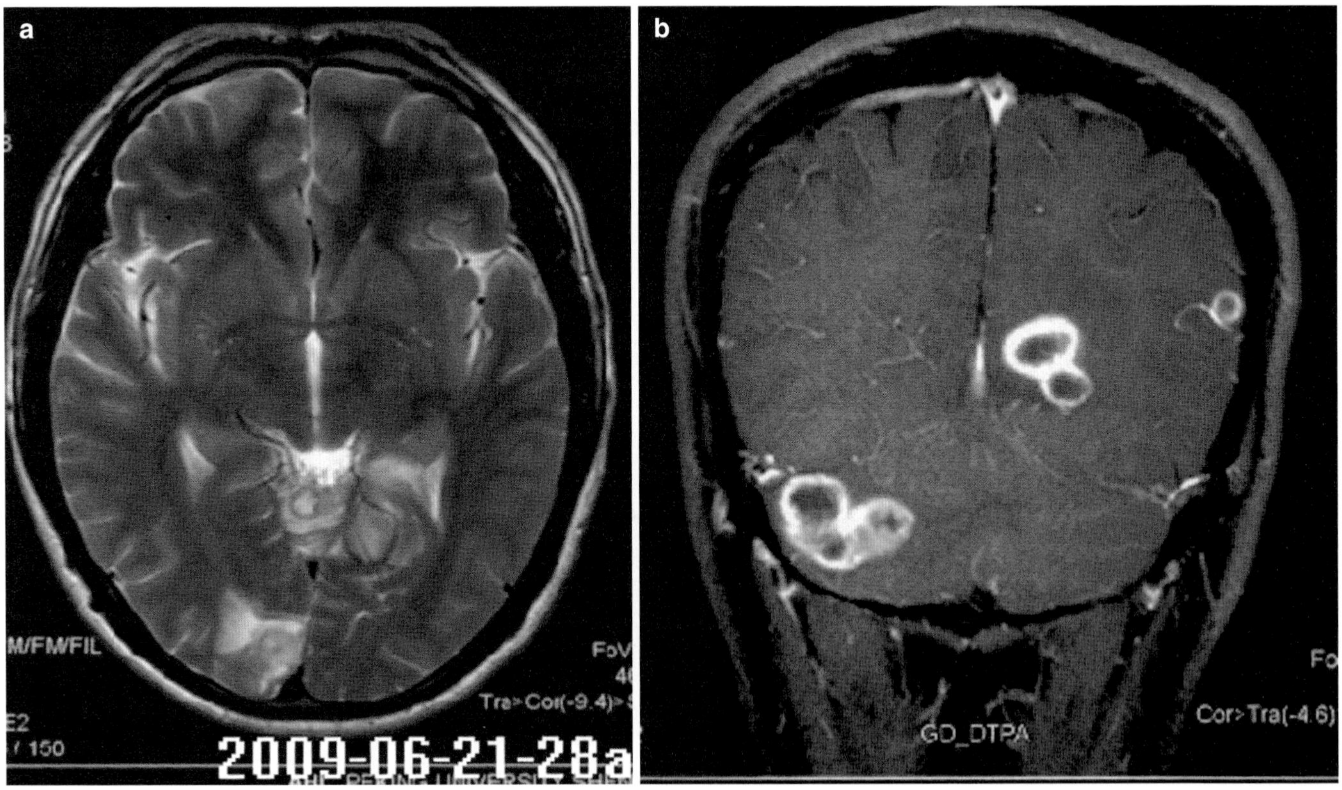

Fig. 8.22 (**a–d**) A female patient aged 46 years with brain tuberculomas. MRI showed multiple nodules in the brain, with obvious ring-shaped enhancement by contrast imaging

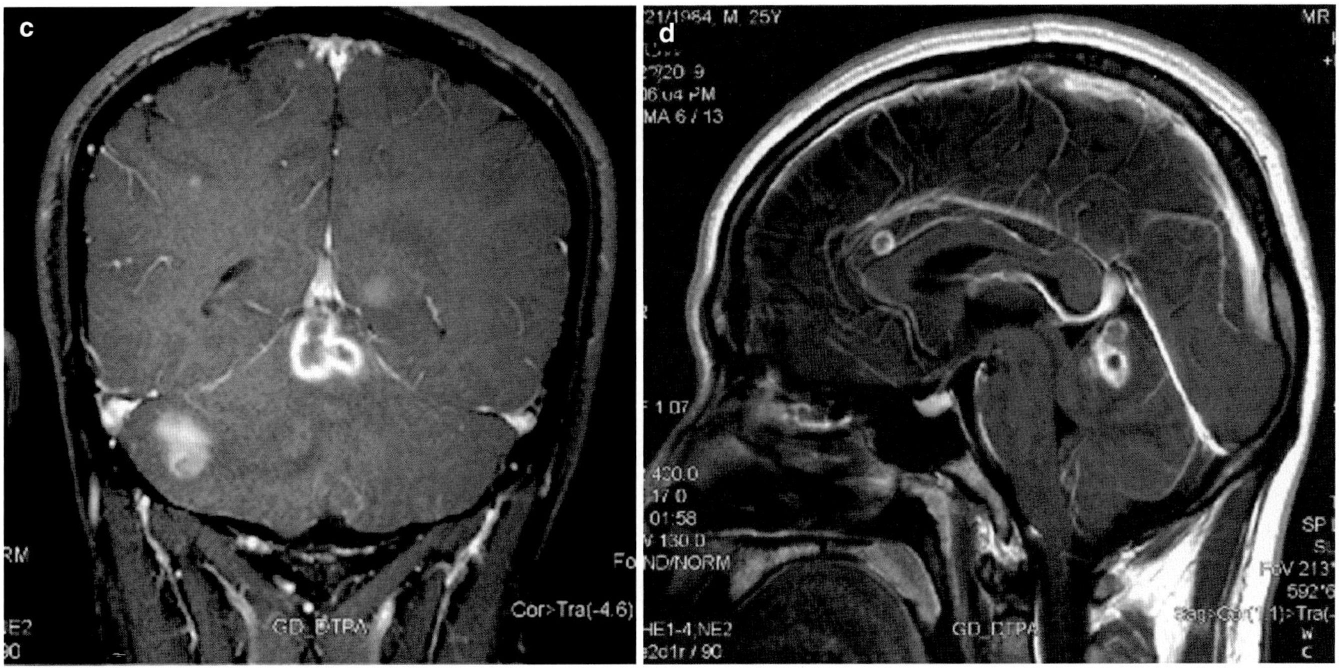

Fig. 8.22 (continued)

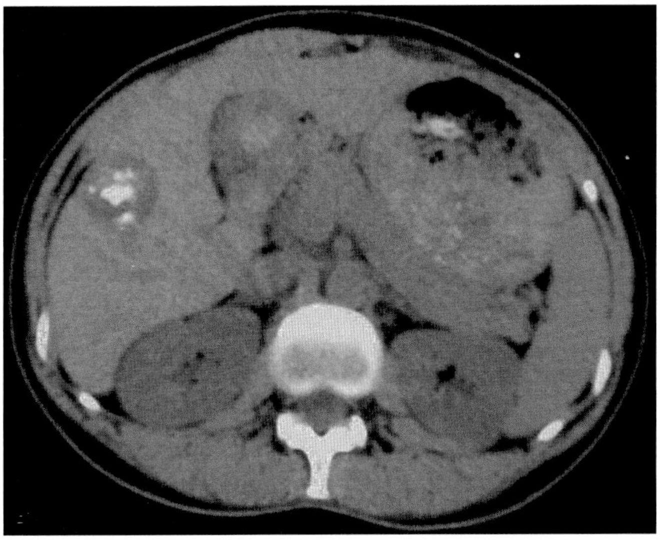

Fig. 8.23 A female patient aged 46 years with hepatic TB. The hepatic soft tissue window by CT scans demonstrates the right hepatic lobe with a round-like opacity with mixed density. In the opacity, there were low-density opacity and scattering spots of calcification. The boundary of most lesions were clearly defined, regular, and intact

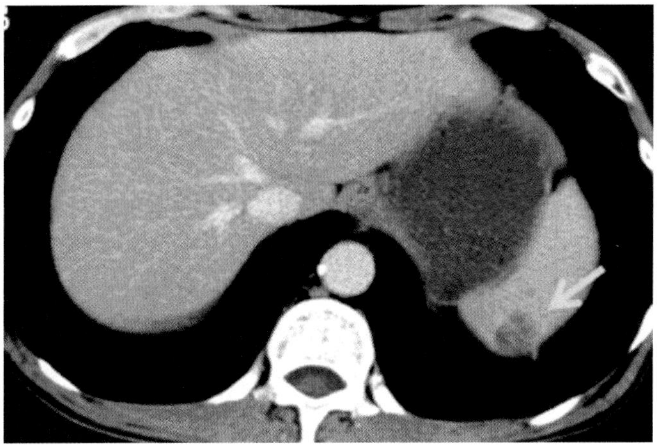

Fig. 8.24 A male patient aged 54 years with splenic TB. Contrast CT scans displayed irregular enhancement around the intrasplenic lesions

Splenic Tuberculosis by Radiology

1. Enlarged spleen can be detected.
2. Nodular splenic TB is radiologically demonstrated with nodular opacity with low or equal density and poorly defined boundary. Contrast scans commonly display no enhancement of the lesion but rarely ring-shaped enhancement.
3. Abscess splenic TB is displayed with singular or multiple round-like low-density lesions in the spleen. Contrast scans demonstrate marginal enhancement (Fig. 8.24).
4. Spots or small nodular calcification is demonstrated in the spleen.

8.6.1.8 Renal and Adrenal Tuberculosis

Renal TB by Radiology

1. Renal TB at its early stage may show no abnormality by radiology. And CT/MRI is superior to intravenous pyelography in demonstrating the advanced lesions.

2. Local outline of the kidney protrudes outward, or the kidney is enlarged. Renal arterial stenosis induced by fibrosis of renal TB lesions can cause atrophy and thinning, predominantly the renal cortex.
3. The renal parenchyma is demonstrated with multiple round and oval liquid-like low-density opacities in different sizes, with quite poorly defined boundaries. These lesions are actually liquefied caseous necrosis (Fig. 8.25).
4. The renal parenchyma is demonstrated with spots and small nodular or eggshell-like calcification.

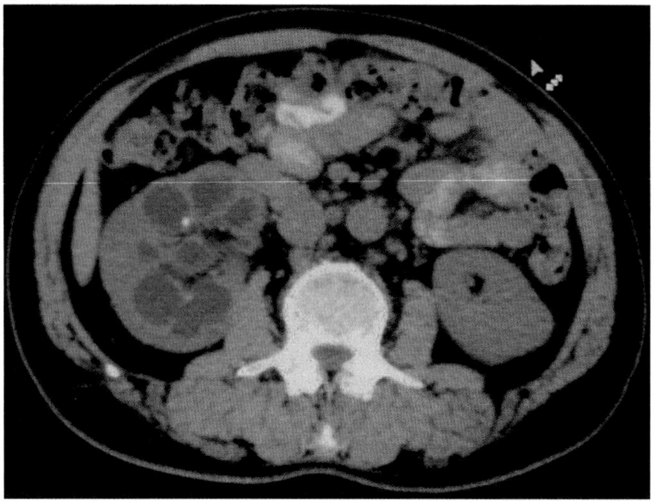

Fig. 8.25 A male patient aged 53 years with right renal TB. The renal soft tissue window by CT scans showed enlarged right kidney with wave-like boundary. The right renal parenchyma was displayed with multiple oval cystic fluid-like low-density opacities, with different sizes and quite unclearly defined boundaries. One cystic fluid-like low-density opacity was demonstrated with marginal calcification

5. The renal pelvis wall can be detected to be thickened. In some cases, linear and short curved linear opacity of calcification can be detected at the renal pelvis wall.
6. The ureteral wall of the affected kidney side is demonstrated to be thickened. And the renal pelvis and the ureter are demonstrated to be dilated with effusion (Fig. 8.26).
7. Contrast enhanced CT can show smaller lesions which do not demonstrate apparent enhancement at early dynamic phase stage and therefore is useful to differentiate from neoplasm as neoplasm may demonstrate early enhancement. Meanwhile, contrast enhanced CT can be used to assess the renal function of affected side.

Adrenal Tuberculosis by Radiology

Based on pathology or clinical staging, the development of adrenal TB can be divided into the caseation and the calcification stages or acute and chronic stages. At different stages, the radiological demonstrations vary. At the caseation stage, adrenal TB is radiologically demonstrated with enlarged bilateral adrenal glands and formation of lump. The long axis of the lump is consistent with the long axis of the adrenal gland, and the density of the lump can be even or uneven. At the margin or center of the lump, there may be spots of calcifications. By contrast scans, the lump may be demonstrated with ring-shaped enhancement (Fig. 8.27). During the calcification stage, adrenal TB shows spots of calcifications in partial or whole adrenal gland as well as slightly enlarged adrenal gland (Fig. 8.28). Adrenal TB with an illness course of less than 1 year is demonstrated with enlarged bilateral adrenal glands, but their outline can still be defined. Adrenal TB with an illness course of 1–4 years also presents enlarged bilateral adrenal glands, but the outline can be

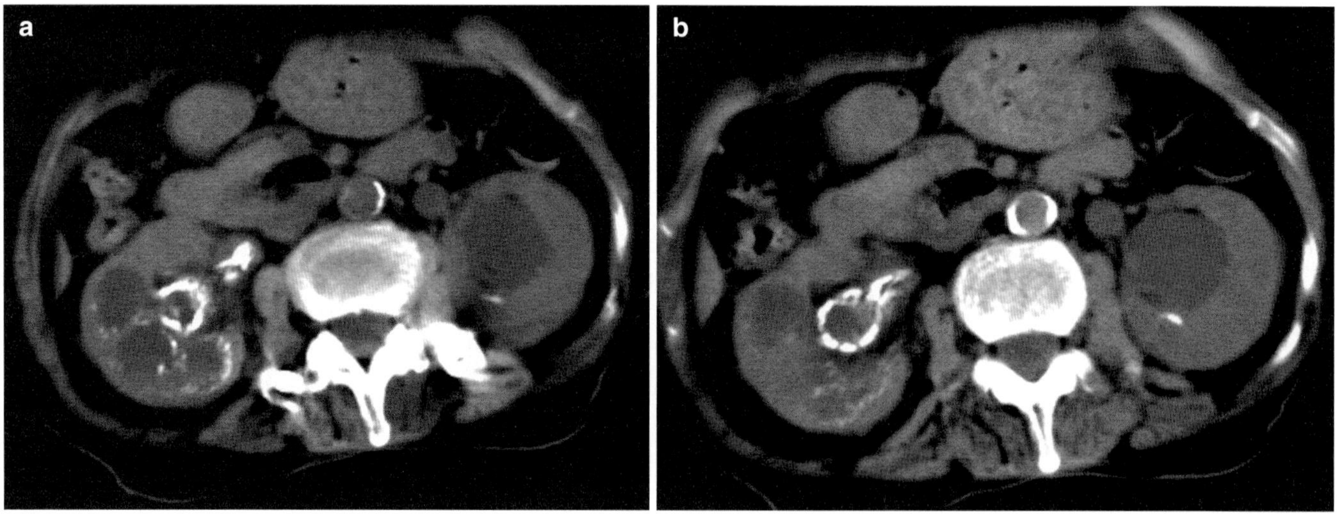

Fig. 8.26 (**a**, **b**) A female patient aged 64 years with bilateral renal TB. Both kidneys were demonstrated with severe effusion. The right renal pelvis and renal calices were displayed to be enlarged, with extensive marginal calcification

hardly defined. Adrenal TB with an illness course of above 4 years mostly presents normal-sized or shrinkage of adrenal glands and rarely cord-like irregular enlargement of the adrenal glands.

8.6.1.9 Spinal Tuberculosis

Spinal TB by Radiology (Fig. 8.29)

1. Bone destruction

   Vertebral bone destruction is common in cases of spinal TB, but bone destruction is rare at the spinal accessories. The lesions of bone destruction are irregular with worm-bitten-like margins. In some bone destruction lesions, there are smaller fragment opacities of sequestrum.
2. Narrowed intervertebral space

   Bone destruction at the superior or inferior margin of the adjacent vertebrae causes flattened vertebral body of the diseased vertebra. It further destructs the adjacent intervertebral disks to cause narrowing of the intervertebral space.
3. Paravertebral soft tissue swelling

   Around the diseased vertebra, soft tissue swelling can be detected, with internal liquid-like low-density area and poorly defined boundary. The swell is commonly accompanied by spots and patchy mass of calcifications.
4. Spinal canal involvement

   After bone destruction occurs in the vertebral body and spinal accessories, caseous lesions, sequestrum fragments, and granulation tissue extend into the adjacent spinal canal to cause secondary spinal canal stenosis.
5. Lumbar spinal TB

   Swelling of unilateral or bilateral psoas is commonly detected. In some cases, the swollen psoas is demonstrated with focalized low-density abscess.
6. MRI findings

   MRI can well display the range of lesions, which are mostly demonstrated with hypointense T1WI signal and mixed hyperintense T2WI signal. MRI can also well display the lesions of intervertebral disk, which are mostly demonstrated with hypointense T1WI signal and uneven mixed hyperintense T2WI signal. MRI can show abnormities in paravertebral soft tissue as well as location, size, and range of cold abscess. Paravertebral soft tissue lesions are mostly demonstrated as hypointense T1WI signal and

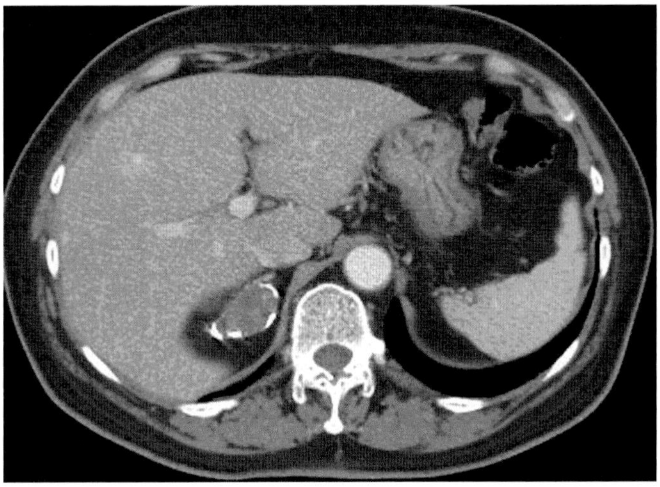

Fig. 8.27 A male patient aged 32 years with right adrenal TB. CT scan showed enlarged adrenal gland with abnormal morphology. The lesions were displayed with slightly low-density and marginal ring-shaped calcification

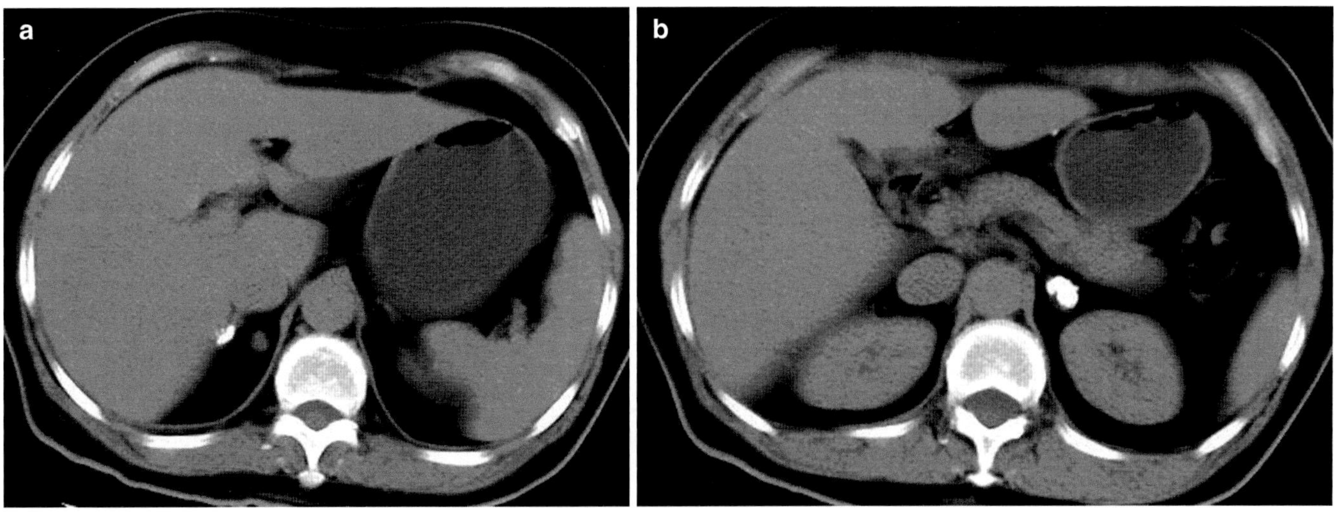

Fig. 8.28 (**a**, **b**) A male patient aged 39 years with bilateral adrenal TB. (**a**) The right adrenal gland was displayed with lateral strip-like calcification. (**b**) The left adrenal gland was demonstrated with nodular calcifications at the adrenal lateral and medial limbs and abnormal morphology

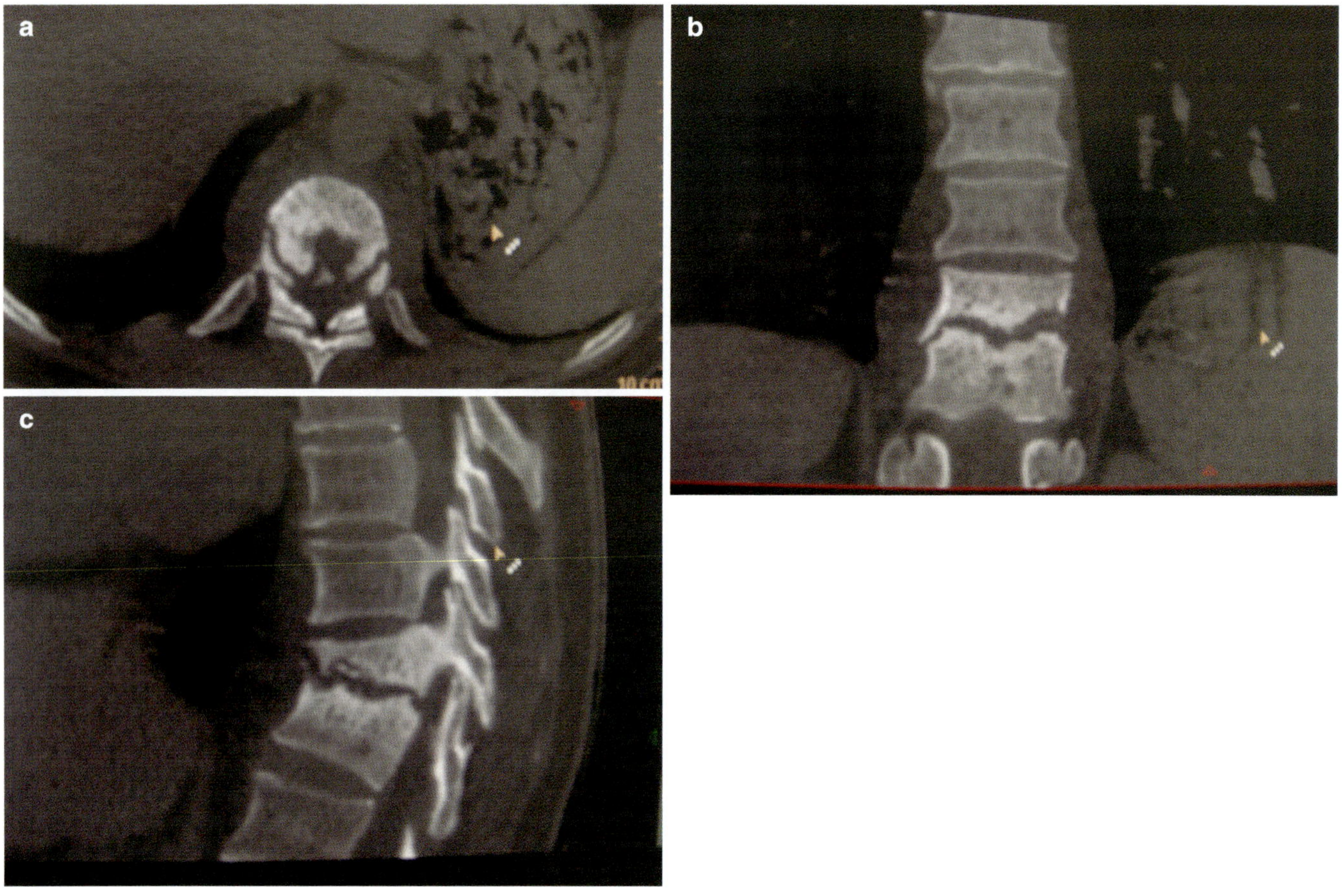

Fig. 8.29 (**a–c**) A female patient aged 46 years with thoracic spinal TB. Bone destruction was displayed between two adjacent thoracic vertebrae, with worm-bitten-like margin. The upper diseased vertebra was demonstrated with small fragments of sequestrum. The intervertebral space was shown to be narrowed, and slight spinal kyphosis was observable with the intervertebral space as the center. The paraspinal soft tissue was demonstrated with spindle-shaped abscess opacity

uneven mixed T2WI signal, sometimes even hyperintense T2WI signal. MRI can display the extent and range of involvement in the spinal cord and can facilitate in assessing the occurrence of ischemia and degeneration.

8.6.2 Atypical Pulmonary Tuberculosis by Radiology

Along with the increasing incidence of TB and its increasing drug resistance and due to inappropriate anti-TB treatment, some patients are radiologically demonstrated with atypical signs, resulting in misdiagnosis and delayed treatment. The radiological atypicality includes atypical location and/or morphology of the lesions.

8.6.2.1 Atypical Radiological Signs of Primary Pulmonary Tuberculosis

Primary complex is demonstrated with no typical signs of dumbbell-like sign or bipolar sign induced by intrapulmonary primary TB lesions, hilar lymphoid TB, and draining lymphatic TB. The intrapulmonary primary TB lesion shows nodular and flaky opacity and accompanying mediastinal lymphadenectasis, with no draining tubes connecting the two lesions (Fig. 8.30). Intrathoracic lymphoid TB shows hilar lymphadenectasis and multiple lesions of mediastinal lymphadenectasis. Otherwise, intrathoracic lymphoid TB shows only singular enlarged mediastinal lymph node or multiple enlarged lymph nodes. Enlarged lymph nodes integrate with each other, with poorly defined boundaries (Fig. 8.31).

8.6.2.2 Hematogenous Disseminated Pulmonary Tuberculosis

Hematogenous disseminated pulmonary TB is rarely displayed with atypical radiological signs. In rare chronic cases, due to diffuse distribution of the lesions, miliary nodules integrate into multiple large nodules or masses. In addition to intrapulmonary large flake of primary lesion, it may be misdiagnosed as intrapulmonary malignancy with extensive metastasis in lungs (Fig. 8.32).

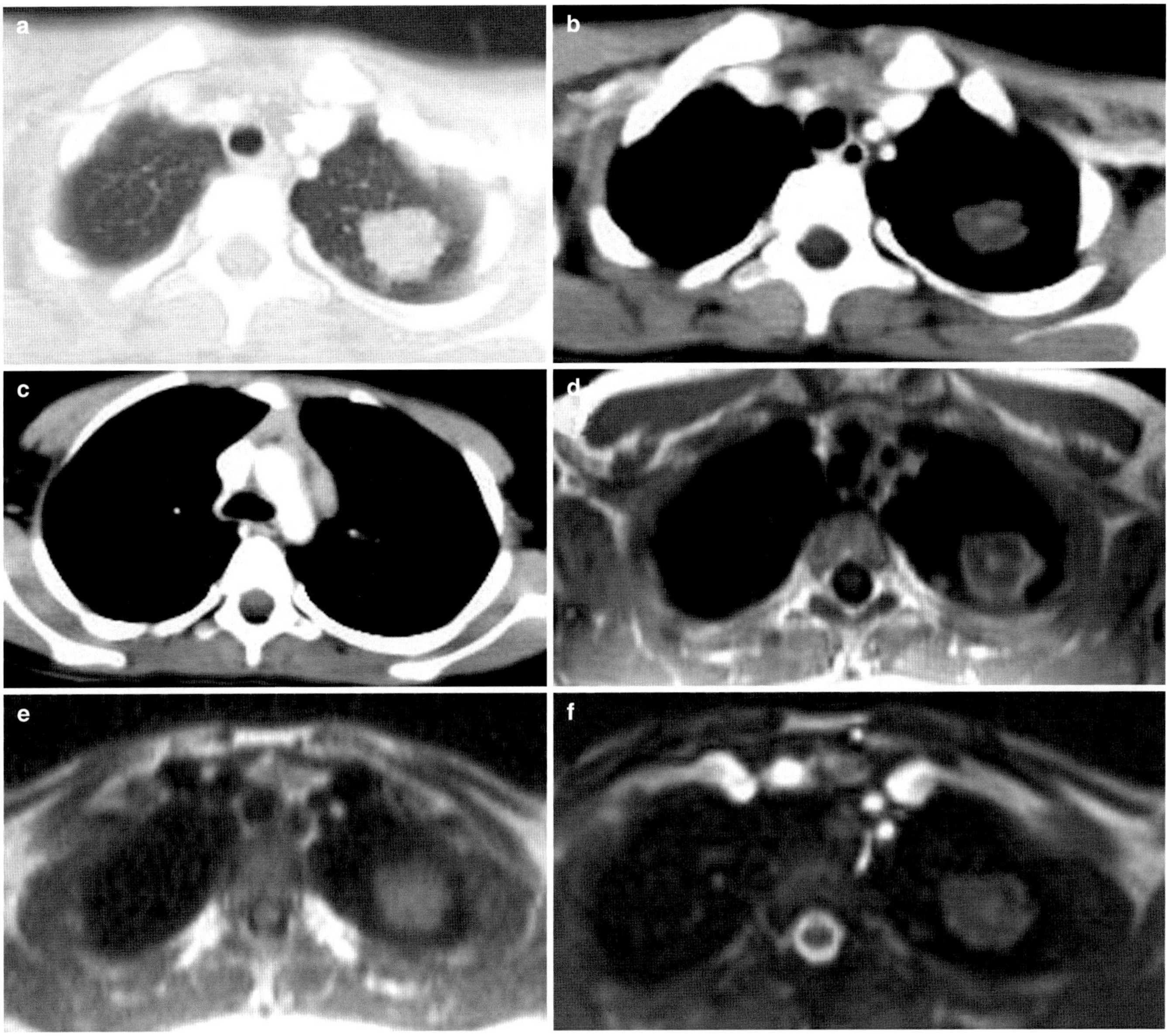

Fig. 8.30 (**a–f**) A boy aged 9 years with pathologically defined primary complex after surgery. CT scan showed round-like mass at the apex of left lung. Contrast scan demonstrated slight ring-shaped enhancement. Multiple enlarged lymph nodes were shown adjacent to the aortic arch with even enhancement. MRI displayed moderate and slightly high T1WI and T2WI signals. Contrast MRI displayed obvious ring-shaped enhancement

8.6.2.3 Atypical Radiological Signs of Secondary Pulmonary Tuberculosis

Secondary pulmonary TB is commonly displayed with atypical radiological signs. Some lesions are displayed with atypical location, occurring at the basal segment of the lower lung or the right middle lung lobe, with mass opacity that is slightly or moderately enhanced by contrast scan (Fig. 8.33). Some lesions are also displayed with secondary mediastinal lymphadenectasis (Fig. 8.34). Some lesions, although occurring at the upper lung, closely adhere to the spine to form singular mass with no satellite lesions around. And in some other cases, secondary pulmonary TB is shown as tuberculoma with solitary pulmonary nodule (SPN) or lump in the lungs, i.e., atypical tuberculoma, whose diameter may be up to above 4.0 cm. Its lesions are mostly found at the parts other than typical locations of secondary pulmonary TB, possibly with accompanying mediastinal lymphadenectasis (Fig. 8.35). Morphologically, the atypical radiological signs include lobulated lesions, lesions with fine spikes, vessel convergence, and pleural indentation. Due to no obvious satellite lesions and no obvious calcifications, the condition tends to be misdiagnosed as peripheral lung cancer

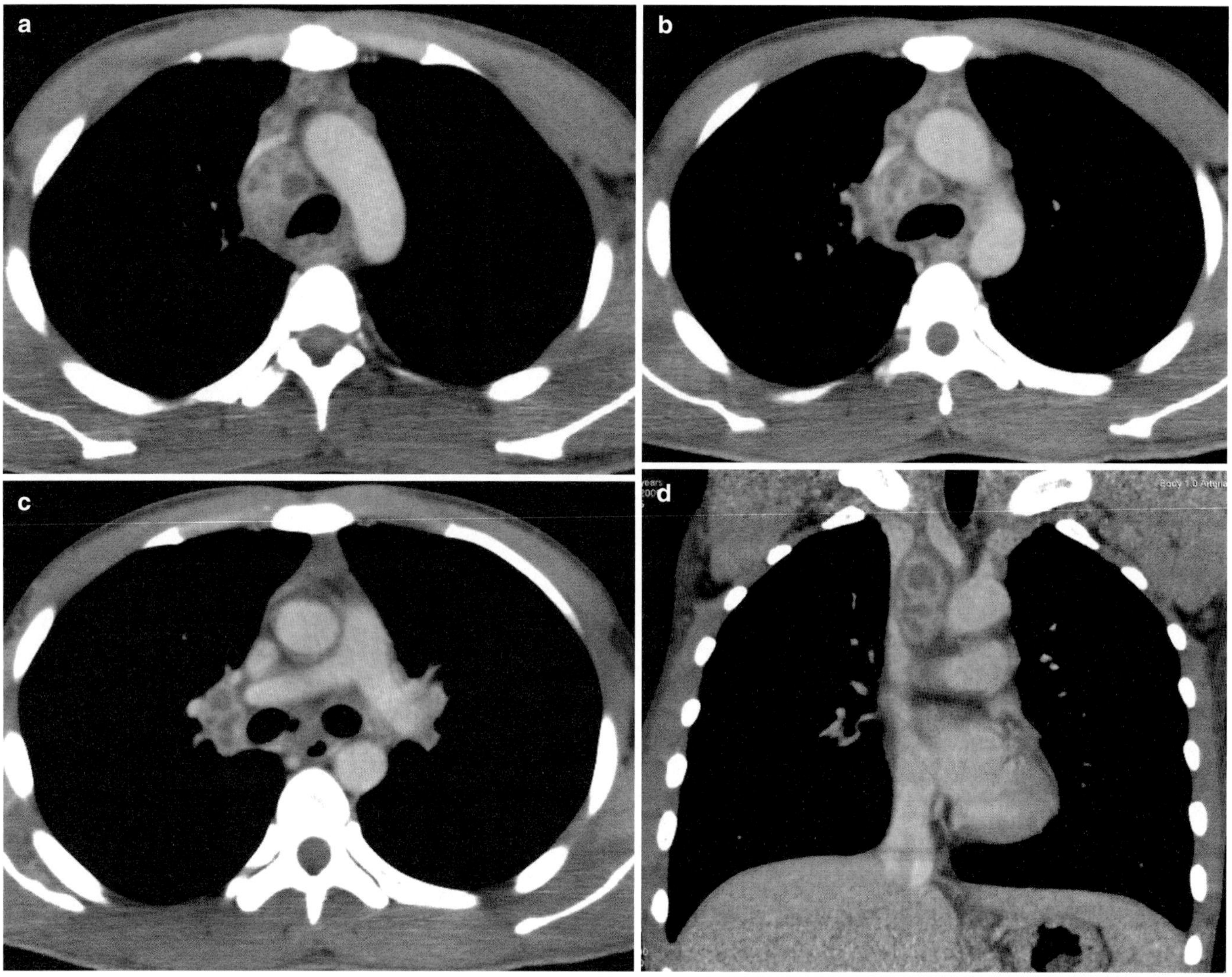

Fig. 8.31 (**a**–**d**) A male patient aged 26 years with pathologically defined mediastinal lymphoid TB after mediastinoscopy. Contrast transverse and coronal CT scans showed the mediastinum and right hilum with ring-shaped enhancement of multiple enlarged lymph nodes, with quite well-defined boundaries

(Fig. 8.36). Contrast delayed scan shows tuberculoma with thin-wall ring-shaped enhancement, which is a specific radiological sign.

8.6.2.4 Secondary Pulmonary TB with Predominant Interstitial Change by Radiology

Secondary pulmonary TB with predominant interstitial change is a special type of secondary pulmonary TB. The radiological signs by HRCT are characteristic, including segmentally distributed lesions and integrated flakes of lesions. Intralobular interstitial abnormalities are the main radiological signs of secondary pulmonary TB with predominant interstitial change. These signs include fine reticular opacity, micronodule, tree-bud sign, and ground-glass opacity. The lesions are mostly distributed in the upper lung or diffusely distributed in both lungs to form snowflakes sign (Fig. 8.37).

8.6.3 Multidrug-Resistant Tuberculosis by Radiology

8.6.3.1 Introduction

Multidrug-resistant tuberculosis (MDR-TB) is resistant to two major potent anti-TB drugs, isoniazid and rifampin. In addition to the two first-line anti-TB drugs, isoniazid and rifampin, extensively drug-resistant tuberculosis (XDR-TB) is also resistant to any one drug of quinolones and at least three second-line injectable anti-TB drugs such as kanamycin, amikacin, and capreomycin.

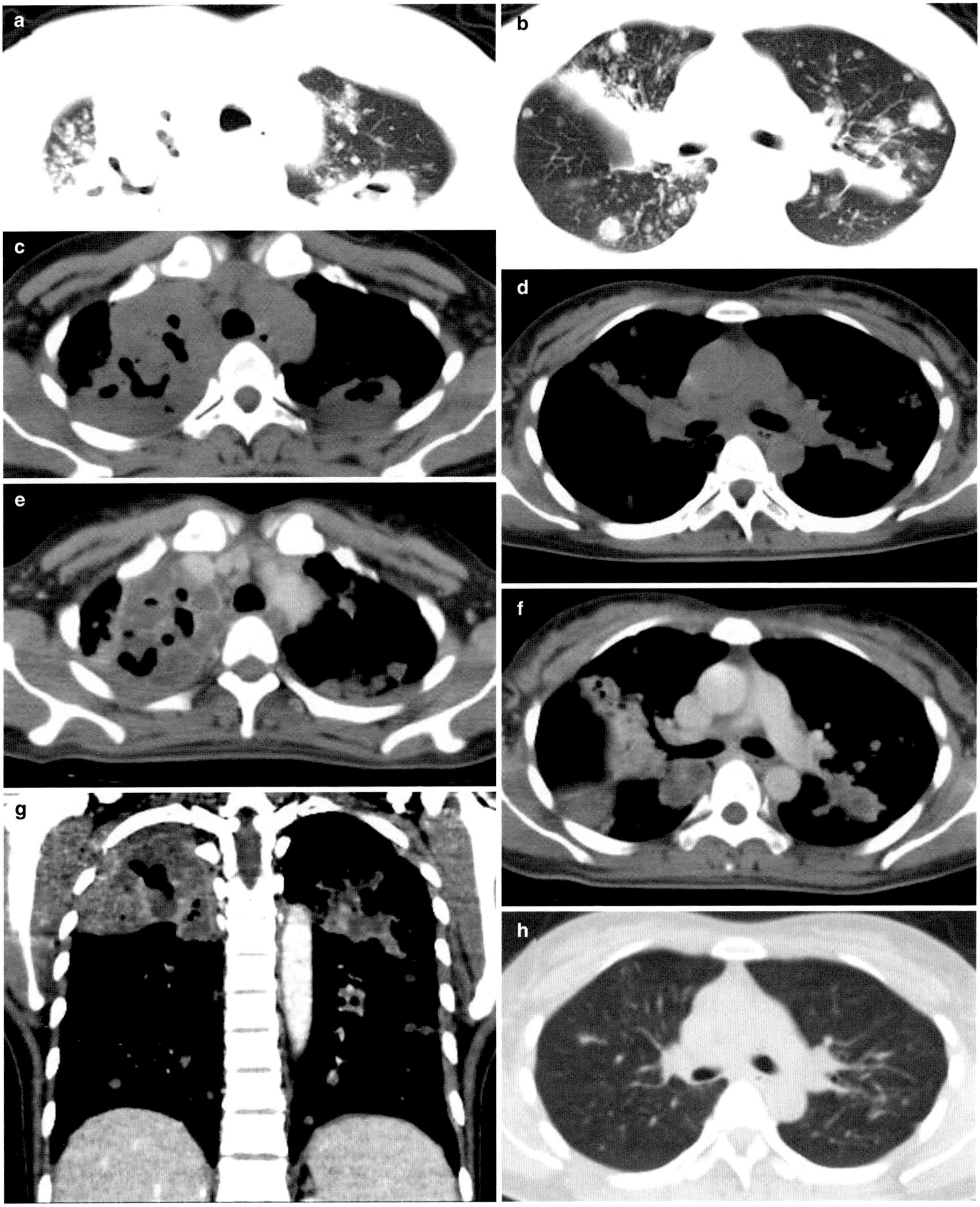

Fig 8.32 (**a–h**) A female patient aged 35 years with pathologically defined pulmonary TB after lung puncture. (**a–d**) The lung and mediastinum windows by plain CT scan showed the left upper lung with mass opacity and cavity and the right upper lung with large flaky opacity as well as accompanying air bronchogram sign and worm-bitten-like cavity. Both lungs were displayed with diffuse miliary nodules, which integrated into larger nodules and masses, with small flaky opacity. (**e–g**) Contrast transverse and coronal CT scans showed ring-shaped enhancement of nodules and masses. (**h**) Reexamination after anti-TB treatment for 6 months displayed obvious absorption of the lesions

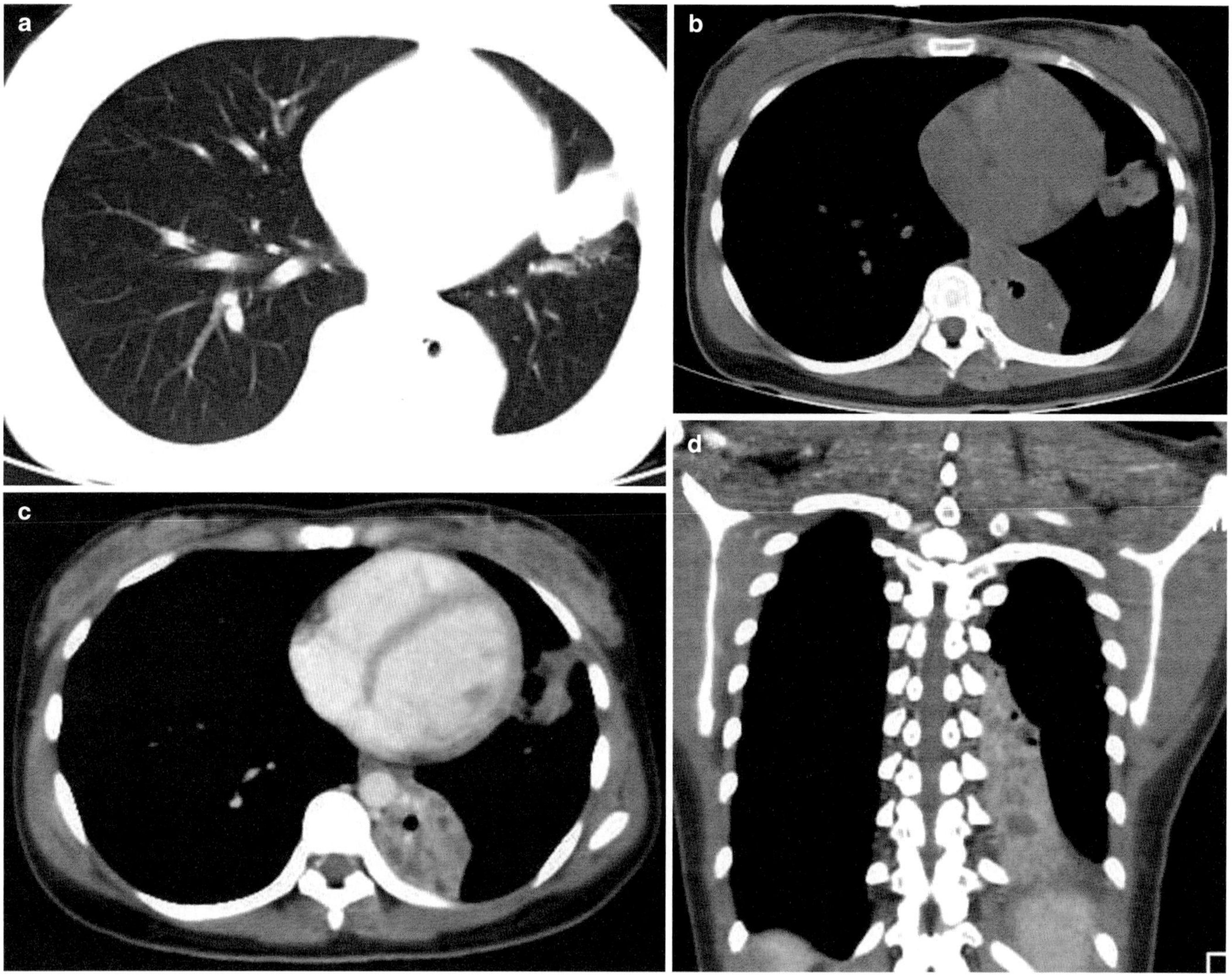

Fig. 8.33 (**a**–**d**) A female patient aged 21 years with pulmonary TB defined by fiber-optic bronchoscopy. (**a**, **b**) The lung and mediastinum windows by CT scan showed mass opacity with soft tissue density adjacent to the heart boundary in the left lower lung, with satellite lesions around. The posterior basilar segment of the left lower lung was displayed with segmental atelectasis, which adheres closely to the spine. (**c**) Transverse CT scan showed slight enhancement of the mass opacity adjacent to the heart boundary in the left lower lung. (**d**) Coronal CT scan showed significant enhancement of the segmental atelectasis at the posterior basilar segment of the left lower lung

Infection of drug-resistant TB has various reasons. And the following populations are vulnerable to the infection:

1. Patients with TB receiving inadequate or not standard therapies or patients with poor compliance of persistent drug use. These are the main reasons responsible for infection of drug-resistant TB;
2. Patients with a case history of contact to patients with drug-resistant TB. This is the main reason responsible to infection of primary drug-resistant TB.
3. Patients with active TB but ineffective treatment.
4. Migration is also an important factor. Patients with a history of contact to patient with active TB living in prevailing region of drug-resistant TB or with a history of living in prevailing region of drug-resistant TB are more likely to be infected.
5. Individuals with a history of hospitalization, imprisonment, and living in a place with long-term monitoring device or drug-giving facilities and those homeless living in sanctuaries.
6. HIV-infected patients.

8.6.3.2 Radiological Demonstrations

The most characteristic sign of MDR-TB by CT scans is multiple cavities (Fig. 8.38). Compared to drug-sensitive tuberculosis (DS-TB), multiple cavities in cases of primary MDR-TB are more likely to be detected, with larger volume.

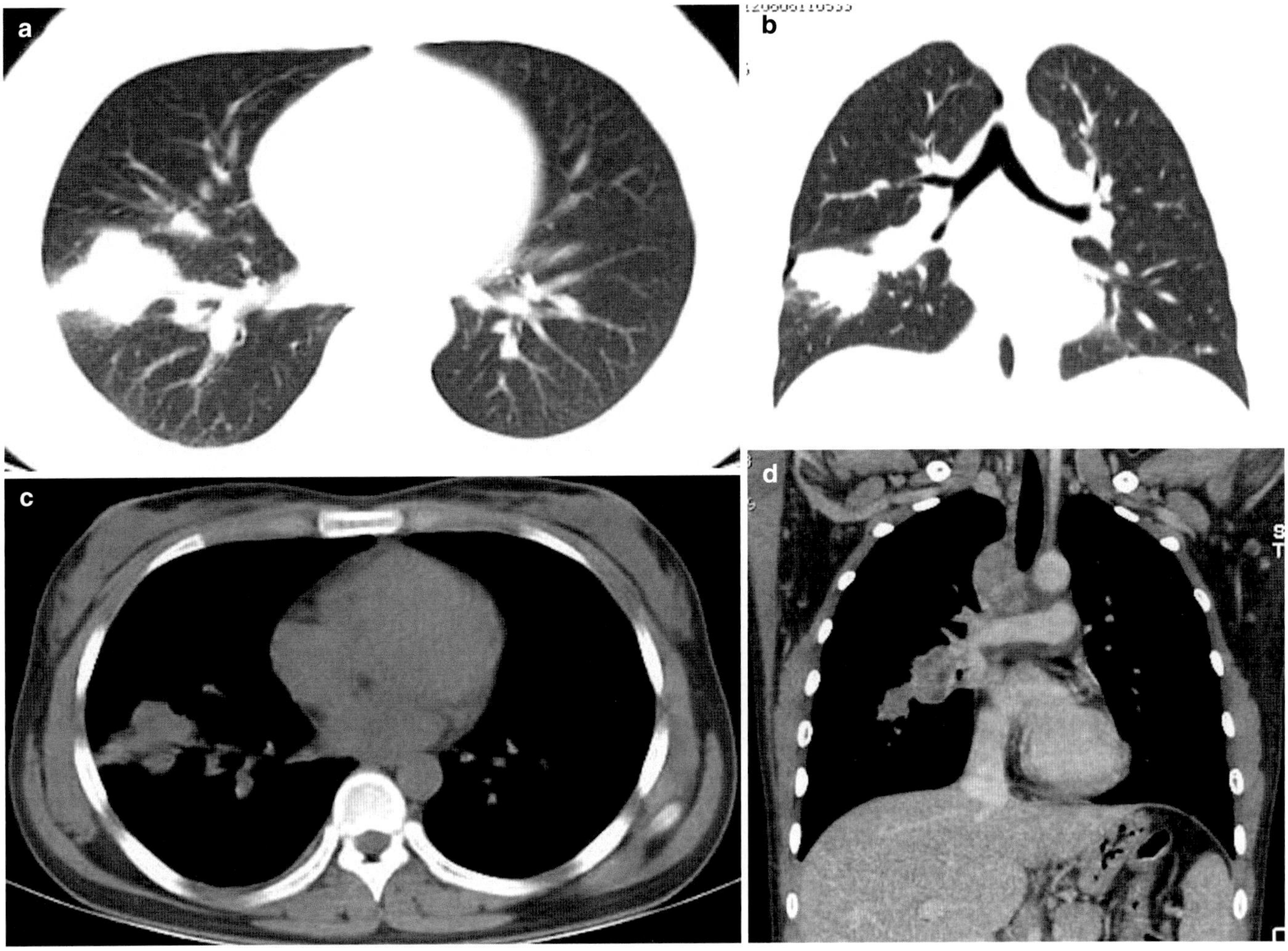

Fig. 8.34 (**a–d**) A female patient aged 17 years with pathologically defined pulmonary TB after percutaneous lung tissue puncture for biopsy. (**a–c**) Plain CT scan showed irregular mass with soft tissue density and quite clearly defined boundary, which closely adhered to the right oblique fissure of the right lower lung. (**d**) Contrast coronal CT scan showed significant ring-shaped enhancements of the mass opacity in the right lung and multiple enlarged mediastinal lymph nodes

In addition, multiple large nodules and ground-glass opacity are more extensively distributed. And more segments contain multiple clusters of small nodules. Radiological signs of MDR-TB and DS-TB show no substantial difference. However, multiple cavities and some chronic conditions, such as bronchiectasis and granuloma with calcification, are more common in cases of MDR-TB (Fig. 8.39). In patients with MDR-TB, pulmonary parenchymal lesion has a higher incidence rate, and more lung segments are involved. In cases with liquefied contents discharged into the bronchus, they are disseminated rapidly in the bronchi of both lungs, especially the unaffected lung tissue (Fig. 8.40).

Compared to DS-TB, large nodules, bronchiectasis, and multiple cavities have higher incidence rates in MDR-TB, with more cavities and segmental small nodules as well as more extensive parenchymal lesions. Cavities and multiple nodules are the main abnormalities radiologically demonstrated in the lungs of patients with XDR-TB and MDR-TB, which are more common in young adults. Therefore, acid-fast staining positive in combination with radiological signs of multiple cavities and multiple nodules in young adults constitutes the basis for suspected diagnosis of MDR-TB or XDR-TB.

8.6.4 Nontuberculous Mycobacterial Lung Disease by Radiology

8.6.4.1 Introduction

Nontuberculous mycobacteria (NTM) refers to mycobacteria in the genus *Mycobacterium* other than *Mycobacterium tuberculosis* complex (including *M. tuberculosis*, *M. bovis*, *M. Africa*, and *M. murine*) and *M. leprae*. Until now, a total of 154 species of NTM as well as 13 subspecies have been

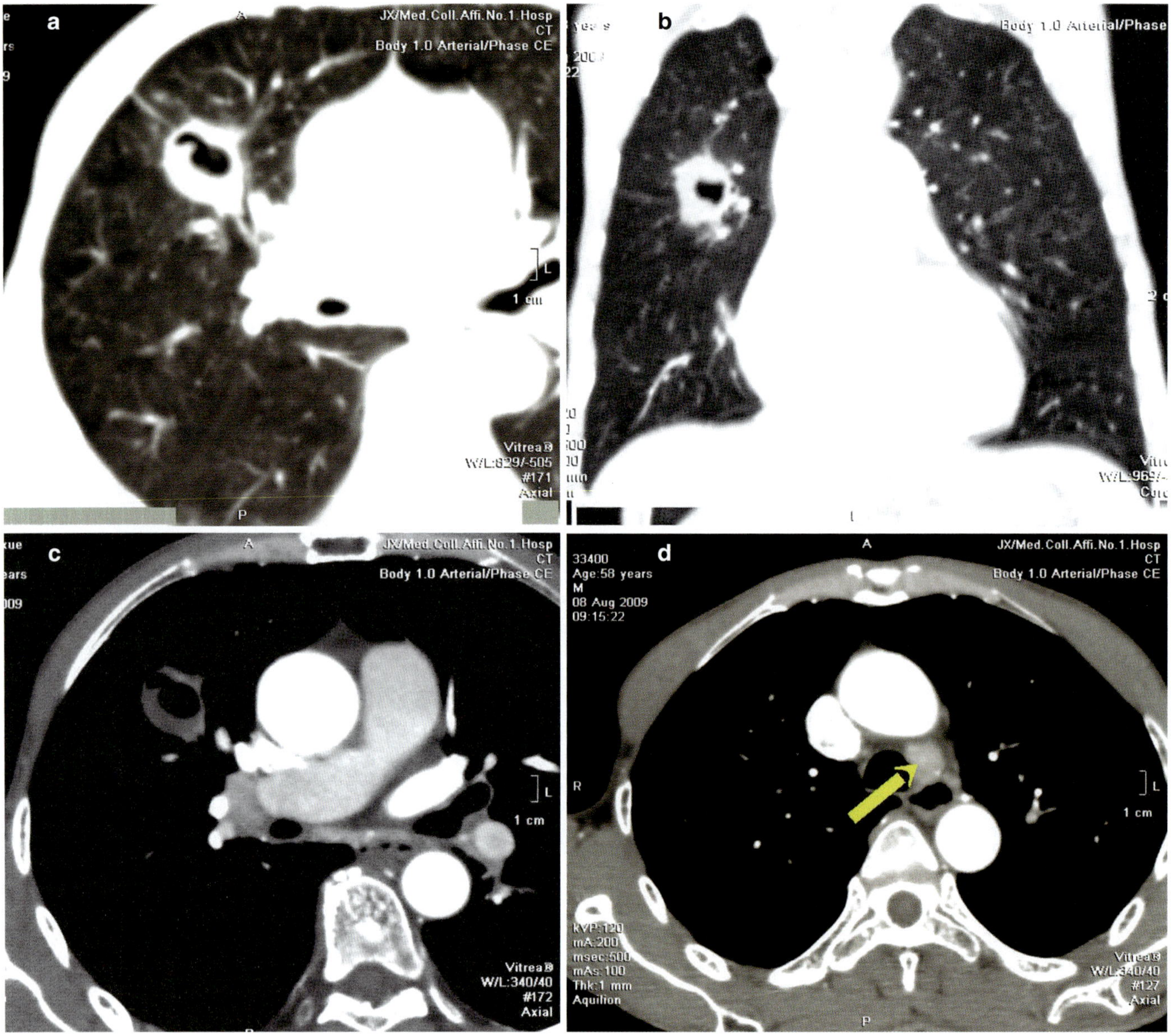

Fig. 8.35 (**a–d**) A male patient aged 58 years with pathologically defined tuberculoma in the right upper lung and accompanying mediastinal tuberculous lymphadenitis after surgery. (**a**, **b**) CT scan showed solitary nodular opacity in the anterior segment of the right upper lung, with slight lobulation and short spikes. Fissure-like cavity was also demonstrated. (**c**, **d**) Contrast scan showed slight enhancement of the lesions in the right upper lung. The mediastinal aorta and pulmonary artery window demonstrated enlarged lymph nodes with significant and homogeneous enhancement

identified. Some of them are pathogenic bacteria or conditional pathogenic bacteria. NTM can invade human tissues and organs such as lungs, lymph nodes, bones, joints, skin, and soft tissues. It may induce systemic disseminated disease. Infection of NTM in lungs is the known as NTM lung disease. It is more common in elderly patients with pulmonary diseases, patients with HIV/AIDS, patients with long-term use of immunosuppressants, and patients after organ transplantation. NTM can also infect humans together with *M. tuberculosis* to cause mixed infection. In recent years, the occurrence of NTM infection has been increasing, and it has been one of the important diseases threatening human public health.

8.6.4.2 Radiological Signs by CT

1. Multiple cavities.

   Multiple cavities, especially thin-walled cavities, are common, with different sizes and smooth inner walls. The surrounding infiltrative lesions are mild (Figs 8.41 and 8.42).

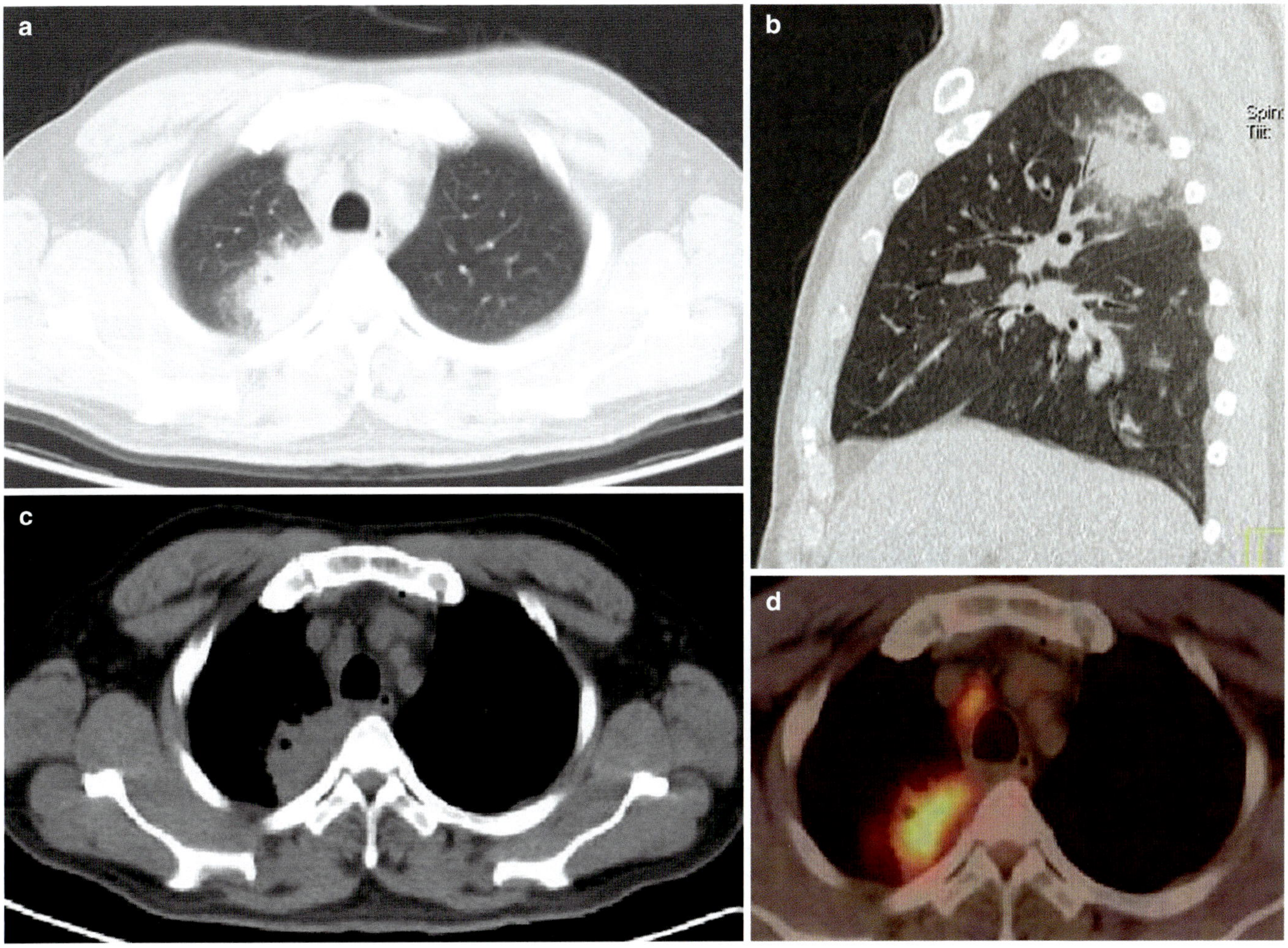

Fig. 8.36 (**a**–**d**) A male patient aged 40 years with pathologically defined pulmonary TB after percutaneous lung puncture for biopsy. (**a**) The lung window presented mass-like opacity that closely adhered to the spine with poorly defined boundary and internal vacuolation. (**b**) Sagittal scan displayed air bronchogram sign in the lesion. (**c**) Vacuolation was displayed in the lesion, and an enlarged lymph node was detected posterior to the tracheal precaval vein. (**d**) PET/CT fusion image showed nodular opacity induced by abnormal concentration of radionuclide in the lesion, with an SUVmax value of 5.9. The enlarged lymph node posterior to the tracheal precaval vein was also shown with nodular opacity induced by abnormal concentration of radionuclide

2. High incidence rate of bronchiectasis

   The incidence rate of bronchiectasis is high. The dilated bronchi are surrounded by small nodular opacities, ground-glass opacities, and flaky opacity (Fig. 8.43).
3. Small consolidation in the lungs

   The lungs are displayed with small consolidation, with air bronchogram sign inside (Fig. 8.44).
4. Involvement of the apex of upper lung lobe

   The lesions commonly involve the apex of the upper lung lobe, which is predominantly unilateral. The quantity of lesions in the right lung is two times as many as those in the left lung. The acinar nodular opacity, namely, the tree-bud sign, is commonly located under the pleura (Fig. 8.45).
5. Around the irregular transparent areas, there are clustered and linear opacities, which radiate from the transparent areas.
6. Multiple radiological signs may coexist. For instance, the radiological signs of bronchiectasis, tree-bud sign, small nodules, consolidation, and ground-glass opacity can be simultaneously demonstrated (Fig. 8.46).
7. The illness course is relatively long. Pleural thickening is obvious in the affected parts.

Radiological signs of NTM lung disease are nonspecific, resembling radiological signs of pulmonary TB. Radiology plays a role in implicating the diagnosis and the definitive diagnosis should be based on sputum culture and biopsy.

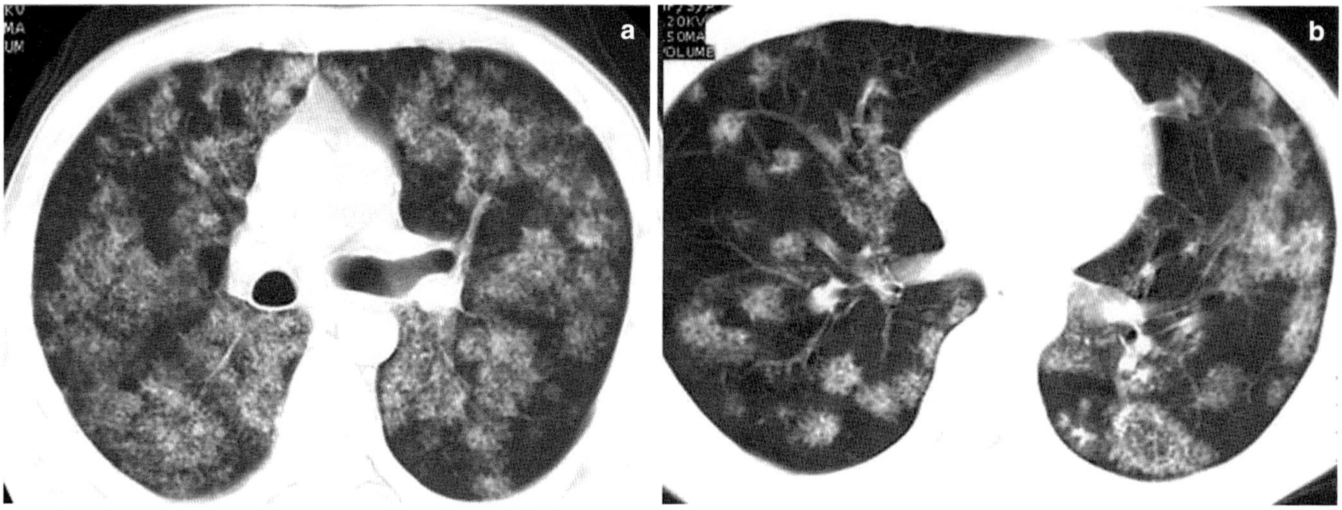

Fig. 8.37 (**a**, **b**) A male patient aged 44 years with pulmonary TB of both lungs. The lung window by CT showed intralobular fine reticular opacity, micronodule, tree-bud sign, and ground-glass opacity in both lungs. The lesions distributed segmentally with flaky integration to form snowflakes sign

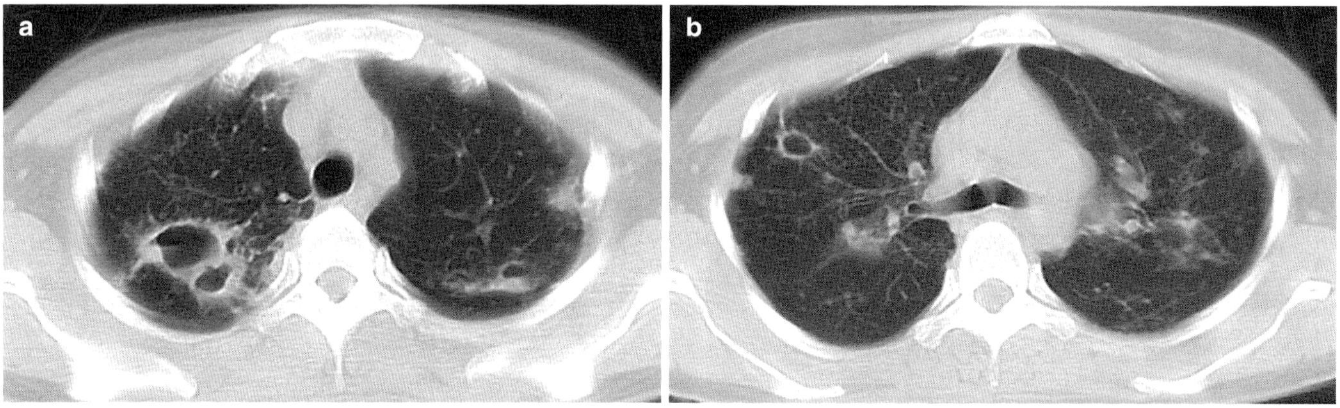

Fig. 8.38 (**a**, **b**) A female patient aged 30 years with MDR-TB. Sputum culture demonstrated the growth of *M. tuberculosis*, which showed resistance to isoniazid, rifampicin, and levofloxacin. CT scan showed multiple cavities in the right upper lung and patchy and nodular opacities in the left upper lung, with accompanying cavities

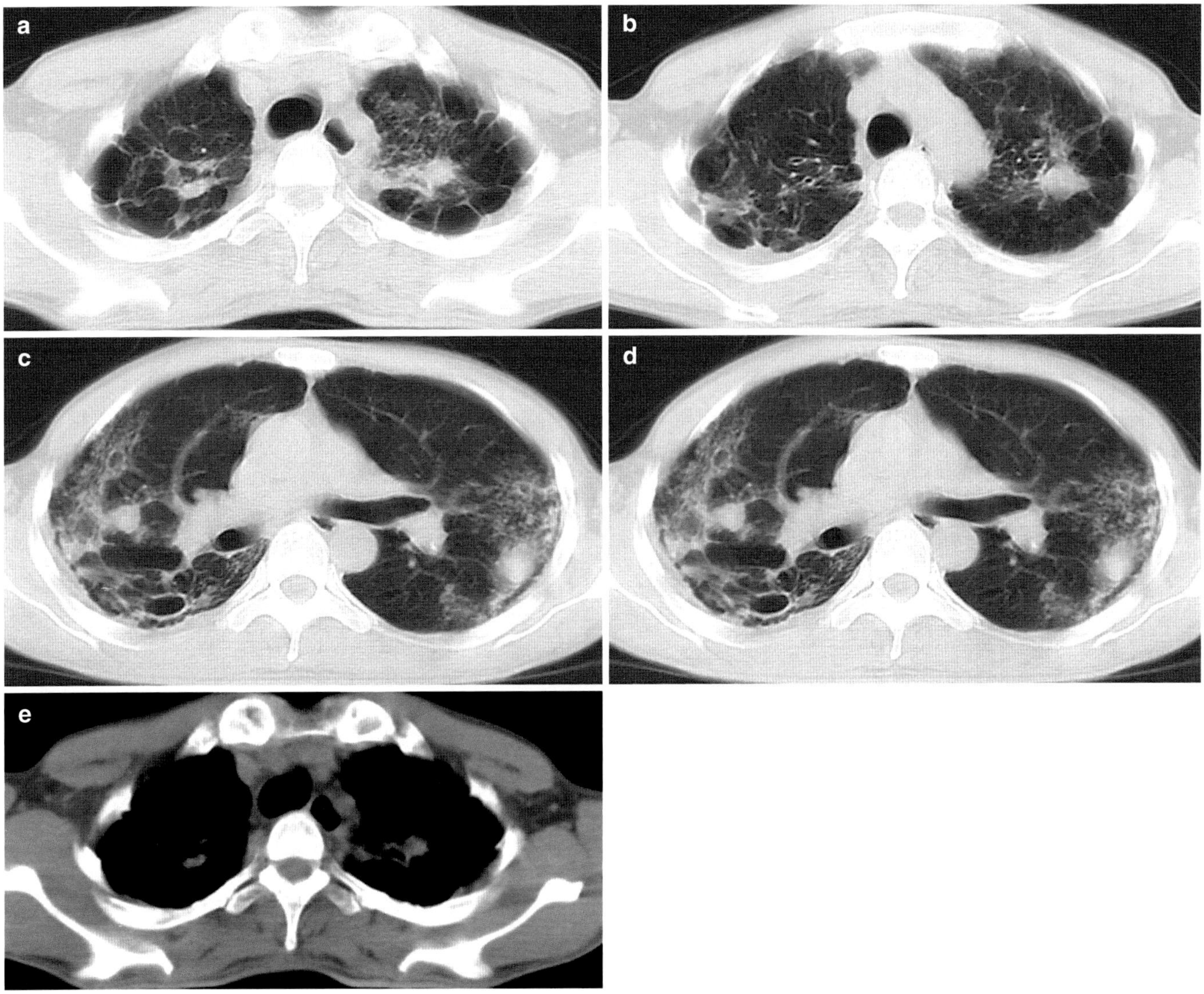

Fig. 8.39 (**a–e**) A male patient aged 32 years with MDR-TB. Sputum culture demonstrated the growth of *M. tuberculosis*. The lung window by chest CT scan displayed multiple irregular cavities and nodules in both lungs, with accompanying grid-like opacity. The lesions were mainly distributed under the pleura

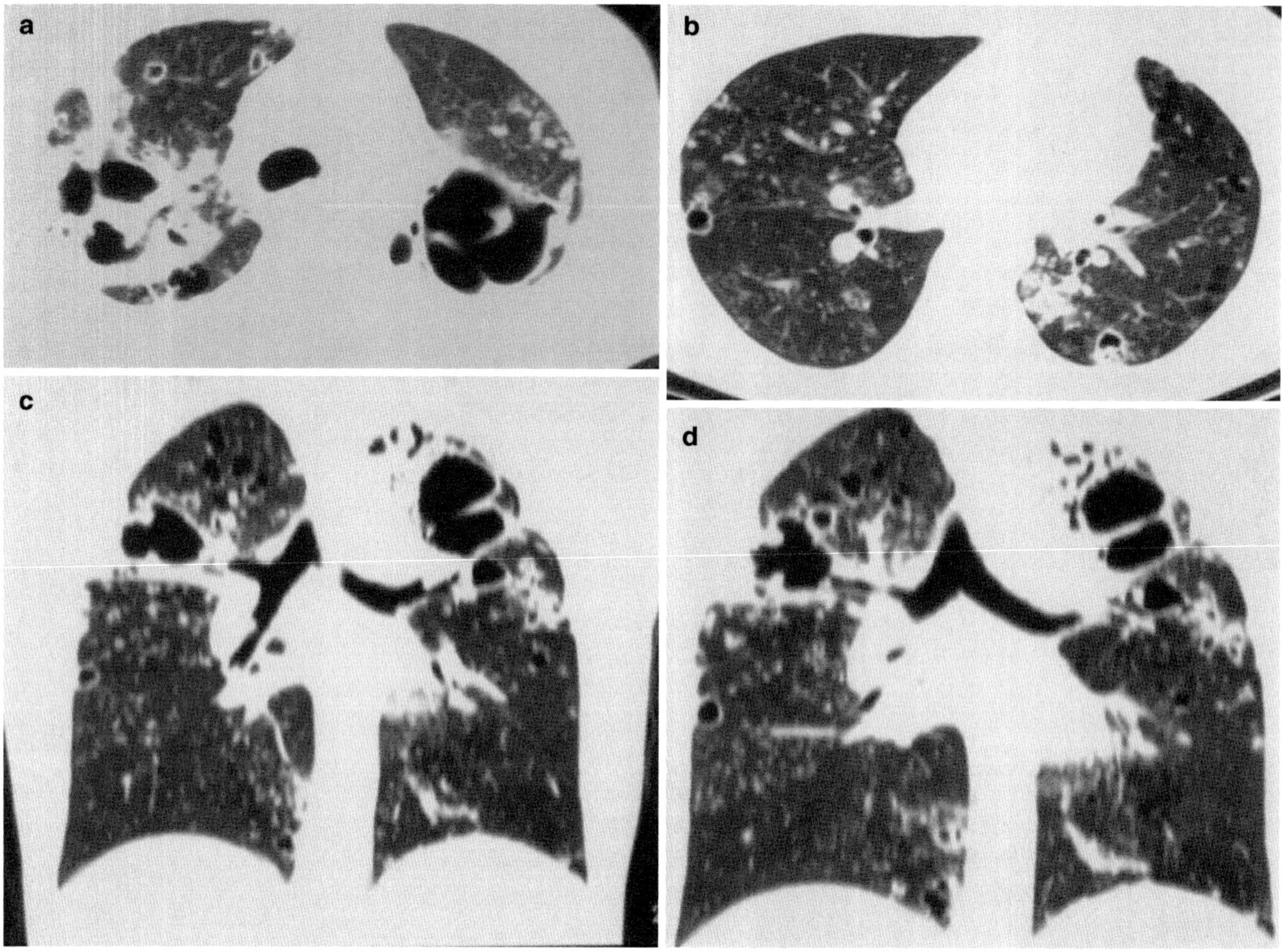

Fig. 8.40 (**a–d**) A male patient aged 68 years with MDR-TB. Sputum culture demonstrated the growth of *M. tuberculosis*, which showed resistance to isoniazid and rifampicin. The middle and upper lung fields of both lungs were displayed with multiple cavities and nodules. Reconstructed image showed well-defined inner wall of the cavities

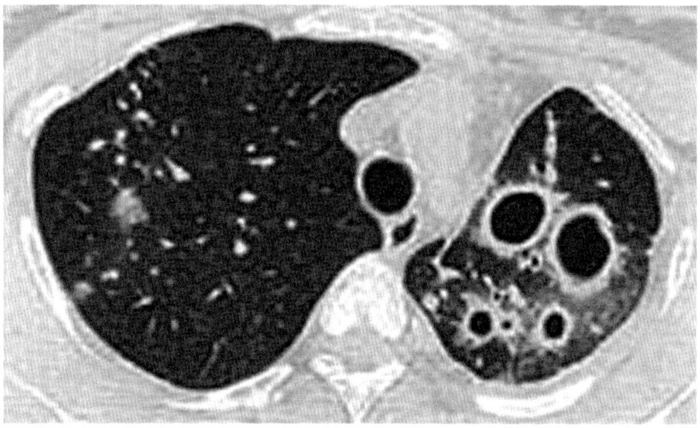

Fig. 8.41 NTM lung disease. Multiple thin-walled cavities were shown in the left upper lung. Small nodular and small flaky infiltrative lesions were displayed in the right upper lung

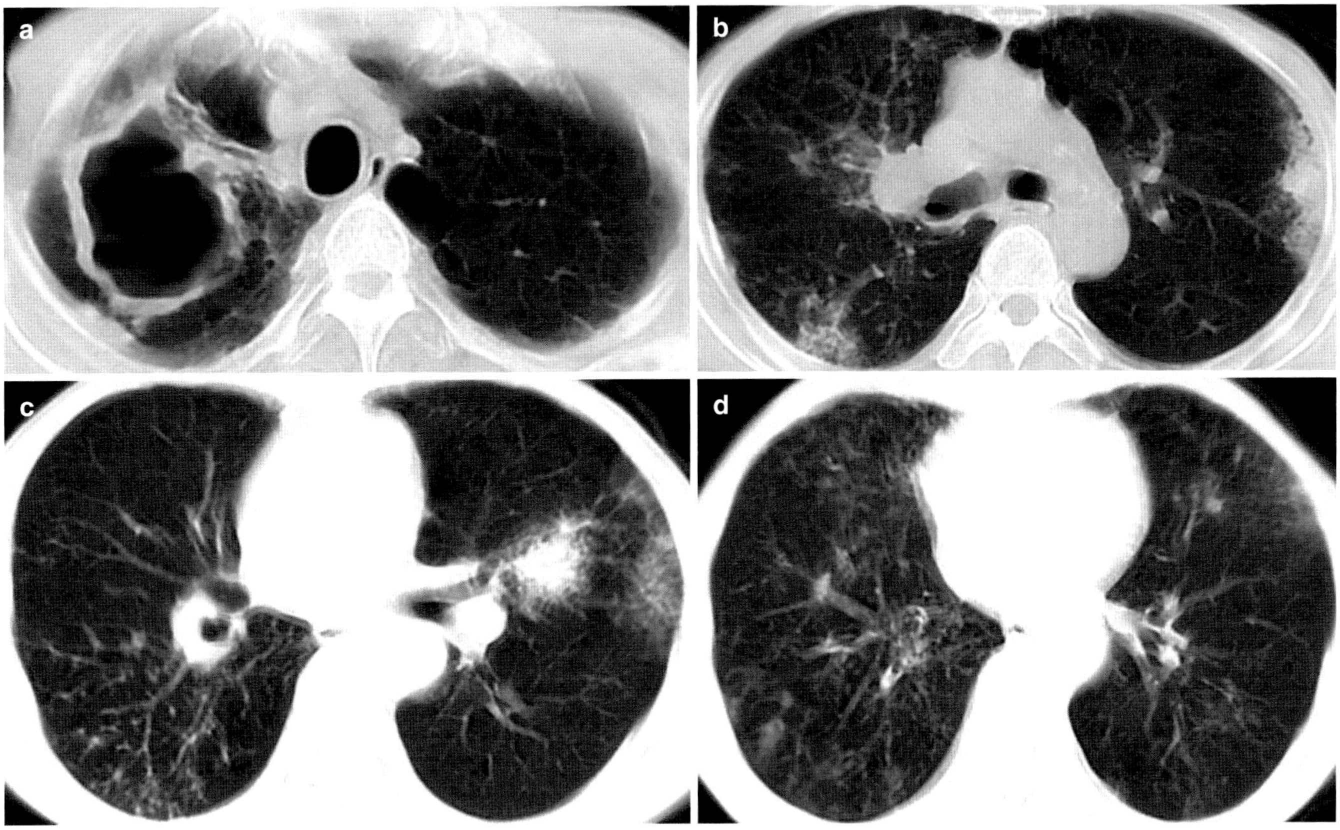

Fig. 8.42 (**a**–**d**) A male patient aged 68 years with HIV infection. By sputum culture, the diagnosis was NTM lung disease. (**a**) The lung window displayed a large thick-walled cavity in the right upper lung lobe, with irregular inner wall. Adjacent to the cavity, strips and nodular opacities were observable. (**b**, **c**) The lung window showed nodular opacities in the dorsal segment of the right lower lung lobe and in the lingual segment of the left upper lung lobe. Some of the nodular opacities integrated into patches. (**d**) The lung window displayed thickened and deranged lung markings at the lower lobe of both lungs

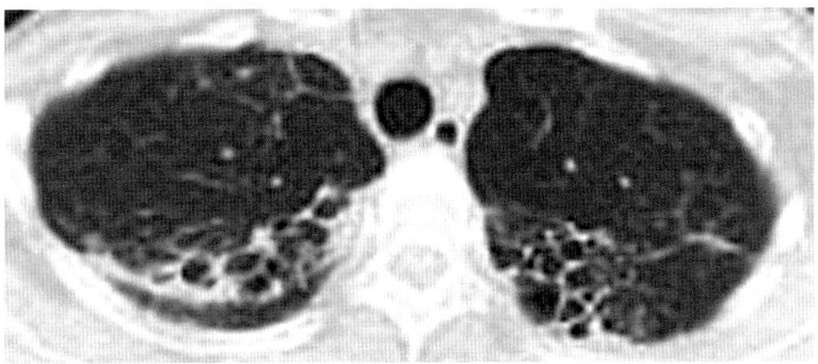

Fig. 8.43 NTM lung disease. Both upper lungs were displayed with bronchiectasis, which was surrounded by patchy infiltration, small nodules, and fibrous cord-like opacity

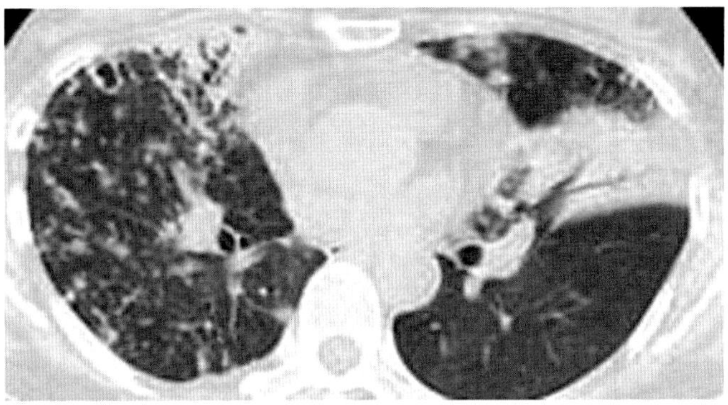

Fig. 8.44 NTM lung disease. Bronchiectasis was shown in the lingual segment of the left upper lung and in the right middle lung lobe. Bronchiectasis was accompanied by small flaky consolidation and air bronchogram sign in the left upper lung

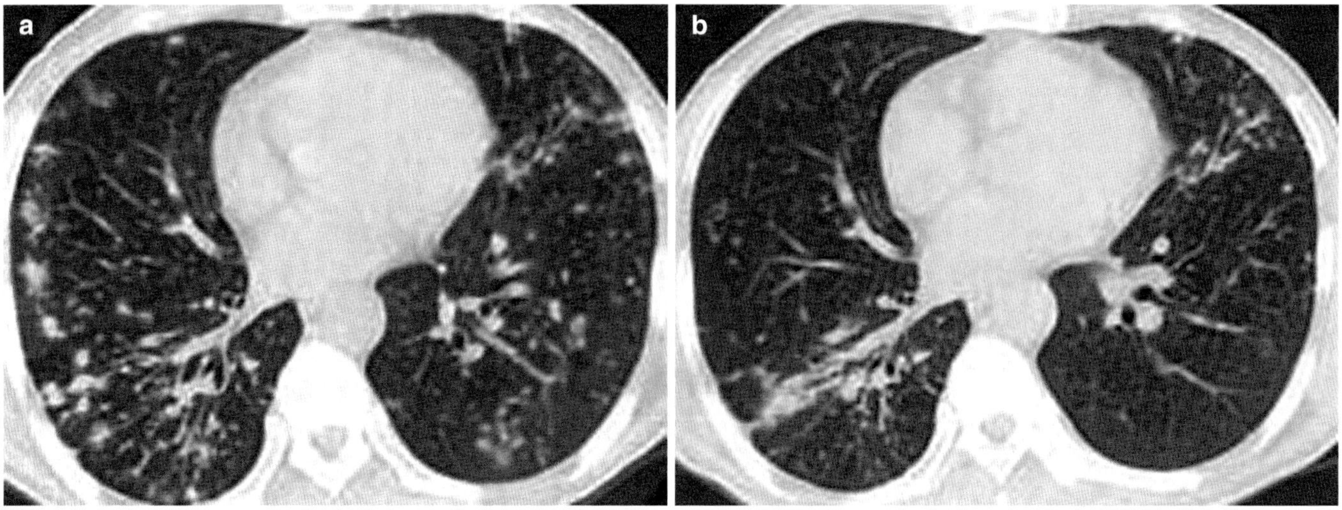

Fig. 8.45 (**a**, **b**) NTM lung disease. (**a**) The middle and lower parts of both lungs were displayed with scattering patches and nodules, namely, the tree-bud sign. The opacities were mostly distributed under the pleura. Bronchiectasis was shown in the right lower lung and in the lingual segment of the left upper lung. (**b**) The lesions were demonstrated to be absorbed after treatment

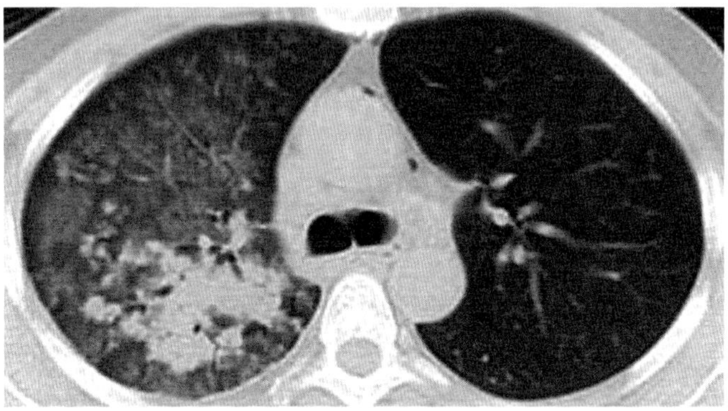

Fig. 8.46 NTM lung disease. The right upper lung was displayed with consolidation, surrounded by ground-glass opacity

Further Reading

1. Corbett EL, Watt CJ, Walker N, et al. The growing burden of tuberculosis. Arch Intern Med. 2003;163(9):1009–21.
2. Wang L, Liu J, Chin DP, et al. Progress in tuberculosis control and the evolving public-health system in China. Lancet. 2007;369(9562):691–6.
3. Philips JA, Ernst JD. Tuberculosis pathogenesis and immunity. Annu Rev Pathol. 2012;7:353–84.
4. Chen JB, Huang TH, Chen YY, et al. Comparison of 3 laboratory tests for diagnosis of tuberculosis and drug resistance of M. tuberculosis. International Journal of Laboratory Medicine. 2012;33(4):420–3.
5. Schluger NW, Burzynski J. Recent advances in testing for latent TB. Chest. 2010;138(6):1456–63.
6. Harari A, Rozot V, Enders FB, et al. Dominant TNF-alpha + Mycobacterium tuberculosis-specific CD4+ T cell responses discriminate between latent infection and active disease. Nat Med. 2011;17(3):372–6.
7. Rekha RS, Kamal SM, Andersen P, et al. Validation of the ALS assay in adult patients with culture confirmed pulmonary tuberculosis. PLoS One. 2011;6(1), e16425.
8. Du G, Qiu L, Shen L, et al. Combined megaplex TCR isolation and SMART-based real-time quantitation methods for quantitating antigen-specific T cell clones in mycobacterial infection. J Immunol Methods. 2006;308(1–2):19–35.
9. Wei H, Wang R, Yuan Z, et al. DR*W201/P65 tetramer visualization of epitope-specific CD4 T-cell during M. tuberculosis infection and its resting memory pool after BCG vaccination. PLoS One. 2009;4(9), e6905.
10. Kaur D, Guerin ME, Skovierová H, et al. Biogenesis of the cell wall and other glycoconjugates of Mycobacterium tuberculosis. Adv Appl Microbiol. 2009;69:23–78.
11. Hoffmann C, Leis A, Niederweis M, et al. Disclosure of the mycobacterial outer membrane: cryo-electron tomography and vitreous sections reveal the lipid bilayer structure. Proc Natl Acad Sci U S A. 2008;105(10):3963–7.
12. Zuber B, Chami M, Houssin C. Direct visualization of the outer membrane of mycobacteria and corynebacteria in their native state. J Bacteriol. 2008;190(16):5672–80.
13. Lienhardt C, Glaziou P, Uplekar M, et al. Global tuberculosis control: lessons learnt and future prospects. Nat Rev Microbiol. 2012;10(6):407–16.
14. Kaur D, Guerin ME, Škovierová H, et al. Biogenesis of the cell wall and other glycoconjugates of Mycobacterium tuberculosis. Adv Appl Microbiol. 2009;69:23–78.
15. Ma Y, Zhu LZ, Pan YX. Tuberculosis. People's Health Publishing House, Beijing; 2006.
16. Huang XR, Zhu WK, Lu PX, et al. Clinical significance of embolizations of nonbronchial systemic arteries for diagnosis and treatment of patients with tuberculosis and hemoptysis. Radiologic Practice. 2011;26(9):923–7.
17. Lu PX, Zhu WK, Yu WY, et al. Radiological signs of AIDS complicated by pulmonary tuberculosis and its relationship with CD4 cell count. Chin J Tuberculosis and Respiratory Diseases. 2005;28(1):13–6.
18. Liu Y, Zhan NY, Li HJ, et al. Clinical treatment of AIDS complicated by disseminated penicillium marneffei infection and the outcomes: report of 8 cases. Chin J Infectious Diseases. 2005;23(4):256–9.

19. Yuan J, Yu WY, Hu YW, et al. Clinical data of AIDS complicated by tuberculosis: analysis of 23 cases. Chin J Tuberculosis and Respiratory Diseases. 2004;27(11):767–70.
20. Zhe WK, Huang XR, Lu PX, et al. Diagnostic value and occupational protection of CT guided lung puncture for biopsy in patients with AIDS complications. Radiologic Practice. 2009;24(10):1064–6.
21. Yu WY, Liu Y, Liu Z, et al. Changes of immunity in patients with AIDS complicated by pulmonary tuberculosis. J Clinical Pulmonary Medicine. 2003;8(4):310–1.
22. Zhu WK, Lu PX, Yu WY, et al. CT findings in patients with AIDS complicated by pulmonary tuberculosis and its relationship with CD4 cell count. Chin J Medical Radiol. 2007;15(4):256–9.
23. Deng YY, Dong QL, Lu PX, et al. Radiological signs of pulmonary mycosis in non-HIV infected and HIV-infected patients: a comparative study. International Journal of Infection. 2009;9(3):152–6.
24. Yu WY, Liu Y, Zhu WK, et al. Clinical data of military pulmonary tuberculosis in AIDS patients. J Clinical Pulmonary Medicine. 2008;13(5):537–8.
25. Liu Y, Yu WY, Lu PX, et al. Clinical study of the immune functions in patients with AIDS complicated by pulmonary tuberculosis. Bulletin of Chinese Anti-tuberculosis Association. 2005;27(1):47–50.
26. Yuan H, Peng C, Lu PX, et al. CT manifestations of miliary pulmonary tuberculosis in AIDS patients. Radiologic Practice. 2009;24(10):1061–3.
27. Zhu Y, Zhang ZY, Shi YX, et al. Development of radiological diagnosis for AIDS complicated by drug sensitivity and multidrug resistant tuberculosis and extensive drug resistance tuberculosis. Radiologic Practice. 2011;26(9):941–3.
28. Lv SX, Jiang KM. X-ray signs of nontuberculous lung disease: report of 39 cases. J Clinical Pulmonary Medicine. 2003;8(2):145.
29. Horwttz MA. Recombinant BCG, expressing Mycobacterium tuberculosis major extracellular proteins. Microbes Infect. 2005;7(5–6):947–54.
30. Grode L, Seller P, Baumann S, et al. Increased vaccine efficacy against tuberculosis of recombinant Mycobacterium bovis bacille Calmette-Guerin mutants that secrete listeriolysin. J Clin Invest. 2005;115(9):2472–9.
31. McShane H, Pathan AA, Sander CR, et al. Recombinant modified vaccinia virus Ankara expressing antigen 85A boosts BCG-primed and naturally acquired antimycobacterial immunity in humans. Nat Med. 2004;10(11):1240–4.
32. Vilaplana C, Montane E, Pinto S, et al. Double-blind randomized. Placebo-controlled phase I clinical trial of the therapeutical antituberculous vaccine RUTI. Vaccine. 2010;28(4):1106–16.
33. Von Reyn CF, Mtei L, Arbeit RD, et al. Prevention of tuberculosis in Bacille Calmette Guerin primed, HIV infected adults boosted with an inactivated whole–cell mycobacterial vaccine. AIDS. 2010;24(5):675–85.

Index

P.-X. Lu, B.-P. Zhou (eds.), *Diagnostic Imaging of Emerging Infectious Diseases*, DOI 10.1007/978-94-017-7363-8

Printed by Printforce, the Netherlands